# THE MENOPAUSE *Wellness* MANUAL

*You are not alone. Joy and vitality can blossom again.*

JULIE ROBERTSON

**The Menopause Wellness Manual**
by Julie Robertson
Published by Write Wild Books Press
First published in the United Kingdom in 2025

ISBNs:
Paperback: 978-1-7394150-4-4
eBook: 978-1-7394150-5-1

# THE MENOPAUSE *Wellness* MANUAL

WRITE WILD BOOKS
PRESS

# *Dedication*

For my late Mum – Where love began and will live on forever in our hearts.
For my late Dad, whose guiding hand is always on my shoulder.
For Craig, my anchor and soulmate, my world.
For Moira Skene and John Hamilton, whose light continues to guide and inspire me.

And to every woman navigating the challenges of hormonal changes in midlife—this book is for you. You deserve to feel vibrant, seen, and empowered; this is your time. Let's embark on this journey together—I'll be with you every step of the way.

# *Disclaimer*

The information contained in this book is intended solely for general educational and informational purposes. It is not a substitute for professional medical advice, diagnosis, or treatment. You should always consult your own doctor or other qualified healthcare professional with questions or concerns regarding any medical condition or treatment. Reading this book, you acknowledge that the author will not be held liable for any loss, harm, or damage arising from reliance on the information contained within.

Every effort has been made to ensure the information is accurate and up to date at the time of publication. However, the author does not provide any warranties or representations, expressed or implied, regarding the completeness, reliability, suitability, or availability of the information contained within this book. The case studies included in this book are drawn from real-life experiences. They have been shared with explicit permission, anonymised to protect identities, or they represent composite scenarios inspired by actual events. These case studies are intended solely for educational and illustrative purposes and should not be interpreted as medical advice or specific guidance for individual circumstances. Always consult with a qualified healthcare professional for personalised advice.

You should not rely on the information in this book as an alternative to professional medical advice. Never delay seeking professional medical advice, disregard medical advice, or discontinue medical treatment based on the information in this book.

Nothing in this disclaimer will limit or exclude liability for death or personal injury resulting from negligence, fraud, or fraudulent misrepresentation. This disclaimer does not limit any liabilities in a way that is not permissible under applicable law or exclude liabilities that cannot be legally excluded.

# Contents

# *The Unexpected Visitor*

Can I tell you a tale?
Of a midlife female
Who happens to be me—
A sight I didn't foresee.

It hides out of sight,
Waiting till night,
Then overnight, it seems,
While I'm comfy in dreams,
With no warning at all,
It grows long and tall.

It's as strong as an ox
A stubborn little fox
Growing at super speed,
Determined to lead.

So, with no further ado,
Let the battle begin,
Between me and this huge
Hair on my chin.

**Julie Robertson**

# *Introduction*

You Are Not Alone.

*Imagine a world where menopausal women are revered for their unique insights and celebrated for the wealth of wisdom they offer.*

*Imagine embracing the lessons, from global cultural traditions and the natural world, to foster a society that honours and uplifts women during their menopausal journey.*

*Imagine how this shift would cultivate a deeper sense of connection and harmony across generations, recognising the invaluable contributions of women in this transformative stage of life …*

Have you read this far and already want to throw the book away, shouting, 'I can't imagine any of this … I want to, but I can't. It's *un*imaginable!'?

Then what's happened is that you've lost your joy during menopause – and you are not alone. You need – you *deserve* – help to navigate the physical, emotional, and psychological aspects of menopause, to rekindle your joy and find renewed purpose and passion in this new phase of life.

I'm Julie.

And I've written this book for you – to take your hand and gently remind you that you aren't alone. Menopause can feel alienating, confusing, and stressful, but together, we can make this journey easier. To help you recognise the tools you need to take control of your health and hormones, I want to share my story – the research, challenges, and victories – with you.

I've split the book into four parts, because let's face it, finding the time to read a whole book – and doing it with brain fog or pain or anxiety – is daunting. Not only that but different information is relevant to different people. So, *Part One* is an explanation of all things menopause and *Part Two* discusses the very many symptoms and what we can do about them. These sections are in bitesize pieces so you can dip in and out; they may be all you need right now. *Part Three* is a slightly deeper dive, a little more general detail about maintaining a healthy lifestyle alongside the menopause. In *Part Three* I treat you like the intelligent woman you are, arming you with a fuller understanding of the science behind my nutritional advice. *Part Four* is a selection of personally recommended recipes.

I hope this book becomes a source of comfort, understanding, and empowerment as you, like me, reclaim your joy in menopause.

*Because you are not alone.*

# *Part One*

## Understanding Menopause

# *Chapter One*

## Julie's Joy

You might be asking, rightly, who is she? Why is she qualified to write this book? Well, here's a snapshot of my story:

From a young age, I've always loved sport, health and fitness, which led me to study for a Bachelor of Science degree in Nutrition and Dietetics at Robert Gordon University in Aberdeen. Whilst I enjoyed learning about nutrition, I realised I missed sport and fitness, so, after graduation, I moved back home and started to work in a fitness club, where I was able to combine two of my great passions – nutrition and fitness. Working in the club, I fell in love with the environment: the camaraderie, the incentive, and the profound impact health and fitness could have on people's lives. I even met my two best friends there, Heather and Arlene, and they have been by my side, supporting me, ever since. Even when I am battling severe anxiety, the gym has always been my haven, a place where I feel comfortable, confident, and fully myself.

After the unexpected closure of the gym, I decided I wanted a new challenge and started working for British Telecom (BT). During my time there, I had the privilege of meeting some truly fabulous women of all ages. We shared countless laughs, supported one another through tears, and celebrated many milestones together. Not long after I started at BT, I met Craig. A year later, we moved into our first flat. Craig proposed to me on our first anniversary, and we celebrated our marriage in 1999—a very happy time indeed.

At the age of thirty-one, I began experiencing issues with vertigo, which had a significant impact on my confidence. I never knew when an attack of dizziness might strike, and the uncertainty was overwhelming. However, after undergoing numerous tests for vertigo and various issues with my ears, I was left without any clear answers. I eventually resigned myself to the idea that this was just something I had to live with—a world that always felt slightly off balance, out of kilter, and just a little harder to navigate.

After the closure of BT, I returned to fitness and began working at Curves, a ladies' gym. I loved being part of such a supportive team of staff and members. One person who left a lasting imprint on my heart was Moira, whom I had the great privilege of working alongside. Moira is sadly no longer with us, but she was one of the kindest and most genuine people I've ever met. She had a unique ability to make everyone feel included, seen, and valued, and her warmth touched everyone around her, including me. Moira's presence was a blessing, and her memory continues to inspire me every day.

At the age of thirty-five, while still employed at Curves, I began noticing unsettling changes in my body. I was constantly achy, struggled with sleep, and my periods had become irregular and unpredictable. Although I had managed to overcome the severe anxiety brought on by vertigo, my anxiety levels suddenly skyrocketed again. I put on a brave face, but deep down, I was terrified of the changes happening to my mind and body. My self-care fell by the wayside. Months would go by without a period, only to be followed by a month of debilitating pain. I kept pushing my worries deeper and deeper, trying to ignore what was happening. Looking back now, I realise this was perimenopause.

Life took a difficult turn after we decided to relocate to Aberdeen in 2010. My health, physically and mentally, started to take a downward turn and I went from being around people constantly to becoming a virtual recluse in a new city. My hair was falling out, my weight plummeted, and my periods stopped. I assumed it was stress, but, as my physical health deteriorated further and my mental health reached crisis point, it became clear something much bigger was happening. With the loving support of my husband, I sought medical help to learn I had gone through perimenopause and was now in menopause at forty years old. I was prescribed HRT. The reality that I would never have a family hit me hard. For me, menopause signalled ageing. I felt a great sense of loss – for myself and for my husband – and grief for the children we would never have. This was it: it would always be just the two of us.

It took time, but HRT helped me, and eventually my mental health started to improve. I became a volunteer at Northeast Sensory Services, working in the gym to help clients who were hearing and sight impaired. Their perseverance and positive outlook on life greatly motivated me. I will always be eternally grateful that they demonstrated to me how to live life regardless of the difficulties it presents.

Looking back, I see how isolated I felt at that time. While my friends were having babies and nurturing their beautiful families, I was going through an internal perimenopause. I repressed my feelings and continued to fight silently through the insomnia, vertigo, thinning hair, anxiety, sadness, and the sense that I was going insane. I started researching my own symptoms and the relationship between the brain and body because I was determined to discover exactly what was wrong with me. At a time where resources were limited, I spent hours in libraries, studying everything I could on menopause. That's how I began to put together my menopause toolkit – a collection of practical information and methods that helped me through this transition.

One of the main tools that made a difference for me was Reiki. My first session was an experience that changed my life. The constant strain and my endless, rushing thoughts began to ease. Finally, it was as if I could feel my body again. The tight ball of hysteria I had become accustomed to carrying around began to loosen, and, for the first time in what seemed like forever, I had a sensation of calm. This session inspired me to learn more about Reiki, and I studied under the lovely Elizabeth Harley, to earn my certificates as a Reiki 1, 2, and Master Practitioner. Reiki turned into a source of comfort and support for me, particularly when my lovely dad passed over in 2017. Through our regular Reiki shares, I was able to connect with some incredibly remarkable women: Susan B, Susan M and Linda who I believe I was always meant to meet. My gratitude for having met them will last a lifetime.

One day, while walking to my gym volunteering role, I noticed a sign in a shop window advertising for a shop assistant. At the time, I was just beginning my Reiki training, and I thought this opportunity might be a perfect fit. The only problem? I had absolutely no experience. Despite that, I decided to apply. I was offered an interview and met the manager, Lynne. From the moment I walked in, she made me feel so welcome and she took a real chance on me, hiring me even though I lacked experience.

It was there that I met the two Alisons and Carol, and, along with Lynne, these wonderful women have since become some of my closest friends. What they may never fully realise is just how much they helped Craig and me feel at home in a new city. I always think of the saying: "People may forget what you said, but they'll never forget how you made them feel." These incredible women truly took me under their wings, made me feel included, and welcomed me as part of their team. Their kindness, warmth, and generosity of spirit left on me an impact I will never forget.

As I continued my life's path, my passion for nutrition called to me once again. We moved to Edinburgh, and, at the age of fifty-two, I enrolled to study for a Diploma in Naturopathic Nutrition at the College of Naturopathic Medicine. Going back to studying was scary – the menopausal brain fog was constantly with me – and I wondered how I would cope. However, I met three friends for life: Cate, Gill, and Jane, whose support and kindness has been a true gift. I am forever grateful to have met these wonderful women in the later part of my life; their friendship shone a bright light in a very dark time. We encouraged one another through weekly exam classes, which we kept up during the challenges of the pandemic. It was a proud moment when we all received our Diplomas in Naturopathic Nutrition - with distinction!

After graduation, and motivated by my personal experience, I founded Harmony Health & Menopause with the dream of supporting women in managing their own menopausal journeys. To deepen my understanding and provide the best possible support, I took a step further in my journey and enrolled in a health coaching course, completing my Zest4life training in Health Coaching Skills for Nutrition Professionals. This training offered fresh insights into how to genuinely connect with and guide women through the challenges of menopause. It demonstrated to me that true support goes beyond offering advice—it's about building a partnership where women feel truly heard, valued, and empowered.

From the beginning, when I was at my lowest, my mission became taking care of myself so that I could take care of others. "Learn to love yourself again, and then help others do the same", is what I kept telling myself. One pivotal moment happened at a Bonds of Sisterhood circle at Perth Wellness Centre, led by the amazing two Julias. When I was having trouble speaking during our group session, they suggested I write my thoughts down in a journal. Once I started, I couldn't stop. It was lightbulb moment. I have always loved to write, and this gave me the push I needed: writing could be my way to help even more women on their menopause journeys. Excited, I signed up for a writing programme in Perth, facilitated by the inspirational Sarah Clayton, who gave me the tools I needed to find my voice again. The course was life-changing, and, because of Sarah's continuing support as my writing coach, I realised that writing a book was not just a dream, it was possible.

*"Empathy has no script.*
*There is no right way or wrong way to do it.*
*It's simply listening, holding space, withholding judgement, emotionally connecting, and communicating that incredibly healing message of 'You are not alone'."*

*Brené Brown*

Guided by the overarching principle that "you are not alone", this book serves as the manual I wish I'd had during my journey through early menopause and into post-menopause. Through it, I hope to guide you, the reader, to decipher the language of menopause, empowering you to make informed choices, seek support, and embark on a transformative educational journey toward menopausal joy.

Before we start, I would like to take a moment to express my heartfelt gratitude to my husband, Craig, who has played an instrumental role in helping me rediscover my joy. Early in my journey, he experienced the pain, in many ways, of losing the woman he married. He saw the haunted look in my eyes and watched as the challenges of early menopause created a growing distance between us. That distance impacted every aspect of our relationship, and it wasn't easy for either of us.

Yet, through it all, Craig has remained steadfast, offering his love and support even when things felt uncertain. With time, and the help and understanding we both needed, we found our way back to one another. Celebrating our 25th Silver Anniversary was a true testament to the strength of our bond and a reminder of the joy and love we have built together.

The song below perfectly captures how I feel about Craig and the pivotal role he played in helping me find my way back to myself. Every time I hear it, I'm overwhelmed with emotion—it reminds me of how he stood by me through everything, and never gave up on me, even when I struggled to find my own strength.

From the bottom of my heart, thank you, Craig, for your patience, your unwavering support, and for loving me back to joy.

**Loved Me Back to Life**

*I was walking dead, stuck inside my head*
*I couldn't get out, turn the lights down*
*The voices inside were so loud*
*Need a jump start, Catatonia*
*I couldn't feel, I wish that I could disappear*
*The voices inside were so real*

*But you stood by my side*
*Night after night*
*Night after night*

*You loved me back to life*
*From the coma*
*The wait is over*
*You loved me back to life*

**Celine Dion**

# *Chapter Two*

## The Universal Menopause

*"There are only two mammals who have evolved to survive after their childbearing years: toothed whales and humans."*

*Dr Jen Gunter, OB/GYN*

The menopause isn't exclusive to humans. Females of certain toothed-whale species, such as short-finned pilot whales, false killer whales, killer whales, narwhals, and beluga whales, also experience menopause. These menopausal whales often live up to forty years longer than their breeding counterparts, which is thought to provide evolutionary advantages. The cessation of breeding allows them to invest more time and resources into the well-being of their offspring and grand calves.

Older female toothed whales play a pivotal role in their communities by offering intergenerational support. They engage in behaviours such as sharing food, imparting knowledge about the ecosystem and its potential dangers, and assisting in the care of their grand calves. This matrifocal social structure, where the oldest female leads and organises the group, is particularly observed among beluga whales and narwhals. These matriarchs' wisdom and experience are invaluable to the survival and success of their pods.

Across different cultures, menopause is perceived and interpreted in ways that reflect the unique beliefs, traditions, and values of each society. In China, menopause is associated with the concept of a "second spring", symbolising a belief that women enter a new phase of vitality and wisdom. Similarly, in Japan, menopause is viewed as a significant life transition, referred to as "kounenki", which emphasises ageing gracefully. Japanese culture holds high regard for the elderly, valuing wisdom and experience, and sees menopause as a time for self-reflection, self-care, and embracing a new chapter in life.

In contrast, the UK and Western cultures have historically discussed menopause with less openness and cultural significance. However, attitudes are shifting and there is a growing recognition of menopause's impact on women's lives. Despite the varied cultural perspectives, the commonality lies in recognising menopause as a transformative phase, offering opportunities for self-care, self-acceptance, and empowerment. This universal view underscores the importance of menopause as a natural and empowering stage in a woman's life.

**But universal or not, how many of us know what menopause really is?**

Feeling completely out of control and angry for no apparent cause at all? Crying for no apparent reason while watching a puppy commercial? Are you still awake at 3 a.m., staring at the ceiling as though it's the most fascinating thing ever? Does it appear as though your body has chosen to dry out and heat up and you have lost any sense of humour? Do your mood swings have you thinking of trying out for a soap opera? Or do you simply feel as though you've accidentally landed in the wrong body – like an alien from another planet?

Why does it seem like your body is rebelling? Though you've undoubtedly heard jokes, horror stories, and whispers, when it comes to you, it's not anything to laugh at. Menopause can feel like an unexpected rollercoaster ride, for which you haven't bought a ticket. Sweaty nights, mood swings, brain fog, weight gain, and the sensation that you are *actually* losing control over the very body you've inhabited for so many years.

Sound familiar? Greetings from the Wild West of menopause, when everything feels out of control, and nothing makes sense. Although it's a perplexing and daunting experience, you are not going mad, and you are not alone. Menopause does not mean that you, your joy, vitality, or happiness will end. Even though there has been a significant shift, you can still take charge if you know what's going on.

Together, let's explore the underlying causes of this hormonal rollercoaster and find strategies for coping with it – and that means launching into the science. Ready? Let's go!

## The science of menopause

Menopause, derived from "meno" for menstrual cycle and "pause" indicating cessation, and is confirmed when a woman hasn't had a period for 12 consecutive months. Women are born with a finite number of eggs stored in our ovaries and menopause occurs when the ovaries cease releasing those eggs every month, leading to a reduction in hormones such as oestrogen, progesterone, and testosterone.

As a natural part of biological ageing, menopause signifies the conclusion of reproductive capability, marked by a profound transformation stemming from the loss of ovarian activity. The body undergoes both physical and emotional shifts, with hormone fluctuations affecting every cell, organ, and system. The lead-up to menopause, known as the perimenopausal phase, is characterised by variable hormone levels and a gradual decrease in ovarian function.

*'The Middle is messy, but it's also where the magic happens."*

*Brené Brown*

This transition, potentially lasting several years, presents a variety of symptoms. In the United Kingdom, the typical age for menopause is around 51, though experiences can differ widely. During perimenopause, individuals may experience diverse symptoms as their bodies adapt to changing hormone levels, underscoring the intricate relationship between reproductive hormones and overall well-being.

Understanding the scientific basis of menopause is crucial for effectively managing this transition and its associated symptoms. It's important to acknowledge that, while most people undergoing menopause identify as women, menopause can also impact individuals with various gender identities, including those assigned female at birth who may identify as transmasculine, intersex, or non-binary. Recognising the broad spectrum of menopausal experiences fosters inclusivity and affirms the journeys of all individuals during this significant life phase.

Menopause is increasingly understood as a complex and individualised phenomenon· Projections suggest that by the year 2025, approximately 1.1 billion women worldwide will be postmenopausal.

As women transition through menopause, they encounter a variety of physiological changes that can profoundly influence their daily lives, affecting personal, social, and occupational spheres. A study by the British Menopause Society, concluded that 47% of women surveyed had needed to take a day off work due to menopausal symptoms. A significant number also reported a decrease in social engagement and an impact on their intimate lives. Notably, 10% of women have felt compelled to resign from their jobs as a direct result of the challenges presented by menopausal symptoms. It all highlights the need for increased awareness and support during this pivotal life stage·

By learning about menopause, you're already on the path to feeling more in control; you're taking a powerful step toward understanding your body's needs. At times, the hormonal shifts can feel overwhelming – like finding your footing on shifting sands. But remember, your body is constantly communicating with you. By tuning in, you can support it in ways that bring balance and well-being. Menopause is just one chapter of your life, and, though it brings challenges, it's also an opportunity to learn more about your body and reclaim your sense of balance and well-being.

*"The best years are yet to come. Menopause is just the start of living your truth, boldly and beautifully."*

*Anon*

# *Chapter Three*

# Hormones – the Hidden Key

*Have you ever wondered what's really driving the changes in your body as you approach menopause?*

Hormones. Yes, those tiny, powerful chemical messengers, hormones, are at the heart of it all. They're the invisible force shaping everything from your mood to your metabolism, from sleep patterns to skin health.

Let's explore the world of hormones together. By understanding how they shape your daily well-being, you'll be empowered to make choices that genuinely support your health and bring you more in tune with your body. Ready to discover the impact of hormones on your vitality, mood, and overall health? Let's begin.

## Hormones are the body's communication network

The human body isn't a collection of independent organs but an interconnected system where every organ influences the others. Hormones act as messengers, coordinating communication between organs and tissues. They travel in the bloodstream, binding only to cells with specific receptors – like keys fitting into locks – to trigger responses essential for harmony and optimal function.

Our bodies constantly strive for homeostasis, a state of balanced internal conditions that allows us to function optimally. This balance regulates essential parameters like temperature, pH, blood sugar, and hormone levels. Without homeostasis, the body's cells, tissues, and organs cannot operate efficiently, leading to dysfunction and disease.

This equilibrium is managed by two primary systems: the endocrine system, with its hormone-secreting glands, and the central nervous system (comprising the brain and spinal cord), working together to maintain balance. Imagine your body as a tireless cheerleader, regulating everything from breathing to heartbeat without expecting gratitude. Yet sometimes, it's essential to pause and listen to what your body is telling you. As a Cherokee proverb wisely states:

*"If you listen to your body when it whispers, you won't have to hear it scream."*

Tuning into these signals early can help address issues before they escalate.

## Hormones oversee many vital functions:

- Reproductive cycles and sexual health
- Heart rate regulation
- Body temperature maintenance
- Mood and stress responses
- Metabolism and appetite
- Sleep patterns
- Growth and development

Hormones interact within a complex network, so a change in one can ripple through others, impacting multiple systems. During menopause, fluctuations in sex hormones are particularly impactful, disrupting this harmony.

## Hormones and the menstrual cycle create the rhythmic dance of fertility

Our hormones, particularly oestrogen and progesterone, are like our body's internal guides, influencing not only our reproductive health but also our overall well-being. For women who haven't yet reached menopause, the cyclical nature of these hormones orchestrates the menstrual cycle, a delicate and rhythmic process that prepares the body for a potential pregnancy each month.

The menstrual cycle is divided into four distinct phases, each marked by unique hormonal shifts:

**Menstrual phase**

The cycle begins with a drop in oestrogen and progesterone, leading to the shedding of the uterine lining, which we experience as menstruation.

**Follicular phase**

The hypothalamus signals the pituitary gland to release Follicle Stimulating Hormone (FSH), which encourages the ovaries to prepare follicles containing immature eggs. As these follicles mature, they release oestrogen, thickening the uterine lining in preparation for a potential pregnancy.

**Ovulation**

Rising oestrogen levels prompt the release of Luteinising Hormone (LH) from the pituitary gland, which triggers ovulation – the release of an egg – ready for fertilisation. This is the phase where conception is possible.

**Luteal phase**

After ovulation, the leftover follicle transforms into the corpus luteum, which produces progesterone to stabilise the uterine lining, preparing it to support a possible pregnancy. If pregnancy doesn't occur, the corpus luteum breaks down, causing another drop in oestrogen and progesterone, which triggers the next menstrual cycle.

Each of these phases is a part of the intricate, miraculous process that our bodies go through. However, when hormones fall out of balance, as they sometimes do, it can lead to a range of conditions. Many of us have experienced symptoms of Premenstrual Syndrome (PMS) with its blend of water retention, headaches, mood swings, and more. Conditions like fibroids, endometriosis, and Polycystic Ovary Syndrome (PCOS) may also arise from hormonal imbalances, presenting additional challenges. Knowing that these symptoms can stem from the natural shifts in our cycle can help us approach them with compassion and understanding.

## Nature's monthly health check

Your menstrual cycle is more than just a routine; it's a window into your overall health – a natural "report card" reflecting how your body is functioning. Each month, it quietly offers insights into your well-being, influenced by factors like stress, nutrition, sleep, and exercise. As you approach perimenopause, tuning into these subtle changes becomes even more valuable. They can be the early whispers of hormonal shifts, gently guiding you to pay closer attention.

Keeping a simple menstrual diary or using a tracking app to log changes in timing, flow, or symptoms can offer a sense of clarity. This helps you stay connected to your body, allowing you to notice patterns and anticipate perimenopausal shifts with greater ease. By tracking these changes, you're not only gathering insights but empowering yourself to work closely with your healthcare provider to craft a care plan unique to you.

## Take control with confidence

Embracing this journey through your cycle – and eventually into perimenopause and beyond – may feel daunting, but it's also an opportunity for self-empowerment. Tuning into your body's natural rhythms gives you a sense of control, helping you navigate changes with compassion and confidence. Each phase of your cycle has something to teach you, and, by listening, you're nurturing yourself in the most supportive way. Trust that your body knows the way and remember – you're never alone in this journey.

# Chapter Four

## "Where did I leave the car keys?"

*Does anybody actually understand this torturous stage called perimenopause?*

What even is perimenopause, and why does it feel like my body has suddenly decided to go rogue? Before I experienced it myself, I couldn't have told you either. I mean, we've all heard of menopause but perimenopause? I didn't even know it existed!

Like many women, I was caught off guard when I started having symptoms – anxiety, vertigo, mood swings, and periods that were suddenly all over the place. I thought I was too young for menopause and had no idea there was an in-between stage that could make me feel so out of sorts. Looking back, I realise how much easier it might have been if I had known that what I was experiencing was part of the perimenopause journey. I could have approached it differently, maybe with a little more self-compassion and a lot less fear.

Because here's the thing: this is where it all begins. And for many women, this stage can be confusing, frustrating, and, at times, overwhelming. If you're anything like me, you might be feeling lost or even a little panicked by all the changes happening in your body and mind. But I want to repeat – you're not alone.

So, let's dive into the details of perimenopause. I promise, with the right strategies, you can move through this phase with more confidence, less frustration, and a greater sense of control over your well-being. You've got this, and I'm here to guide you every step of the way.

## What exactly is perimenopause?

Perimenopause is the transitional period leading up to menopause. It's marked by fluctuating hormone levels and a series of physiological changes as the ovaries gradually wind down their reproductive function. During this time, ovarian function begins to decline, and your hormone production alters – mainly in terms of oestrogen and progesterone. But it's not a straightforward decrease like you might imagine; it's more like a hormonal rollercoaster with unexpected dips and peaks that keep you guessing.

This phase usually begins in your forties, or like me, can sneak up on you as early as your thirties, sometimes even sooner. Perimenopause is its own separate stage, and you can still get pregnant during this time. It can last anything from a few months to as long as a decade: the timeline is never set in stone.

## What's happening to your hormones?

The key players here are oestrogen and progesterone, and during perimenopause their levels are fluctuating wildly.

**Progesterone**

This is the first to dip. The biggest hormonal change during early perimenopause is a drop in progesterone. This is due to having shorter luteal phases (the second half of your menstrual cycle after ovulation) and more anovulatory cycles, which means you're not ovulating every month. Without ovulation, there's no progesterone being produced that cycle. This imbalance is what often causes mood swings, anxiety, and those heavier periods.

**Oestrogen**

Is the most unpredictable. Some months it's high, other months it's low, and it can spike unexpectedly. This rollercoaster is responsible for symptoms like hot flushes, night sweats, and breast tenderness.

**Testosterone**

Often thought of as a "male" hormone, this is also in the mix, affecting everything from your energy levels to libido. As it declines, you might notice you feel more tired or have less interest in sex.

This hormonal turmoil is why perimenopause can feel like a minefield. It's not just a steady decline, it's a constant ebb and flow, which can leave you feeling unsteady and, frankly, frustrated.

**Signs of perimenopause**

Because your hormones are fluctuating so dramatically, the symptoms can be just as unpredictable. Some of the most common signs include:

**Irregular periods**

Shorter, longer, heavier or lighter. Maybe you're caught off guard by sudden flooding periods or random spotting. No two months are the same.

**Hot flushes and night sweats**

Your body's thermostat seems to be on the blink.

**Mood changes**

Anxiety, irritability, or bouts of depression crop up unexpectedly.

**Sleep disruption and fatigue**

Finding it hard to fall or stay asleep, then feeling wiped out even after a good night's sleep.

**Brain fog**

Memory lapses and trouble focusing – the "what was I saying again?" feeling.

The list goes on: weight changes, thinning hair, skin issues and weight gain. In addition to hormonal changes, perimenopause is characterised by shifts in reproductive anatomy and physiology. Alterations in the uterine lining, vaginal tissues, and cervical mucus can contribute to symptoms such as vaginal dryness, irritation, and discomfort during intercourse.

The truth is, no two women experience perimenopause the same way, and that's what makes it so confusing and, at times, isolating. One woman might breeze through with just a few mild hot flushes, while another is hit with intense mood swings, brain fog, and fatigue that leaves her exhausted. It's frustrating because what you're going through can feel unpredictable and, worse, invisible to others. Even you might be left wondering, "Is this really perimenopause, or is something else going on?" It's important to check in with your healthcare provider just in case there's something else at play. Hormonal changes can mimic other health issues, so ruling out other possible conditions will give you peace of mind. Think of it as covering all bases, allowing you to move forward with clarity and confidence by knowing exactly what's going on with your body.

When that body is sending mixed signals and every day feels different, it's easy to feel overwhelmed and uncertain. I remember feeling lost myself, trying to figure out whether my anxiety, sleep issues, and sudden shifts in energy were related to hormones, or if something was seriously wrong. But here's the thing: *you* know your body better than anyone. So, when things start to feel off, trust that instinct and be confident you're not imagining it. Perimenopause can show up in countless ways, and recognising these changes is the first step toward feeling more in control.

*"Why didn't anyone warn me that perimenopause would feel like puberty all over again, but with more responsibilities and less fun?"*

## Preparing for perimenopause

It's never too early – or too late – for preparation. Supporting your body before and during menopause is all about being proactive, but for many of us, the first signs of perimenopause come as a surprise. Ideally, preparation should start well before any symptoms show up, but life doesn't always work like that, does it? For me, it wasn't until I was right in the thick of it – confused, overwhelmed, and dealing with a barrage of unexpected changes – that I started looking for answers.

That's where this book comes in. I want to help guide you with practical nutrition and lifestyle tips, whether you're planning ahead or already deep into the perimenopause challenge. By understanding what's happening with our hormones at this stage, we can recognise the signs and feel less blindsided.

Remember, it's not about going through this alone. With the right knowledge, the support of your family and friends, and working alongside your healthcare providers, you can get through this – and come out stronger on the other side. I've got you!

# *Chapter Five*

## Is Post-Menopause Really a Thing?

*"So many women I've talked to see menopause as an ending. But I've discovered this is your moment to reinvent yourself after years of focusing on the needs of everyone else. It's your opportunity to get clear about what matters to you and then to pursue that with all of your energy, time and talent."*

*Oprah Winfrey*

Post-menopause is definitely a thing! Technically speaking, menopause is defined as that one day when you've gone a full year without a period. After that, welcome to post-menopause, the stage spanning the rest of a woman's life – in the modern era, women often live over a third of their lives in post-menopause.

This is the time when hormonal fluctuations stabilise, potentially reducing or eliminating symptoms of perimenopause and menopause. Hurrah! It is often described as the final chapter in our hormonal journey, but I've found that it's really the beginning of a whole new, empowering phase of life. Now is the time to apply everything you've learned about your body, your health, and your well-being. It's a chance to redefine self-care and support your changing needs, embracing the wisdom you've gained along the way.

Post-menopause, in my view, is a time when self-care becomes more important than ever. The hormonal rollercoaster might still be running, but I've learned to recognise the signs, understand what my body needs, and take proactive steps – both physically and mentally – to bring myself back into balance. It's a stage of life that calls for more than just riding out the waves, it's about actively guiding your ship through these changing waters.

Take a moment and ask yourself: "What really matters to me, and how can I bring a little more of that into my life today?" You've done so much to get here, and now it's time to honour everything you've learned and use it to support yourself in the way that feels right for you. This new chapter is about recognising and embracing what truly nurtures your soul. Keep moving forward with awareness and confidence – this is your time to thrive!

For me, it hasn't always been easy, there have been plenty of moments when the ups and downs caught me off guard. I was considered to be in post-menopause at age 40, and I can say that, while some of the more intense symptoms improved with Hormone Replacement Therapy (HRT), there are still some lingering ones like anxiety and all-over skin dryness. But over time, I've started to honour my body and listen more deeply to what it needs. I've realised that I'm happiest when I prioritise things that bring me calm and peace, like walking in nature, sitting by the sea, or attending women's circles and meditation groups. And if I fancy a nap, I take a nap. I still love socialising, but now it's more of a relaxed afternoon out – lunch or coffee on a Saturday instead of a night out dancing. I have to admit that I look forward to getting home to my PJs, cup of tea in hand, just in time for *Strictly Come Dancing*. Oh, how things have changed!

But post-menopause does come with its own challenges. It's important to recognise that women may still face long-term effects of decreased oestrogen, such as a higher risk of osteoporosis and heart disease. We may also be susceptible to health issues stemming from immune and metabolic dysfunction and neurodegenerative diseases. So, understanding the impact of declining oestradiol levels on age-related health decline is crucial.

Women today face numerous challenges that affect their mental and physical health, shaped by distinct lifestyles and increased longevity in both professional and personal life. The "sandwich generation", for example, deal with the dual responsibilities of caring for children and ageing parents while maintaining their careers. This contributes layers of complexity to the menopausal experience. Managing stress and fatigue simultaneously during menopause not only tests resilience but also challenges the ability to cope effectively with stress.

"*For many women who have been caring for and putting others first, midlife is the time when there's finally space to start thinking about you. You may feel compelled to make room for you, to live with greater purpose, or to answer the call to do something big in the world. It's during this time that we can begin to define what legacy we want to leave.*"

*Terri Hanson*

# *Chapter Six*

## Premature and Early Menopause

While menopause is often thought of as a natural transition that occurs around the age of 51 or 52, for some women it comes much sooner or is brought on by medical or surgical interventions. These experiences each carry their own challenges—physical, emotional, and practical.

My own journey has been deeply influenced by a diagnosis of premature menopause as has my family's. My mum, Betty, experienced a very challenging early menopause at a time when "menopause" was never spoken about, let alone understood. No one really knew how to support her, and it must have been incredibly isolating and difficult for her to navigate this life-altering change on her own.

Years later, my older sister, Sandra, faced an early menopause too, and although things had improved slightly, the support and understanding were still very poor, leaving her to navigate many of the same challenges with limited guidance and care. Their experiences have always stayed with me, shaping my desire to ensure that no one else feels as alone as they did. Their strength and resilience inspire me every day, and they are a poignant reminder of why we must continue to advocate for greater awareness and support for all women navigating menopause.

Looking back now, perhaps I should have joined the dots and anticipated that, with the genetic clues I had, my own fertility might end earlier. But, like many women, I assumed I had more time to make choices about my fertility. When that possibility suddenly ended, it was hard to process – it felt like something precious was taken too soon.

My hope is that, by sharing my own story and the information I've gathered, I can offer support and guidance for navigating the unique challenges of premature menopause. Understanding the potential causes can provide clarity and help with emotional acceptance.

Let's explore what happens when menopause doesn't follow the expected timeline and how we can better understand and support these unique journeys.

**Medication-induced menopause**

Certain medications, particularly cancer treatments such as chemotherapy and radiotherapy, can damage ovarian cells, leading to menopause.

### Surgical menopause

Surgical menopause occurs when the ovaries are surgically removed in a procedure called an oophorectomy. This surgery, often performed to treat or prevent conditions such as ovarian cancer or severe endometriosis, leads to an immediate and complete cessation of hormone production, particularly oestrogen and progesterone.

Unlike natural menopause, where hormonal changes occur gradually over time, medication-induced and surgical menopause result in a sudden and abrupt transition. This rapid shift often leads to more intense and immediate menopausal symptoms, such as hot flushes, night sweats, and mood changes, which can significantly affect quality of life. Women experiencing these types of menopauses require tailored support to manage symptoms and mitigate long-term health risks, including bone loss and cardiovascular disease. Seeking guidance from a healthcare professional both before and after treatment is essential for developing a comprehensive care plan that addresses both immediate needs and long-term well-being.

### Early menopause

Early menopause refers to the onset of menopause between the ages of 40 and 45. While some causes are identifiable, including genetic predisposition, surgical removal of ovaries, chemotherapy, or radiotherapy, many cases remain unexplained.

### Premature menopause

Premature menopause is the permanent cessation of ovarian function and menstruation before the age of 40. As with early menopause, it can be linked to surgery (e.g., removal of ovaries), chemotherapy, radiation, or certain medical conditions, although the cause often remains unknown.

**Premature ovarian insufficiency (POI)**

A condition where the ovaries stop functioning normally before the age of 40. The ovaries stop producing eggs years and, in some cases decades, before they should.

A woman with POI may still have periods, even though they might not come regularly, and she may still get pregnant.

POI affects approximately 1 in 100 women under 40, 1 in 1,000 under 30, and 1 in 10,000 under 20. The ovaries may function irregularly, often without a clear cause—around 90% of cases remain unexplained. When a cause is identifiable, it may include:

**Genetic factors**

Genetic conditions such as Turner Syndrome or Fragile X Syndrome can disrupt ovarian function, sometimes resulting in primary amenorrhea or other complications. These conditions highlight the importance of two functioning X chromosomes for ovarian health.

**Iatrogenic causes**

Surgical removal of the ovaries, hysterectomy, radiotherapy, and chemotherapy.

**Autoimmune disorders**

Autoimmune disorders occur when the body's immune system mistakenly targets its own tissues. When this process affects the ovaries, it can lead to the development of POI.

POI doesn't just affect fertility. Its unpredictable hormone production can have profound physical and emotional impacts, including increased cardiovascular risk, decreased bone density, and mental health challenges due to hormonal imbalances.

Premature Menopause and POI are often confused, as both involve ovarian dysfunction before the age of 40. However, they are distinct conditions with differences in causes, symptoms, and outcomes.

## Seeking support

The early onset of menopause often brings a complex set of challenges. Physically, you may face symptoms such as hot flushes, night sweats, and mood swings. Emotionally, it can bring profound grief, particularly around the loss of fertility and the sudden end of a chapter in life that you may not have been prepared for. Coping with these changes requires both medical management and emotional support, alongside access to trusted resources and communities.

For me, grieving the end of my fertility was an integral part of the healing process. It wasn't just my journey; it was one I shared with my husband as we mourned the loss of the family life we had imagined. While it was a deeply emotional time, it also became a chance for us to reshape our path. Together, we found joy and fulfilment in other ways—through travel, meaningful shared experiences, and building a life that reflected our values and dreams.

## The Daisy Network: a community of understanding

One of the most valuable resources available to women navigating early menopause, premature menopause, or POI is The Daisy Network. This dedicated organisation provides education, guidance, and an empathetic community for women dealing with premature menopause and ovarian insufficiency.

The Daisy Network offers:

- **Access to reliable information**
  Navigating the medical aspects of early menopause or POI can be daunting. The Daisy Network provides evidence-based resources on topics such as hormonal health and emotional well-being, helping you make informed decisions about your care.

- **Connection with others**
  Through local networks and meet-ups, The Daisy Network fosters a sense of community. Hearing others' experiences can not only validate your own but also provide practical tips and emotional encouragement. Knowing you are part of a supportive network can be a powerful antidote to the isolation that often accompanies a POI diagnosis.

- **Expert-led webinars and workshops**
  The network organises talks and live chat sessions led by menopause specialists. These sessions offer practical advice and empower you to take charge of your health and well-being.

- **Tailored support for fertility concerns**
  For women affected by premature menopause, concerns around fertility can be especially painful. The Daisy Network provides compassionate resources to help you understand your options and navigate this deeply personal issue with care and support.

Connecting with others who truly understand your experience can be transformative. Joining a supportive community like The Daisy Network provides access to valuable tools, reliable knowledge, and meaningful connections, empowering you to navigate this journey with strength and resilience.

## Moving forward

If you've been diagnosed with premature menopause or POI, it's important to seek the right support—both medical and emotional. Consulting with healthcare professionals, such as a GP, endocrinologist, or menopause specialist, is crucial for managing the symptoms and long-term health risks. They can provide personalised advice and support. Don't hesitate to connect with organisations like The Daisy Network for further guidance.

Remember, this is a chapter of your life—not the whole story. By accessing the right resources, leaning on supportive networks, and giving yourself space, you can find a way forward that feels empowering and fulfilling. There is a community ready to lift you up, share their experiences, and remind you that you are never alone.

Below are some resources to support you further:

- **British Menopause Society (BMS):** BMS offers resources and a directory of healthcare professionals focused on menopause care, helping to improve the standard of care and understanding. https://thebms.org.uk/find-a-menopause-specialist
- **Menopause Matters:** A comprehensive website covering all aspects of menopause, including early menopause, with forums where you can connect and find support. www.menopausematters.co.uk
- **NHS Menopause Clinics:** Many NHS trusts offer specialised menopause clinics for expert advice and support. Your GP can help you locate one near you.

- **Women's Health Concern (WHC):** As the patient arm of the BMS, WHC provides independent advice on a range of women's health issues, including POI.
- **MIND:** This mental health charity provides resources and counselling services to help cope with the emotional impact of premature or surgical menopause.
- **NICE guideline:** Menopause: diagnosis and management. www.nice.org.uk/guidance/ng23
- **National Menopause Society:** Established to create a positive change in how people perceive, understand and experience Menopause. https://nationalmenopausefoundation.org/
- **The Menopause Society:** To empower healthcare professionals to improve the health of women during the menopause transition and beyond. https://menopause.org

# *Chapter Seven*

## Decoding Oestrogen: Why Does It Matter?

*What's the deal with oestrogen, and why does it seem to have so much power over how we feel?*

Picture this: oestrogen is like that friend who's always been around, keeping everything running smoothly. Then one day, she announces she's going on an extended holiday, and suddenly, everything's out of sync – hot flushes, mood swings and brain fog move in like unwelcome houseguests. Turns out, we never realised how much we relied on her until she started packing her bags! So, what exactly was she up to all those years, and why does everything feel so off without her?

Oestrogen is primarily synthesised in the ovaries from cholesterol. However, it's not limited to these reproductive organs. Tissues such as fat cells, skin, bones, and even the brain can step in and produce oestrogen through a process known as aromatisation, where androgens (like testosterone) are converted into oestrogen. This becomes especially crucial during menopause, as ovarian production slows down. At this stage, your body cleverly adapts, relying on these peripheral tissues to sustain oestrogen levels, even if they're not as high as before.

So, you can already see that oestrogen is a key player in maintaining the overall balance of your body. Because it's a steroid hormone, it can easily cross into cells by binding to its specific receptors – oestrogen receptors (ER) α and β – which are found throughout the body.

**ER-α** is mainly found in tissues such as the breasts and uterus, where it plays a role in stimulating cell growth and proliferation. **ER-β**, on the other hand, is more widely distributed across the brain, bones, and skin. It is essential for tissue maintenance, contributing to the overall structure and function of these systems.

When oestrogen binds to these receptors, it triggers a cascade of genetic events that influence everything from growth to metabolism and reproduction. The wide presence of these receptors throughout the body shows how integral oestrogen is – not only to reproductive health, but to keeping your bones strong, your skin resilient, your heart healthy, and even your brain functioning smoothly.

In premenopausal women, the ovaries produce most of the body's oestrogen, but its influence reaches far beyond reproductive health. Oestrogen supports immune function, cardiovascular health, and central nervous system balance. It plays a crucial role in maintaining bone density, skin elasticity, and cognitive functions such as mood and memory. Oestrogen even supports the mucous membranes, ensuring that everything from your eyes to your intestines stays hydrated and healthy.

However, during perimenopause and menopause, oestrogen levels begin to fluctuate unpredictably. These fluctuations can lead to a variety of symptoms such as hot flushes, night sweats, mood changes, and a gradual decline in bone density. It's easy to feel overwhelmed when these changes start affecting so many aspects of your health, from your mental clarity to your physical strength.

## The different types of oestrogen

- **Estrone (E1):**
  Estrone is the predominant oestrogen during menopause, produced primarily in peripheral tissues like fat cells. It becomes the main circulating oestrogen after the decline of estradiol (E2) levels. While it's less potent, estrone still plays a role in maintaining hormonal balance and supporting physiological functions.

- **Estradiol (E2):**
  The most active and potent form of oestrogen during the reproductive years, estradiol is produced mainly by the ovaries. It's crucial for menstrual regulation, reproductive health, bone density, cardiovascular well-being, and overall energy and mood. When estradiol levels begin to decline during menopause, it can trigger a range of symptoms such as hot flushes, night sweats, and mood swings.

- **Estriol (E3):**
  This form of oestrogen is produced primarily during pregnancy by the placenta. It plays a critical role in supporting foetal development and maintaining pregnancy. Outside of pregnancy, estriol levels are relatively low, but understanding its role can still provide insights into the different ways your body uses oestrogen. Oestrogen is often discussed as if it's a single hormone, but there are actually three primary types found in the body, each produced at different stages of life and serving distinct roles. Let's break them down:

## Oestrogen transport: the role of SHBG

Another factor that significantly influences oestrogen's effectiveness in the body is its transport. This is where sex hormone-binding globulin (SHBG) comes into play.

SHBG is a protein produced in the liver that serves as a carrier molecule for sex hormones like oestrogen and androgens. Since these hormones are not water-soluble, SHBG binds to them and allows them to circulate through the bloodstream, acting as a molecular shuttle.

The binding between SHBG and oestrogen is not a static process, it's dynamic and responsive to various factors such as hormonal levels, diet, and even stress. Changes in SHBG levels can impact the availability of active, "free" oestrogen, influencing how the hormone affects cells and tissues throughout your body. This means that even if your oestrogen levels are within a normal range, high or low SHBG levels can alter the balance, making symptoms more pronounced or even triggering new ones.

## Oestrogen's reach: beyond reproduction

Oestrogen is more than just a reproductive hormone; it influences many areas of our health to keep the body's systems in harmony:

**Menstrual cycle regulation**

Oestrogen thickens the uterine lining, preparing it for pregnancy, and helps the egg mature during ovulation. As levels drop during menopause, these processes change, leading to irregular periods and, eventually, the end of menstruation.

**Bone density maintenance**

Oestrogen helps maintain bone density by regulating bone turnover. When levels decline, bone loss can accelerate, increasing the risk of osteoporosis.

**Cardiovascular health**

Oestrogen supports cardiovascular health by keeping blood vessels flexible and managing cholesterol. As oestrogen levels decline, the risk for heart disease can increase.

**Brain function**

Oestrogen receptors in the brain regulate mood, memory, and cognitive sharpness. Lower levels can contribute to symptoms like brain fog and mood swings.

**Mood regulation**

Oestrogen impacts serotonin, the "feel-good" neurotransmitter. Its decline can lead to mood fluctuations, anxiety, or even depression.

**Metabolism and weight regulation**

Oestrogen helps manage metabolism and fat distribution. With lower levels, many women notice weight gain, especially around the midsection.

**Combating inflammation**

Oestrogen modulates the immune system and reduces inflammation. A decrease can make you more prone to conditions like joint pain.

**DID YOU KNOW?**

A review of over 160 scientific studies found that oestrogen is far more than just a reproductive hormone. It plays a crucial role in protecting long-term health, helping to reduce the risk of chronic conditions like osteoporosis and cardiovascular disease

## Oestrogen detoxification

As your body transitions through perimenopause and menopause, maintaining balanced oestrogen levels becomes increasingly important. Whether the oestrogen is naturally produced or comes from hormone replacement therapy (HRT), it needs to be processed and eliminated efficiently. If not managed well, it can lead to oestrogen dominance – a state where the body has more active oestrogen than it requires, which may contribute to symptoms like breast tenderness, mood swings, and weight gain. This highlights why optimising your body's oestrogen detoxification pathways is essential.

Oestrogen detoxification is a multi-step process, with the liver and gut playing key roles. Once oestrogen has done its job – whether regulating bone density, stabilising mood, or supporting other bodily functions – it must be metabolised and safely removed from the body. Think of it like a highly efficient processing line: the liver and gut work together to break down, neutralise, and eliminate oestrogen. If this process doesn't run smoothly, it can cause a backlog, leading to potential imbalances and increased risk of certain health concerns.

Let's explore how oestrogen detoxification works and how you can support your body in maintaining optimal hormonal health.

## Step 1: The liver's role in oestrogen detoxification – breaking down the process

### Phase 1 Detoxification

In this initial stage, oestrogen is chemically altered, creating intermediate metabolites. These metabolites can sometimes be more reactive and potentially harmful than the original hormone, making it crucial that Phase 2 steps in quickly to neutralise them. A diet rich in antioxidants, such as berries and green tea, can support Phase 1 by protecting against potential oxidative stress from these metabolites.

### Phase 2 Detoxification

Here, the liver binds these intermediate metabolites with water-soluble compounds, making them easier for the body to excrete. Amino acids like glutamine, glycine, taurine, and cysteine, along with sulphur-containing foods such as garlic and cruciferous vegetables, play crucial roles in this stage. If Phase 2 lags behind Phase 1, these reactive intermediates may build up, potentially causing cellular damage and contributing to hormone-related issues. Incorporating foods that support Phase 2 detoxification, like leafy greens and broccoli, can help keep this process running smoothly.

## Step 2: Understanding oestrogen metabolites – not all oestrogen is created equal

When the liver processes oestrogen in Phase 1, it converts it into one of three main metabolites. The balance of these metabolites is crucial because they can either protect or potentially harm your body. Here's a quick breakdown:

- **2-Hydroxyestrone (2OH):** a relatively weak and stable metabolite, often considered protective when properly methylated. Supporting this pathway is beneficial for overall health.
- **4-Hydroxyestrone (4OH):** this more unstable metabolite can form reactive quinones, which may cause oxidative stress and damage to DNA, posing potential health risks.
- **16-Hydroxyestrone (16OH):** a potent metabolite with a high affinity for oestrogen receptors that can promote cell growth. While beneficial for bone health, excessive levels may pose risks to tissues like the breast.

Ideally, the liver should produce more 2OH, as it is less harmful. However, certain lifestyle factors, such as diet, environmental toxins, and stress, can influence which pathway your liver favours. Appropriate dietary and lifestyle adjustments will encourage healthier oestrogen metabolism.

## Step 3: Optimising oestrogen metabolism – your action plan

Here's how you can support your body's ability to metabolise oestrogen safely and effectively and improve your overall hormonal health.

Promote the protective 2-Hydroxyestrone (2OH) pathway by including cruciferous vegetables like broccoli, cauliflower, kale, and Brussels sprouts in your diet. These foods promote the activity of the enzyme CYP1A1, which favours the production of 2OH. Likewise, consider adding ground flaxseeds to your food, as they also support this beneficial pathway by promoting the production of protective metabolites.

Support the protective 2/4 Methoxyestrone (MeOH) pathway with an adequate intake of magnesium (found in leafy greens, avocados, and nuts) and B vitamins (B6, B12, and folate from meat, legumes, and leafy greens) to enhance the conversion of 4OH into the less harmful 4-MeO by supporting the activity of catechol-O-methyltransferase (COMT). Secondly, since stress can reduce its efficiency in detoxifying oestrogen, take steps to minimise any stresses in your life!

Minimise the problematic 4-Hydroxyestrone (4OH) and 16-Hydroxyestrone (16OH) pathways by reducing exposure to environmental triggers like polycyclic aromatic hydrocarbons (PAHs) found in charred or grilled meats, tobacco smoke, and certain pollutants, which can activate the enzyme CYP1B1.

## Step 4: The gut's role in phase 3 detoxification – the final countdown

The gut is more than just a digestive organ, it's a key player in regulating our overall health and hormone function. One of its most critical roles is maintaining a balanced ecosystem of microorganisms, known as the gut microbiome. This diverse community of bacteria, viruses, fungi, and other microbes is not only essential for digestion and immune health but also significantly influences hormonal balance.

When the gut's ecosystem is disrupted (a condition known as dysbiosis), it can have a knock-on effect on the entire body, leading to hormonal imbalances and other health concerns. Factors like poor diet, chronic stress, or gastrointestinal conditions can all contribute to dysbiosis, making it harder for your body to function optimally.

The gut is intricately linked to oestrogen metabolism through a specialised collection of bacteria known as the estrobolome. This helps break down and manage oestrogen compounds, preparing them for final elimination from the body. However, when the gut's microbial balance is disrupted, certain enzymes like beta-glucuronidase, can become overactive. Elevated levels of this enzyme can reactivate oestrogen that was neutralised, sending it back into circulation. This can result in more active oestrogen than the body needs, leading to symptoms such as bloating, fatigue, and mood swings.

So, when gut health is compromised, especially within the estrobolome, it can significantly impact your hormonal balance, making an already challenging menopausal transition even more difficult.

## The pathway as production line

Think of maintaining hormonal balance as managing a production line. Phase 1 and Phase 2 of oestrogen detoxification work hard to process oestrogen metabolites, efficiently preparing them for removal. But if Phase 3 – the gut – is not functioning optimally, it can lead to a backlog, causing oestrogen to accumulate, much like a traffic jam at the end of a busy road. Imagine it as a blocked exit, preventing oestrogen from leaving the body smoothly. The liver, already working hard to manage this flow, must now cope with the additional strain of processing the overflow. To keep everything running smoothly and maintain hormonal harmony, it's essential that Phase 3 is well-prepared and functioning effectively to ensure the entire detoxification process stays on track.

Remember, small changes make a difference as MJ's story below demonstrates. Consider adding nutrient-rich vegetables like broccoli or Brussels sprouts to your meals, swapping white rice for brown for more fibre, or starting your day with flaxseeds and berries in yoghurt to support gut health. Try incorporating liver-friendly foods such as beetroot, eggs, or nuts to aid oestrogen detoxification.

**MJ'S STORY**

I came to see Julie because I was struggling with low energy, mood swings, and that dreaded mid-afternoon slump. I'd lost the motivation to do my weekly hill walks, which were my go-to for clearing my mind and boosting my mental health after a tough week at work. I'd also put on weight around my middle, had dark circles under my eyes, and found myself waking up every night around 3 a.m.

Julie took a detailed health history and reviewed my 3-day food diary, then came back with a plan that included simple, manageable steps to support my liver. These changes were as straightforward as drinking more water, adding a cup of cruciferous vegetables to my meals, adding a source of protein to every meal, and cutting back on caffeine. Within just a week, I noticed a big difference – I was sleeping more soundly, waking up less frequently, and had more energy for my hill walks at the weekend.

It's amazing how small, targeted changes can make such a noticeable difference!

Each small choice brings you closer to balance and well-being. So, ask yourself, which step could you take today?

# *Chapter Eight*

## When the Scales Tip: Understanding Oestrogen Dominance

*"It's not the changes that define us – it's how we choose to respond to them. Our journey to balance is not a sprint, but a series of thoughtful, nurturing choices."*

Oestrogen dominance is an area where there has been some confusion. It isn't a medical term, but it refers to a state where oestrogen levels are out of balance with progesterone levels. This typically happens when oestrogen is relatively high compared to progesterone, a situation that's particularly common during perimenopause, because hormonal fluctuations are more frequent. Even if progesterone levels are within a normal range, an imbalance can still exist if oestrogen levels are elevated. Contributing factors include inefficient clearance of oestrogen from the body and exposure to environmental sources of oestrogen.

As we've seen, oestrogen is vital for many bodily functions, such as regulating the menstrual cycle and supporting tissue growth, but, equally, having too much can create problems. High levels of oestrogen are linked to hormone-sensitive conditions like fibroids, ovarian cysts, and an increased risk of hormone-dependent cancers such as breast and ovarian cancer. Symptoms of oestrogen dominance include heavy or irregular periods, breast tenderness, PMS, headaches, reduced libido, and difficulties with conception.

This imbalance arises from several factors. One of the primary causes is anovulatory cycles (cycles without ovulation), which are common in perimenopause. When ovulation doesn't occur, progesterone production drops, shifting the balance in favour of oestrogen. Another significant factor is the liver's ability to process and clear excess oestrogen. If the liver is sluggish or overburdened by toxins, it can lead to an accumulation of oestrogen in the body.

Additionally, stress plays a crucial role in hormone imbalances. During chronic stress, the body prioritises producing cortisol, the stress hormone, over other hormones like progesterone. This results in a further drop in progesterone levels and exacerbates the oestrogen-progesterone imbalance. This connection highlights how deeply emotional and hormonal health are intertwined.

## Environmental oestrogens: unseen disruptors of hormonal health

Have you ever wondered how everyday products might be affecting your hormones?

In today's world, we are exposed to external sources of oestrogen more than ever before. Known as environmental oestrogens or xenoestrogens, these compounds mimic your body's natural oestrogen, disrupting the delicate hormonal balance. Unlike your body's own oestrogen, these imposters can bind to hormone receptors – sometimes even more strongly than your body's oestrogen does – leading to various symptoms and potential long-term health concerns.

Environmental oestrogens enter our bodies through food, water, air, and even personal care products. They're hidden in cosmetics, plastics, and pesticides, making them hard to avoid completely. Once inside the body, these synthetic compounds don't break down easily and tend to accumulate in fat cells. This build-up adds stress to your liver, which works hard to eliminate them. Unlike naturally occurring hormones, which the body can metabolise efficiently, these synthetic compounds disrupt your hormonal balance and strain your liver's detoxification processes.

Common sources of environmental oestrogens include:

**Cosmetics and personal care products**
Parabens and phthalates, often found in skincare and beauty products, are absorbed through the skin.

**Plastics**
Bisphenol A (BPA), found in water bottles and food packaging, can leach into food and beverages, especially when heated.

**Pesticides and herbicides**
Non-organic produce may be contaminated with hormone-disrupting chemicals.

**Household products**
Solvents and volatile organic compounds (VOCs) from items like flooring, paints, and cleaning products can contaminate indoor air.

When xenoestrogens accumulate, they interfere with your body's natural hormone transport and function. They can occupy the binding sites of Sex Hormone Binding Globulin (SHBG) – the protein that helps transport oestrogen and testosterone – making it less effective. As xenoestrogens build up in fat cells, they further strain your liver, slowing its ability to detoxify the body and creating a cycle of toxin accumulation and hormonal disruption.

While you may not be able to eliminate all environmental oestrogens, there are several steps you can take to reduce your exposure:

**Opt for organic produce**
Prioritise organic fruits and vegetables, especially those known to have low pesticide residues.

**Choose hormone-free animal products**
Select organic or hormone-free meat and dairy to avoid synthetic hormones used in farming.

**Use natural cleaning products**
Replace chemical-heavy cleaners with natural alternatives like vinegar, baking soda, and essential oils.

**Switch to paraben and phthalate-free personal care products**
Look for natural or organic skincare, haircare, and cosmetic products.

**Minimise plastic use**

Store food in glass or stainless-steel containers and avoid heating food in plastic. Beeswax wraps are a great alternative to cling film.

**Filter your water**

Use water filtration systems to reduce contaminants, including xenoestrogens, from your drinking water.

**Limit contact with thermal paper receipts**

These often contain BPA, which can transfer to your skin, so handle them sparingly.

What simple swaps can you make today to protect and support your health in the long run?

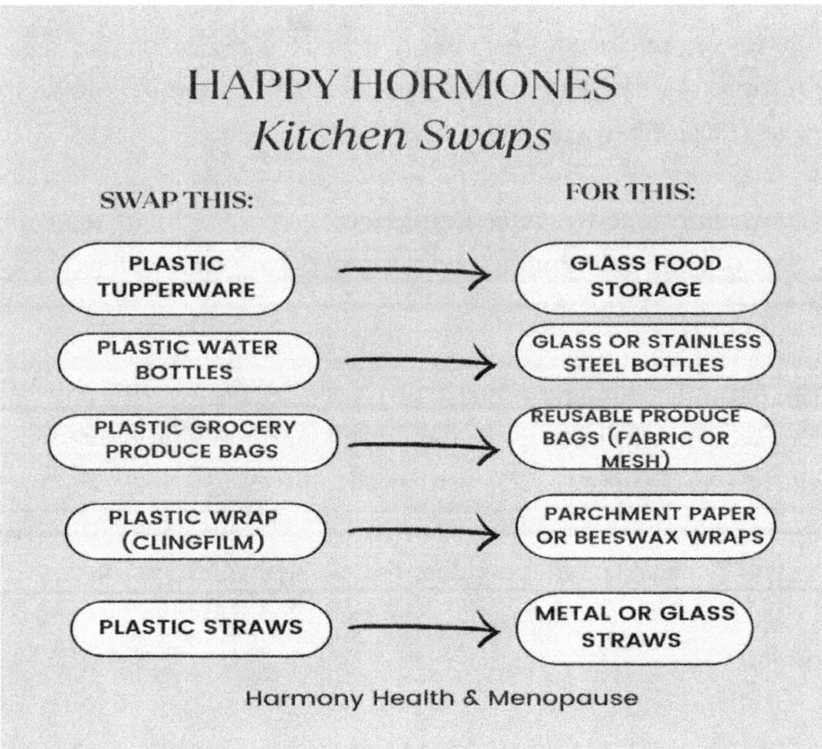
HAPPY HORMONES
Kitchen Swaps
SWAP THIS:
FOR THIS:
PLASTIC TUPPERWARE
GLASS FOOD STORAGE
PLASTIC WATER BOTTLES
GLASS OR STAINLESS STEEL BOTTLES
PLASTIC GROCERY PRODUCE BAGS
REUSABLE PRODUCE BAGS (FABRIC OR MESH)
PLASTIC WRAP (CLINGFILM)
PARCHMENT PAPER OR BEESWAX WRAPS
PLASTIC STRAWS
METAL OR GLASS STRAWS
Harmony Health & Menopause

Bringing all the information in this chapter together, it becomes clear how essential it is for your body to effectively metabolise and eliminate oestrogen during the hormonal shifts of perimenopause and menopause. This process is vital for managing both natural oestrogen and synthetic forms, such as those used in Hormone Replacement Therapy (HRT). When your detoxification pathways are functioning at their best, they help regulate hormonal fluctuations, reduce discomfort, and support your overall health and vitality.

## Key strategies for optimising detoxification

### Support your liver

Your liver plays a central role in hormone metabolism. Cruciferous vegetables like broccoli, cauliflower, and Brussels sprouts contain powerful compounds, such as indole-3-carbinol (I3C) and sulforaphane, which help convert oestrogen into less harmful metabolites like 2-hydroxyestrogen. Aim for two cups of these vegetables daily. Additionally, B vitamins—such as folate (leafy greens), vitamin B6 (pork, oats), and vitamin B12 (meat, eggs)—along with minerals like magnesium, zinc, and selenium, are essential for enzyme activity in oestrogen metabolism. To further support liver detoxification, include antioxidant-rich foods such as leafy greens, citrus fruits, and berries in your diet.

### Increase fibre intake

A diet rich in fibre promotes a healthy gut microbiome, supports digestion, and aids in the removal of excess oestrogen from the body. Incorporate fibre-rich foods such as chickpeas, lentils, carrots, onions, and sweet potatoes. Adding flaxseeds or chia seeds to your breakfast, swapping white rice for whole grains like quinoa, and including extra servings of leafy greens or fibrous vegetables at each meal can make a significant difference.

### Stay hydrated

Drinking at least two litres of filtered water daily supports toxin elimination, including excess oestrogen. Aim for pale-coloured urine as a guide to adequate hydration.

### Minimise hormone disruptors

Reduce exposure to endocrine disruptors by avoiding plastic containers, cling film, and heating food in plastic containers. Choose glass or stainless-steel alternatives and switch to eco-friendly cleaning and personal care products. Limiting processed foods, refined sugars, and unhealthy fats also reduces the burden on the liver, supporting its ability to detoxify and metabolise hormones effectively.

### Reduce alcohol intake

UK guidance recommends 14 units of alcohol per week and studies show that even moderate alcohol intake can increase oestrogen levels and decrease progesterone in perimenopausal women. To reduce intake, try alternating alcoholic drinks with sparkling water or diluting wine with water to create a refreshing spritzer.

**AVOIDING ALCOHOL MAY IMPROVE:**

Sleep quality

Blood sugar levels and cravings

Weight management

Mood stability

Energy levels

Nutrient absorption

Hot flushes and other vasomotor symptoms

## The path to balance

Optimising oestrogen metabolism during menopause is about equipping yourself with the knowledge and tools to make intentional, mindful changes that support your well-being. Think of your body as a thriving garden: by adding fibre-rich foods, staying hydrated, and nourishing your liver, you provide the foundation for achieving balance and vitality. Even small, consistent shifts—such as choosing non-toxic products or swapping plastic for glass—can bring noticeable improvements over time.

For example, one client began by simply adding a handful of leafy greens to her meals each day. Within a few weeks, she experienced improved digestion and greater energy. Another client transitioned to paraben-free skincare products and found her skin clearer and more radiant than it had been in years. These seemingly small changes can create a ripple effect, delivering meaningful and lasting benefits.

The journey to balance isn't about quick fixes or drastic changes—it's a steady process of making thoughtful, nurturing choices. Every step you take supports not only your health today but also your resilience and vitality for the years ahead.

# *Chapter Nine*

## The Silent Drop: How Progesterone Shapes Your Perimenopause

*Ever found yourself wondering why you suddenly feel more anxious, or your once-regular menstrual cycle has turned unpredictable?*

These shifts are not uncommon and might be linked to progesterone. As it quietly decreases during perimenopause, it can disrupt the delicate balance of your entire hormonal landscape. Let's explore why this "silent drop" plays such a big role in your health.

Progesterone is a steroid hormone, which is primarily produced by a specialised structure in the ovary called the corpus luteum. It is the main hormone produced after ovulation, when the follicle that released the egg transforms into the corpus luteum – a small, temporary endocrine gland with a big job.

The corpus luteum forms in the ovary following ovulation and is derived from the remnants of the ovarian follicle that previously housed the developing egg. Its primary role is to produce progesterone, which stabilises and prepares the uterine lining (endometrium) for the possible implantation of a fertilised egg. Progesterone supports the thickening and maintenance of this lining, creating a nourishing environment in the early stages of pregnancy. If the egg is fertilised and pregnancy occurs, the developing embryo releases a hormone called human chorionic gonadotropin (hCG). This hormone signals the corpus luteum to continue producing progesterone until the placenta can take over hormone production, about 8–12 weeks into pregnancy. This is this hormone Healthcare Providers measure to confirm a pregnancy. If pregnancy does not occur, the corpus luteum breaks down after about 10-14 days, leading to a sharp drop in progesterone levels. This decline triggers menstruation, signalling the body to shed the uterine lining and begin a new menstrual cycle.

## The many roles of progesterone

While progesterone's key function is often associated with pregnancy, its influence extends across many areas of women's health. Here are some of its most significant roles:

**Hormonal balance maintenance**
Progesterone works closely with oestrogen to maintain equilibrium throughout the menstrual cycle. It counteracts oestrogen by downregulating oestrogen receptors (ER), ensuring that hormone levels remain balanced to support reproductive processes.

**Bone health support**

Alongside oestrogen, progesterone helps maintain bone density and strength by regulating bone remodelling. This is especially important during the menopausal transition when lower progesterone and oestrogen levels increase the risk of bone loss, osteoporosis, and fractures.

**Calming the brain**

Progesterone has a calming effect on the brain by interacting with gamma-aminobutyric acid (GABA) receptors, a neurotransmitter that promotes relaxation within the central nervous system. By enhancing GABA activity, progesterone can help alleviate anxiety, improve mood stability, and promote restful sleep.

**Supporting insulin sensitivity**

Progesterone plays a role in supporting insulin signalling, which helps regulate glucose metabolism and maintain stable blood sugar levels. This is crucial for metabolic health and reducing the risk of insulin resistance.

**Regulating fluid balance**

Progesterone acts as a natural diuretic, helping the body manage fluid balance by promoting the excretion of sodium and water. As progesterone levels drop during menopause, this balance can be disrupted, leading to fluid retention, bloating, and weight fluctuations.

During perimenopause, progesterone levels often decline due to cycles without ovulation (anovulation). Without ovulation, there is no corpus luteum to produce progesterone, leading to irregular periods and shortened luteal phases. This decline shifts the ratio of progesterone to oestrogen, creating a state known as oestrogen dominance.

Although both hormones drop during menopause, progesterone decreases more sharply, resulting in a hormonal imbalance that underlies many of the challenges women face during this transition. Symptoms of oestrogen dominance may include weight gain, reduced libido, sleep disturbances, and the development of fibroids.

As this imbalance progresses, women may experience irregular periods, spotting, and heavy bleeding due to unregulated uterine lining growth, which is driven by oestrogen. Emotional symptoms, such as increased anxiety and mood swings, often arise because of progesterone's reduced calming effect on the brain's GABA receptors. The loss of this natural tranquilliser leads to heightened emotional sensitivity and more frequent mood fluctuations. Understanding these hormonal shifts provides valuable insight into managing the symptoms of perimenopause.

Supporting progesterone production through mindful nutrition and lifestyle choices is key to maintaining hormonal balance, especially during perimenopause and menopause.

Here are actionable steps you can take to support optimal progesterone levels:

## Balance blood sugar

**Why?** When blood sugar drops too low, the body releases cortisol (a stress hormone) to raise glucose levels. Since progesterone acts as a precursor for cortisol, frequent blood sugar dips force the body to prioritise cortisol production over progesterone, which can lead to an imbalance.

**How?**

- Include protein (chicken, eggs, legumes) and healthy fats (extra virgin olive oil, avocado, nuts, and seeds) with each meal and snack
- Reduce refined sugar intake; focus on whole, unprocessed foods
- Take a brisk walk after meals to help stabilise blood sugar
- Avoid frequent snacking; aim for balanced meals to reduce sugar dips

## Include foods rich in vitamin B6, vitamin C, magnesium, and zinc

**Why?** These nutrients are essential for progesterone production: Vitamin B6 supports hormone synthesis; magnesium regulates enzymatic activity needed for hormone production; Vitamin C acts as an antioxidant, helping reduce oxidative stress; and zinc supports progesterone receptor formation.

**How?**

- Vitamin B6: sunflower seeds, avocados, sweet potatoes, chickpeas, salmon, and chicken
- Vitamin C: red peppers, tomatoes, kiwi, and broccoli
- Magnesium: dark green leafy vegetables, almonds, avocado, and legumes
- Zinc: oysters, pumpkin seeds, sesame seeds, chickpeas, and almonds

## Include healthy fats

**Why?** Monounsaturated and polyunsaturated fats are essential building blocks for hormone synthesis. These fats contribute to the formation of cholesterol, which serves as the precursor to progesterone, ensuring a steady supply for hormone production.

**How?**

- Incorporate monounsaturated fats like avocados, olives, and olive oil into your meals
- Include polyunsaturated fats like fatty fish (salmon, mackerel), flaxseeds, chia seeds, and walnuts

## Reduce stress

**Why?** Chronic stress can elevate cortisol production, diverting resources away from progesterone synthesis. Cortisol and progesterone share a common precursor (pregnenolone), so when stress demands cortisol, progesterone production may suffer.

**How?**

- Prioritise self-care: dedicate time each day to activities that relax and rejuvenate you, such as meditation, mindfulness or yoga
- Set boundaries: learn to say no to overwhelming commitments and create space for activities that support your well-being

## Choose gentle exercise over intense workouts

**Why?** Intense exercise can trigger a stress response, increasing cortisol levels. Elevated cortisol diverts the body's focus away from producing progesterone, prioritising stress adaptation over reproductive health.

**How?**

- Walking: a thirty minute walk each day can help reduce stress and support hormonal balance
- Yoga: a combination of stretching, strength-building, and mindfulness, yoga can help manage stress while improving flexibility
- Swimming: a low-impact, full-body exercise, swimming supports physical health without overstressing the body
- Pilates: strengthens core stability and muscle tone with gentle, low-impact movements

## Limit caffeine and avoid it on an empty stomach

**Why?** Caffeine, particularly when consumed on an empty stomach, can trigger the release of cortisol. This stress hormone's production can be prioritised over progesterone, leading to imbalances.

**How?**

- Eat a protein and healthy fat breakfast (e.g. vegetable omelette, scrambled eggs, avocado on sourdough, or full-fat Greek yoghurt with nuts and berries) before having your coffee
- Gradually reduce your daily caffeine intake
- Opt for herbal teas or decaffeinated coffee

Think of progesterone as that calming friend who has always helped keep things in check – making sure emotions stay level, sleep comes easily, and stress doesn't spiral out of control. But, as menopause approaches, that friend starts showing up less and less, leaving you feeling a bit off-balance and overwhelmed. It's no wonder things feel more chaotic! But just because she's not as present doesn't mean you have to face this transition alone. With a few supportive tweaks to your daily habits, can still find your centre.

**RC'S STORY**

I've recently started HRT, a bit blindly if I'm honest.
I have many if not all of the symptoms of the perimenopause and of course I have been suffering from these cluster migraines for a few years now, so this is hopefully going to help both.
I've had no education from my GP but from a little research myself, instigated this treatment in the hope it would help but with no real idea of what was happening and why.
One chat with Julie and I had a better understanding of what was happening to my body and why! It honestly blew my mind. I also had many tips on how I could help myself.
Why do our health professionals not educate us on something half the population will go through? Why do they not want us to be able to help ourselves?
I can't recommend Julie enough and would encourage anyone who thinks they might be perimenopausal/ menopausal to seek help, whether that be from their GP or from a professional who can educate us. As Julie will tell you – we are not alone.

# *Chapter Ten*

## The Hormone Symphony: Beyond Oestrogen and Progesterone

*"When hormones fall into balance, every system in the body works better – sleep becomes restful, energy stabilises, and the mind feels clearer. Balance isn't just a state of being it's the key to thriving."*

By now, you'll have seen how hormones function as a finely tuned system, with each of them playing a unique and critical role in maintaining your health and well-being. When one hormone shifts out of balance, it can create a ripple effect that impacts others, often leading to noticeable physical and emotional changes. This is particularly evident during perimenopause and menopause when hormonal fluctuations are at their peak.

Beyond oestrogen and progesterone, there are several other hormones that play a vital role in female health:

## Testosterone

Androgens such as testosterone are a class of hormones vital for both male and female physiology. While testosterone is often associated with male characteristics, it also plays an essential role in women's bodies. It is primarily produced in the ovaries, specifically within the cells of the ovarian follicles, and also in the adrenal glands, located above the kidneys. This becomes especially important after menopause when ovarian function declines, and adrenal glands become a more significant source of androgens.

Testosterone serves several important functions in the female body:

**Sexual health**
Testosterone plays a vital role in increasing libido and sexual satisfaction by supporting the health of reproductive tissues, including the clitoris and vaginal tissues.

**Bone health**
It helps maintain bone density, reducing the risk of osteoporosis, especially as women age.

**Muscle mass and strength**
Contributes to muscle growth and strength, supporting overall physical resilience and energy levels.

**Mood and emotional well-being**
Influences emotional balance, helping improve mood, reduce anxiety, and increase overall well-being.

**Cognitive function**
Supports memory retention and cognitive health.

## Follicle stimulating hormone (FSH): the egg-preparing hormone

FSH is a key hormone responsible for regulating reproductive processes, especially in preparing the body for ovulation and the menstrual cycle. Its roles are to:

**Stimulate follicle maturation**

FSH initiates the growth and maturation of ovarian follicles, which contain immature eggs. This process is essential for ovulation and overall reproductive health, helping to regulate regular menstrual cycles.

**Stimulate oestrogen production**

As follicles mature, they produce oestrogen. This hormone plays a critical role in thickening the uterine lining in preparation for potential pregnancy. Maintaining healthy oestrogen levels is essential not only for reproductive function but also for mood stability, bone health, and skin integrity.

**Timing**

FSH secretion peaks during the early phase of the menstrual cycle (the follicular phase), signalling the ovaries to prepare for ovulation. By understanding how FSH levels fluctuate throughout the cycle, women can better manage their reproductive health and hormonal balance.

## Luteinising hormone (LH): the "ovulation trigger" hormone

LH plays a vital role in the female reproductive system by triggering ovulation and supporting the early stages of pregnancy. LH works closely with FSH to ensure healthy ovulation and hormone production. It matters because:

**Triggers ovulation**
LH is responsible for releasing a mature egg from the ovary during ovulation, which is a critical aspect of fertility. Monitoring LH levels can help women better understand their ovulation patterns.

**Corpus luteum formation**
After ovulation, LH helps form the corpus luteum, a structure that produces progesterone. Progesterone supports the uterine lining, prepares the body for potential pregnancy, and plays a role in regulating menstrual cycles.

**Timing**
LH surges mid-cycle, usually around day 14 in a 28-day cycle, which triggers ovulation. Understanding LH timing is essential for fertility awareness, whether you are trying to conceive or monitor your menstrual health.

## Ghrelin: the "hunger hormone"

Ghrelin, often called the "hunger hormone," is a peptide hormone predominantly produced in the stomach. Its primary function is to regulate appetite by sending signals to the brain when the stomach is empty, prompting the sensation of hunger. Ghrelin levels typically rise before meals, encouraging food intake to ensure the body meets its energy requirements. Once you start eating and your stomach is full, ghrelin levels drop, diminishing the sensation of hunger. Its key functions are to: initiate hunger by signalling to the brain's hypothalamus; stimulate appetite; regulate energy balance by ensuring energy levels are replenished, particularly in times of low-calorie intake or fasting; and to enhances growth hormone secretion, which affects muscle mass and fat distribution.

Ghrelin is crucial for maintaining energy homeostasis, but in some individuals, especially those who diet or restrict calories, ghrelin levels may remain persistently high, making weight management more challenging. This can lead to increased hunger, cravings, and difficulty adhering to dietary changes.

## Leptin: the "satiety hormone"

Leptin, often referred to as the "satiety hormone", is primarily produced by the body's fat cells and plays a critical role in appetite regulation and energy homeostasis. It works by communicating with the brain, specifically the hypothalamus, to signal that the body has adequate energy stores, thereby reducing appetite and curbing food intake. When leptin levels are high, it helps suppress hunger, making it easier to feel full and maintain a healthy weight.

Its key functions are to: suppress appetite, sending signals to the brain when energy reserves are sufficient, helping to prevent overeating; regulate energy balance by reducing food intake when body fat stores are adequate; support weight management by managing hunger.

Leptin is essential for long-term regulation of food intake and body weight. Higher levels of leptin usually signal the body that it has enough energy, curbing the desire to eat. Leptin resistance is a common issue. When the brain becomes resistant to leptin's signals, it falsely perceives that the body is starving, triggering increased hunger and reduced energy expenditure. This condition can lead to a cycle of overeating and weight gain.

Tips for enhancing leptin sensitivity: incorporate Omega-3 fatty acids found in fatty fish and flaxseeds; exercise regularly; avoid processed foods, as diets high in sugar and unhealthy fats can impair leptin signalling.

## Neurotransmitters and hormones

Neurotransmitters are chemical messengers that play a critical role in communication between nerve cells (neurons) in the brain and throughout the body. These substances are released from one neuron and travel across a small gap called the synapse to deliver signals to another neuron or target cell. Each neurotransmitter has specific functions and impacts various physiological and psychological processes, including mood, motivation, memory, sleep, and motor control. Hormones and neurotransmitters work together in a delicate balance. During menopause, as hormone levels fluctuate, these interactions can become disrupted, impacting both mental and physical well-being.

## The four main neurotransmitters:

- **Serotonin ("feel-good")**
  Serotonin supports emotional well-being and regulates mood, digestion, and cognitive functions. It connects the brain's limbic system and forebrain, helping to maintain mood and bodily processes. Serotonin is also a precursor for melatonin: the pineal gland synthesises melatonin from serotonin to signal the brain that it's time to sleep. Healthy serotonin levels often correlate with healthy melatonin levels, improving sleep quality. Low serotonin can lead to poor stress management, sugar cravings, and depressive moods.

- **Dopamine ("motivation and reward")**
  Known as the "reward neurotransmitter," dopamine is essential for reward-seeking, motivation, focus, pleasure, emotional regulation, and decision-making. It also influences motor control, locomotion, learning, working memory, and addictive behaviours.

- **Glutamate ("learning and memory")**
  As the brain's primary excitatory neurotransmitter, glutamate is crucial for learning and memory. It activates many brain areas, including the hippocampus and prefrontal cortex, which are essential for cognitive function.

- **Gamma-aminobutyric acid aka GABA ("emotional stability")**
  GABA is the brain's main inhibitory neurotransmitter. It helps balance brain activity and prevents overexcitation. GABA reduces anxiety, supports motor control, and calms the nervous system, promoting relaxation and emotional stability.

Neurotransmitters interact closely with hormones such as oestrogen and progesterone, which modulate their activity and influence mood, cognition, and brain function. During menopause, hormonal changes significantly affect these neurotransmitters, often leading to mood swings, irritability, and emotional instability.

**The oestrogen-serotonin connection**

Oestrogen plays a key role in regulating serotonin by influencing its receptors and availability. During menopause, the decline in oestrogen disrupts this balance, often causing mood fluctuations, irritability, and symptoms of depression. This underscores how oestrogen's relationship with serotonin directly impacts emotional health.

**The oestrogen-and progesterone-dopamine link**

Oestrogen and dopamine share a close connection, particularly in regulating mood. A decline in oestrogen reduces dopamine activity in the brain, contributing to lower motivation, mood swings, and emotional challenges. Falling progesterone further exacerbates this by disrupting dopamine pathways and intensifying emotional instability.

Progesterone's protective influence on the brain is partly attributed to its metabolite, allopregnanolone. This neuroactive steroid binds to GABA-A receptors, enhancing GABA's calming effects on the nervous system, promoting relaxation and stabilising mood during hormonal shifts.

**Circadian rhythm and sleep: melatonin, cortisol, and growth hormone**

The circadian rhythm, often referred to as the "body clock," is an internal 24-hour cycle that regulates the sleep-wake pattern and synchronises various physiological processes with environmental cues like light and darkness. This finely tuned system ensures that sleep, energy levels, hormone release, and metabolism follow a predictable rhythm. Melatonin, cortisol, and growth hormone work alongside neurotransmitters such as serotonin and GABA to maintain this rhythm, creating a critical link between hormones, neurotransmitters, and overall health.

**Melatonin: the sleep hormone**

Melatonin signals to the body that it's time to sleep, increasing in production during the evening and decreasing with exposure to morning light. Poor sleep hygiene or excessive blue light exposure can disrupt melatonin levels, affecting sleep quality and overall restfulness.

**Cortisol: the morning activator**

Cortisol peaks in the morning to promote wakefulness and declines at night to prepare the body for rest. Chronic stress or irregular sleep patterns can disrupt cortisol's rhythm, leading to heightened stress and impaired daily functioning.

**Growth hormone: the restorative hormone**

Released during deep sleep, growth hormone supports tissue repair, muscle growth, and cellular regeneration. It highlights the importance of restorative sleep for overall resilience and physical recovery.

When these systems are in balance, they help optimise sleep quality, energy levels, and emotional stability. Optimising these processes involves practising good sleep hygiene—avoiding blue light exposure in the evening, maintaining a consistent sleep schedule (even on weekends), and creating a restful sleep environment with dim lighting and a comfortable temperature.

## Empowering holistic health beyond oestrogen and progesterone

Menopause isn't just about changes in oestrogen and progesterone; it's a complex interplay of hormones, neurotransmitters, and lifestyle factors that shape your overall well-being. All of these play a key role in regulating mood, sustaining energy, and promoting physical health.

Understanding this broader perspective empowers you to take control of your health. Menopause offers a chance to prioritise what helps you feel your best. Simple practices like improving sleep hygiene, managing stress, and nourishing your body with nutrient-rich foods create a ripple effect that nurtures both body and mind. Consistently practising these habits can help you regain energy, clarity, and stability.

Your menopause journey is as unique as you are. Every step you take to prioritise your health and well-being is important. Trust in your body's incredible ability to adapt and thrive. Ask yourself:

*What small, intentional change can you make today to feel more balanced and energised tomorrow?*

# *Chapter Eleven*

## The Thyroid: Master Regulator of Metabolism and Energy

The thyroid gland, a butterfly-shaped organ located in your neck, plays an essential role in regulating your body's metabolism and energy production. It produces two primary hormones: thyroxine (T4) and triiodothyronine (T3). T3 is the active hormone that drives metabolic processes, mood regulation, and energy balance. T4 acts as a reserve, converting into T3 when needed, primarily in the gut, liver, and kidneys. This clever system ensures your body has enough thyroid hormone to keep metabolism and other vital functions running smoothly.

Maintaining healthy thyroid function relies on the pituitary gland releasing thyroid-stimulating hormone (TSH), which signals the thyroid to produce and release T4 and T3. Think of TSH as the thyroid's messenger, adjusting the body's needs like a thermostat. When thyroid hormone levels dip, TSH rises to kickstart more hormone production. Conversely, when thyroid hormones are plentiful, TSH levels drop, reducing production. This balance is key for stabilising energy levels, supporting metabolism, and preserving overall hormonal health.

When the thyroid isn't working as it should, it can profoundly affect your body's energy, metabolism, and overall well-being. Hypothyroidism (underactive thyroid) and hyperthyroidism (overactive thyroid) are two common thyroid conditions, each leading to different sets of symptoms and challenges. Both imbalances can severely impact energy levels, mood, and general health.

| **Hypothyroidism** | **Hyperthyroidism** |
|---|---|
| Too little hormone is produced, and your metabolism slows down. | Too much hormone is produced and your metabolism speeds up. |
| **Symptoms** | **Symptoms** |
| • Fatigue<br>• Weight gain<br>• Difficulty concentrating ("brain fog")<br>• Sensitivity to cold<br>• Dry skin and hair loss<br>• Mood changes, including depression | • Weight loss<br>• Heart palpitations or rapid heartbeat<br>• Anxiety or restlessness<br>• Difficulty sleeping<br>• Heat intolerance |

## Causes of hypothyroidism

These can vary, but one of the most common is autoimmune thyroiditis, particularly Hashimoto's Thyroiditis. In this condition, the immune system mistakenly attacks the thyroid gland, causing inflammation and damage that impairs its ability to produce hormones. Both genetic predisposition and environmental factors, such as exposure to toxins, infections, or chronic stress, can contribute to the development of Hashimoto's disease.

Hashimoto's disease is diagnosed through blood tests that detect the presence of specific autoantibodies, particularly thyroid peroxidase (TPO) and thyroglobulin (TG) antibodies. These autoantibodies help confirm the diagnosis and the autoimmune nature of the thyroid dysfunction.

The most common symptoms of Hashimoto's disease and hypothyroidism include:

- **Fatigue**
- **Weight gain**
- **Sensitivity to cold**
- **Constipation**
- **Dry skin and hair**
- **Hair loss**
- **Muscle weakness**
- **Joint pain**
- **Depression and memory issues**
- **Irregular menstrual cycles.**

These symptoms can develop gradually and may be nonspecific, making the diagnosis of hypothyroidism more challenging. Treatment often focuses on maintaining hormone balance and managing symptoms to improve quality of life.

Factors that can disrupt thyroid function include:

**Disrupted TSH secretion**
When the communication between your brain and thyroid becomes impaired, hormone production drops.

**Impaired T4-to-T3 conversion**
Issues in the liver, gut, or other tissues can prevent the conversion of T4 into the more active T3, reducing the effectiveness of thyroid function.

**Decreased hormone utilisation**
At the cellular level, tissues may become less responsive to thyroid hormones, limiting their effect on the body.

**Chronic stress**
Excess cortisol and imbalances in stress hormones like adrenaline can disrupt thyroid function, further affecting the body's overall hormonal balance.

Thyroid function is closely connected to other hormonal systems, particularly the reproductive hormones oestrogen and progesterone. This interaction is crucial for women's health, especially during perimenopause and menopause, as fluctuations in these hormones can significantly affect thyroid function:

**Conversion of T4 to T3**
Hormonal changes during perimenopause can disrupt the conversion of T4 to T3, leading to thyroid hormone imbalances. This imbalance often results in symptoms like fatigue, weight gain, and mood changes, which are often compounded during the transition into menopause.

**Thyroid binding globulin (TBG) levels**

TBG is a protein that binds to thyroid hormones and transports them through the bloodstream. Changes in oestrogen and progesterone levels during perimenopause can alter TBG levels, affecting how much free (active) thyroid hormone is available to the body.

**Thyroglobulin levels**

Thyroglobulin is a protein crucial for T4 synthesis in the thyroid gland. Hormonal fluctuations, particularly during perimenopause, can influence thyroglobulin production, further impacting thyroid hormone levels and contributing to the broader hormonal shifts women experience during this life stage.

As women journey through the menopausal transition, supporting thyroid health is crucial. Menopause and thyroid dysfunction often share similar symptoms, such as fatigue, weight changes, and mood fluctuations, which can magnify each other's effects and make this time of life feel more challenging. The good news? With the right dietary choices and lifestyle, you can optimise your thyroid function and ease these overlapping symptoms. There are simple but powerful strategies to help you thrive through menopause by caring for your thyroid health:

**Recognise symptom overlap**

Regular blood tests and consultations with a healthcare provider can help differentiate between the two and ensure that thyroid imbalances are properly addressed.

**Stress reduction**

Chronic stress can disrupt the hypothalamic-pituitary-thyroid (HPT) axis, which may lead to thyroid issues. Incorporating stress-reducing techniques such as mindfulness meditation, deep breathing exercises, yoga, and regular physical activity can lower stress levels and support thyroid health.

**Prioritise gut health**

The gut-thyroid axis is crucial for regulating thyroid function. A fibre-rich diet from fruits, vegetables, whole grains, and legumes promotes a healthy gut. Additionally, incorporating probiotic-rich foods like yogurt, kefir, sauerkraut, and kimchi helps maintain a balanced gut microbiome, which in turn supports optimal thyroid function.

**Stay hydrated**

Adequate hydration is essential for thyroid hormone production and metabolism. Drinking enough water throughout the day helps support thyroid function and prevents symptoms such as fatigue and brain fog.

**Eat nutrient-dense foods**

A nutrient-rich diet is essential for thyroid health and overall well-being. Incorporate the following foods to provide essential vitamins, minerals, antioxidants, and macronutrients:

- Zinc-rich foods: zinc is vital for thyroid hormone synthesis. Include foods like shellfish, beef, pork, chicken, pumpkin seeds, hemp seeds, and lentils.
- Selenium-rich foods: selenium supports thyroid hormone metabolism and protects the thyroid from oxidative damage. Good sources include Brazil nuts, seafood, sunflower seeds, eggs, and spinach.
- Iodine-rich foods: iodine is essential for the production of thyroid hormones. Ensure your diet includes iodised

salt and seaweed.

- Vitamin A: It is essential for the production of thyroid hormones and acts as an antioxidant, reducing oxidative stress that can harm thyroid cells. Good dietary sources include animal-based foods such as liver, egg yolks, and plant-based sources including brightly coloured fruits and vegetables rich in beta-carotene, a precursor to vitamin A. Examples are carrots, sweet potatoes, and mango.
- B Vitamins: are crucial for thyroid hormone production. Consume whole grains, legumes, leafy greens, nuts, seeds, and animal products.
- Vitamin D: deficiency here is linked to thyroid disorders. Incorporate fatty fish, fortified dairy products, eggs, and mushrooms, and aim for regular sun exposure.
- Essential Fatty Acids (EFAs): Omega-3 fatty acids help reduce inflammation and support thyroid function. Sources include fatty fish, flaxseeds, chia seeds, walnuts, and hemp seeds.
- Magnesium-rich foods: essential for thyroid hormone production. Add avocado, leafy greens, whole grains, nuts, seeds, and legumes to your meals.
- Iron: deficiency can impair thyroid function. Include lean meats, poultry, seafood, legumes, tofu, fortified cereals, spinach, and pumpkin seeds.

## Navigating the role of female hormones in menopause

As you journey through perimenopause and menopause, it's important to understand how your hormones interact to impact your overall well-being. As hormone levels fluctuate during menopause, it's natural for imbalances to occur, and being aware of these changes can help you better manage your symptoms.

I've seen many women face these changes and come out stronger. Clients who once struggled with sleepless nights and emotional ups and downs have learned to listen to their bodies and trust the signals. Remember, your body knows exactly what it's doing. The more you understand the hormonal shifts happening within you, the more empowered you become to take control of your health and vitality.

Maybe it's something as simple as prioritising a bit more rest, adding an extra serving of green vegetables to your dinner, or taking a moment to breathe deeply and release stress. Each little act of kindness to yourself is a way of saying, "I am worthy of feeling well."

**MY PERSONAL THYROID JOURNEY: WHEN KNOWLEDGE ISN'T ENOUGH**

I had just completed my studies in Naturopathic Nutrition – a time that should have left me feeling empowered, energised, and ready to help others. But instead, I found myself barely able to get out of bed, struggling to muster enough energy to hold a simple conversation. Despite all the knowledge I'd gained, I was facing rapid weight gain, debilitating fatigue, and a sense of heaviness that didn't seem to make any sense.

Determined to uncover the root of my symptoms, I decided to test my thyroid levels. The results were eye-opening: my TSH (Thyroid-Stimulating Hormone) was high, indicating that my thyroid wasn't functioning properly. Although I was relieved to finally have some answers, it was a sobering reminder that, even with a health background, it's easy to miss what's happening in your own body.

Further testing showed I didn't have any autoimmune antibodies, so I started on thyroxine, which brought some much-needed relief. While it helped, I've come to realise that managing thyroid health isn't always straightforward. I still experience fluctuations, but over time I've learned to recognise the signs and respond with compassion, reducing stress, and being gentle with myself when my body needs it most.

I share this experience not just as a practitioner, but as someone who knows the frustration, uncertainty, and emotional toll thyroid imbalances can take. My journey has deepened my understanding of this powerful little gland, and I hope that by sharing what I've learned, I can support others on their own path to better thyroid health.

Julie

# *Chapter Twelve*

## To HRT or not to HRT?

*That is the question, and the answer is: after considering all your options and seeking guidance, the choice is completely yours.*

Hormone Replacement Therapy (HRT) is prescribed for the relief of menopausal symptoms. It involves supplementing the body with hormones, primarily oestrogen, and sometimes progesterone, to alleviate symptoms of menopause. Many symptoms, such as hot flushes, night sweats, mood swings, vaginal dryness, and sleep disturbances, are linked to reduced oestrogen levels. That's why oestrogen is the primary component of HRT.

In addition to relieving symptoms, HRT offers long-term health benefits, especially for women experiencing premature ovarian insufficiency (POI), premature menopause, or early menopause. For these women, HRT can significantly reduce the risks of osteoporosis and cardiovascular disease, conditions exacerbated by oestrogen deficiency. However, for some people, HRT may not be an option due to personal preferences or medical reasons.

The key is to seek guidance from healthcare professionals, equip yourself with knowledge, and - most importantly - trust yourself; you are the expert on your own body. You know when something feels off.

When taking oestrogen alone, there's a risk of stimulating the womb lining, which can cause unhealthy thickening and increase the risk of womb (endometrial) cancer. To mitigate this, progesterone or progestogen is typically added, unless the womb has been removed, in which case oestrogen alone is prescribed. For women experiencing persistent low libido, testosterone may also be prescribed to address Hypoactive Sexual Desire Disorder (HSDD). Delivered as a gel, testosterone can help improve sexual desire and energy levels.

There are two types of HRT:

**Regulated body-identical hormones (RBHRT)**
Naturally derived hormones that closely mimic the ones naturally produced by the body. They are prescribed by GPs and include options like micronised progesterone (e.g. Utrogestan) and transdermal oestrogen (applied via patches, gels, or sprays).

**Compounded bioidentical hormones**
Which are custom-made formulations prepared by compounding pharmacies and marketed as being individually tailored to specific needs. However, compounded bioidentical hormones are not regulated.

HRT comes in various forms, allowing for customisation based on personal preferences, lifestyle, and symptom severity. The options are:

| | |
|---|---|
| **Tablets** | Convenient but undergo heavy first-pass liver metabolism. |
| **Patches** | Applied to the skin and replaced every few days, offering a steady release of hormones. |
| **Gels and Spray** | Applied topically, these options allow for precise dosage adjustments and are absorbed directly through the skin. |
| **Mirena Coil** | A small device placed inside the uterus, typically fitted in an outpatient clinic. Both a contraceptive and a hormone-releasing device, it delivers a small amount of progestogen directly to the uterine lining. This helps thin the lining, reducing heavy periods and providing the progestogen component of HRT. |

There are several forms of HRT, each incorporating one of these delivery methods:

## Cyclical sequential combined HRT (SEQUI)

This is for women who still have a womb. Oestrogen alone can increase the risk of uterine cancer by thickening the womb lining, so adding progesterone counteracts this by keeping the lining thin and healthy. For women in perimenopause, when periods are still present, HRT often involves taking oestrogen daily and adding progestogen for 10-14 days each month. This is known as sequential HRT and typically results in a monthly withdrawal bleed for about 85% of women. If periods are becoming irregular or infrequent, another option is long-cycle HRT, where progestogen is taken for two weeks every three months, resulting in a withdrawal bleed approximately four times per year.

SEQUI can be delivered in several ways:

| | |
|---|---|
| **Combined Tablets** | Oestrogen is taken alone for the first 14-16 days of the cycle then a combination of oestrogen and progestogen is taken for the remaining 12-14 days. It typically results in a monthly withdrawal bleed. |
| **Combined Patches** | A single patch provides both oestrogen and progestogen, delivering hormones in a controlled manner throughout the cycle. |
| **Separate Oestrogen and Progestogen** | Separate patches can allow greater flexibility and tailored symptom management. |
| **Oestrogen** | Delivered via a patch, gel, or spray. |
| **Micronised Progesterone** | Taken at bedtime in a dose of 200mg daily for 12-14 days within a 28-day cycle. |

### Continuous combined HRT (CONTI)

This is for women who have not experienced a period for over a year or are aged 54 and above. It combines oestrogen and progestogen daily, eliminating the need for withdrawal bleeding.

### Vaginal oestrogen

This is for women experiencing localised urogenital symptoms such as vaginal dryness, discomfort during sex, or recurrent UTIs. It comes in creams, gels, pessaries, or vaginal rings that provide a direct, localised dose of oestrogen. Vaginal oestrogen is low-risk and can be used alongside systemic HRT or on its own.

Before Starting HRT, the following are important:

**Understanding your risk factors**
Discuss your medical history with your GP to weigh the benefits and risks.

**Trial and error**
It may take time to find the right combination of hormones. Be patient and open to adjustments. If it doesn't feel right, advocate for yourself.

**Regular reassessment**
HRT isn't necessarily lifelong; periodic reviews with your GP can ensure the treatment remains suitable for your needs.

So, whether it's patches, tablets, gels, or no HRT at all, remember that the most important thing is taking care of yourself in every way possible. For me, while experiencing early menopause, HRT was a turning point. However, I also knew it wasn't a magic bullet. I still needed to address other areas of my life, like stress and nutrition, to truly support my health.

Keeping track of your symptoms can make a significant difference. Using a symptom tracker (see Chapter 13) ahead of your GP appointments can help you communicate your experiences clearly. I know from both personal experiences, and from working with so many other women, that by the time your appointment arrives, it can feel overwhelming. You might find yourself in "fight or flight" mode, or so emotionally drained that it's hard to get the words out. Having your tracker and writing down your questions or concerns beforehand can be invaluable.

And just a little piece of advice if you go down the HRT patch route – be prepared for a few unexpected adventures. I can't tell you how many times I've heard stories of patches mysteriously disappearing, only to be discovered later stuck to a rogue pair of trousers, or even ... your unsuspecting partner! Laugh at the hiccups along the way, lean into the support around you, and keep nurturing those pillars of health we've talked about – nutrition, stress reduction, self-care, and finding your joy.

# *Part Two*

## Common Symptoms and How to Navigate Them

# *Chapter Thirteen*

## Menopause Symptom Bingo

*Picture this: it's Friday night, and, instead of going out, you and your friends gather around for a game of Menopause Bingo. No fancy prizes, just the satisfaction of knowing that someone else gets it. Forgetting why you walked into a room? That's a tick! Waking up at 3 a.m. for no apparent reason, drenched in sweat? Cross that one off! Crying over a TV commercial about puppies? Bingo! you shout, while your friend nods in understanding because she cried over a fabric softener ad yesterday.*

The Menopause Bingo jackpot is simply knowing you're not going through this rollercoaster alone. It's about more than just the hot flushes and sleepless nights; it's about laughing with your friends when you all realise you've turned the house upside down looking for glasses that were on your head the whole time.

A frequent question I'm asked is, "Is it normal to feel like a stranger in your own body?" And the answer is absolutely yes.

During perimenopause and menopause, I truly felt as if an alien had taken over my body and was changing every part of who I thought I was. I genuinely didn't recognise myself anymore – physically, emotionally, and mentally. My husband seconds this and often told me it felt like he'd lost the woman he married. These shifts can be so overwhelming, not just for us, but for the people around us.

Menopause brings about a whirlwind of changes. Some are well-known, others can take you completely by surprise. When I first started experiencing menopausal symptoms, I felt disconnected from my own body. I couldn't quite link what was happening to my hormones. It felt as though my body was working against me, without any clear reason why. But as I began to learn more about the influence hormones have on almost every part of our well-being – from sleep and skin elasticity to mood and concentration – I finally began to understand.

Around 90% of women seek advice and support from healthcare professionals for symptoms that can drastically reduce quality of life, highlighting the urgent need for effective interventions. According to Women's Health Concern, up to a third of women may experience severe symptoms that substantially impact their well-being.

The empowering truth is that knowledge is power. By understanding the hormonal shifts behind these changes, you can demystify what's happening and reclaim a sense of control. Yes, menopause presents challenges, but it also offers a powerful opportunity to nurture yourself in ways you may not have had the chance to before.

Each woman's experience of menopause is as unique as her

fingerprint. Your journey through menopause is personal, and no two paths will look the same. You may encounter several symptoms in a day, a week, or even over months – some listed in this book and some that aren't – and that's perfectly okay. It's important to remember that every woman is different, and what you experience is entirely normal for you.

Menopause is associated with a diverse range of over 34 symptoms, which may appear suddenly or seem unrelated to hormonal changes. So, grab your bingo card (and a fan for those hot flushes) and let's dive into the many symptoms that make this life phase feel like a never-ending game. Just remember, you're in good company – and that's the real win!

| | | | |
|---|---|---|---|
| Hot flushes | Night sweats | Concentration difficulties | Vaginal dryness |
| Mood swings/ Irritability | Fatigue | Insomnia | Weight gain |
| Decreased libido | Dizziness/ light-headedness | Depression | Memory lapses |
| Irregular periods | Joint pain | Burning sensation in the mouth | Dry skin |
| Changes in body odour | Hair loss/ thinning | Breast tenderness | Increased urinary frequency/ urgency |
| Dizziness/ Tinnitus | Headaches | Digestive issues | Anxiety |

| | | | |
|---|---|---|---|
| Heart palpitations | Gum problems | Muscle tension/ stiffness | Tingling sensations |
| Electric shock sensations | Itchy skin | Brittle nails | Changes in menstrual flow |
| Increased facial hair growth | Worsening of pre-existing conditions | *...add your own...!* | ...add your own...! |

My starting symptom was vertigo, which I initially blamed on swimming while on holiday. After many tests, with no clear answers, it wasn't until much later that I discovered how falling oestrogen levels can affect the balance centres in the brain, causing dizziness. That was a pivotal moment for me, realising how varied menopause symptoms could be and how they don't always fit the common list.

*I went upstairs to grab something important, but by the time I got there, I couldn't remember what it was. The good news? At least I got my steps in.'*

*'Menopause has made me realise that it's completely normal to cry, laugh, and yell—all in the span of 10 minutes. I like to think of it as emotional multitasking'.*

*'Yesterday, I cried because I couldn't find the matching lid to my Tupperware. Clearly, menopause has made me very passionate about food storage'*

Over the next few chapters, we will explore the most common symptoms, discuss why they happen, and formulate simple, empowering tips to help you through. But first, let me introduce you to The Menopause Symptom Tracker. It's designed to be a simple yet powerful tool to log daily experiences with menopausal symptoms. By using a scale from 0 to 10, you can quantify the impact of each symptom on your life, noting both severity and frequency.

## Here's how it can benefit you:

**Identify patterns**

Tracking helps in recognising triggers and patterns and potential triggers, such as certain foods, activities or stressors, which may exacerbate or alleviate your menopausal symptoms. This awareness empowers you to make informed decisions about lifestyle changes that can positively impact your health.

**Personalised care**

By documenting the severity and frequency of symptoms, you can provide your healthcare provider with valuable information to tailor treatment plans specifically to your needs; this personalised approach can lead to more effective symptom management and improved wellbeing.

**Measure progress**

Over time, tracking your symptoms allows you to monitor the effectiveness of any interventions, whether its dietary modifications, hormone therapy, exercise routines, or stress management techniques. By observing trends and changes in symptoms, you can adjust your treatment plan as needed to achieve better outcomes.

**Enhance communication**

A detailed symptom tracker serves as a communication tool between you and your healthcare provider. By sharing your symptom log during consultations, you ensure that important details are not overlooked, leading to more productive discussions and informed decisions about your healthcare.

**Empowerment**

Taking an active role in monitoring and managing your menopausal symptoms can empower you to regain a sense of control over your health and wellbeing by tracking your experiences and advocating your needs.

Remember to be consistent and thorough in recording your symptoms using the tracker. The more accurate and detailed your documentation, the better equipped you and your healthcare provider will be to address your concerns and optimise your treatment plan.

*"I think of the tracker as my own personal bingo card! It can be particularly useful when I have a consultation with my healthcare provider, as it offers detailed insights into my symptoms and patterns. It's my secret weapon for getting the right support – and maybe even winning at this crazy game called menopause!"*

## Menopause symptom tracker

*Keep track of your menopausal symptoms by recording the severity and frequency of each symptom daily or as needed. Use a scale from 0 to 10, with 0 indicating no symptoms and 10 indicating severe symptoms.*

Date: .......................... Age:.................

| SYMPTOM | SEVERITY (0-10) | FREQUENCY (Number of episodes/days/nights) |
|---|---|---|
| Allergic reactions | | |
| Anger or Irritability | | |
| Anxiety | | |
| Blotting | | |
| Brain Fog | | |
| Breast Tenderness | | |
| Brittle Nails | | |
| Burning sensations in mouth | | |
| Changes in body odour | | |
| Changes in menstrual flow | | |
| Concentration Difficulties | | |
| Decreased Libido | | |
| Depression | | |
| Digestive Issues | | |
| Dizziness | | |
| Dry skin | | |

| | | |
|---|---|---|
| Electric shock sensations | | |
| Fatigue | | |
| Gum problems | | |
| Hair loss/thinning | | |
| Headaches | | |
| Heart Palpitations | | |
| Hot flushes | | |
| Increased facial hair | | |
| Insomnia/sleep disturbances | | |
| Itchy skin | | |
| Joint aches and pains | | |
| Memory lapses | | |
| Mood swings | | |
| Muscle tension/ stiffness | | |
| Night sweats | | |
| Panic attacks | | |
| Tingling sensations | | |
| Vaginal dryness/ irritation | | |
| Weight gain | | |
| Worsening of existing conditions | | |

*Notes/Comments:* *[Make a space for any additional notes or comments about your symptoms, triggers, or any patterns noticed.]*

# *Chapter Fourteen*

# Menstrual Changes and Hot Flushes

## 1. Menstrual changes

*"Have you found yourself surprised by changes in your menstrual cycle as you approach menopause? Perhaps your periods have become lighter, or maybe they're arriving more frequently or skipping a month altogether or have become much heavier and you are experiencing flooding?"*

As menopause approaches, many women experience significant changes in their menstrual cycle. These can include variations in flow (heavier or lighter), changes in the length of bleeding episodes, or even skipped cycles. These fluctuations are primarily driven by hormonal changes – especially the gradual decline in oestrogen and progesterone levels. Research indicates that menstrual cycle length often begins to increase roughly 7.5 years before the final menstrual period (FMP), with more pronounced changes occurring around four years prior. Variability in cycle length becomes particularly common in the two years leading up to menopause when ovulation occurs less frequently or ceases altogether.

This variability is due to the body's shifting balance between oestrogen and progesterone. As we've already seen, oestrogen dominance can lead to heavier and more painful periods, shorter or more frequent cycles, and symptoms resembling PMS, such as bloating, mood swings, and breast tenderness. As oestrogen continues to thicken the uterine lining, menstrual cramps and clotting may also intensify.

Meanwhile, declining progesterone, which normally stabilises the uterine lining, can lead to increased menstrual irregularity. If progesterone levels drop significantly, the uterine lining may thicken excessively, resulting in heavier bleeding. On the other hand, some women may experience lighter or skipped periods, reflecting the body's gradual shift toward the end of its reproductive phase.

## Actionable Tips

Managing these menstrual changes can be challenging, but there are practical strategies to help support your body during this transition:

**Track your menstrual cycle**
Keeping a menstrual diary can be incredibly helpful. By noting changes in flow, cycle length, and duration, you'll gain a clearer picture of your body's new patterns. This information is also invaluable when discussing symptoms with your healthcare provider.

**Manage stress effectively**
Stress can worsen hormonal imbalances, making menstrual changes more pronounced. Incorporating stress-reduction techniques like meditation, yoga, or deep breathing exercises can help restore a healthier hormonal balance.

**Maintain a balanced diet**

A nutrient-dense diet rich in fruits, vegetables, whole grains, and lean proteins can support overall hormonal health. Limiting processed foods, refined sugars, alcohol, and caffeine may help alleviate symptoms like bloating, irregular bleeding, and energy fluctuations.

**Incorporate regular physical activity**

Moderate exercise – such as walking, swimming, or cycling – can help regulate hormones, reduce menstrual discomfort, and improve mood. Aim for at least thirty minutes of activity most days of the week.

**Consider Professional Guidance**

If menstrual changes become extreme or particularly uncomfortable, consult a healthcare professional. They can evaluate your symptoms and may suggest hormone therapies or other treatments to manage heavy or irregular bleeding.

## 2. Hot flushes

Hot flushes are one of the most disruptive and overwhelming symptoms of menopause, affecting up to 80% of women (see CH's story below). They are often described as sudden, intense waves of heat that seem to rise from within, leaving you flushed, sweaty, and uncomfortable. Many women also experience a racing heart, anxiety, and occasionally chills after the heat subsides. The sensation can be so intense that it interrupts daily activities and can lead to night sweats, which disrupt sleep and leave you exhausted the following day.

**CH'S STORY**

At the start of 2020 I started showing symptoms of menopause and was experiencing lots of flushes, lack of sleep which was impacting my exercise and food routine which was making me feel bad about myself and impacting my lifestyle and wellbeing.

For many months I struggled to sleep which was impacting my energy to exercise as I was up almost every night changing bed covers, having showers, and steeping my feet in the bath to try and cool down! Pre-menopause I had a great life and overnight it had turned upside down and I didn't know who to go to for help. I had no downtime and no lifestyle balance!

But why do they happen? The exact cause of hot flushes is not fully understood, but they are believed to be closely tied to the hormonal fluctuations that occur during menopause – especially the decline in oestrogen. Oestrogen is a key hormone that plays many roles in your body, and one of its crucial functions is regulating your internal thermostat, which is controlled by a part of the brain called the hypothalamus. The hypothalamus acts as your body's temperature regulator, constantly working to maintain a stable core body temperature. Under normal circumstances, it keeps your body within a comfortable temperature range by adjusting your blood flow, sweat production, and other mechanisms to keep you cool or warm when necessary.

However, when oestrogen levels start to fluctuate and decline during menopause, the hypothalamus becomes overly sensitive. It's as though your thermostat gets recalibrated, narrowing the range of temperatures it considers "comfortable". This means that even the smallest changes in body temperature, such as drinking a hot beverage or sitting in a warm room, can cause the hypothalamus to overreact. This triggers a chain reaction to cool your body down. Blood vessels near the surface of your skin dilate, causing the flushed red face and chest that often accompany a hot flush. Sweat glands kick into overdrive to cool your body, leading to excessive sweating. In some cases, your heart rate increases, and your body enters a state of heightened anxiety, making the experience even more uncomfortable. Once the episode passes, the sudden drop in temperature can cause chills, adding to the complexity of the experience.

## Actionable Tips

There's no one-size-fits-all solution for hot flushes, but the good news is that by making small adjustments to your daily habits – especially around food and lifestyle – you can reduce their frequency and intensity:

**Examine the foods you eat**
Certain foods and beverages can trigger or intensify hot flushes. Becoming mindful of what you eat can make a big difference.

**Alcohol**
Alcohol dilates blood vessels, which can trigger a sensation of warmth and increase the likelihood of hot flushes. Try replacing alcohol with refreshing mocktails or fizzy Kombucha.

**Caffeine**

Caffeine is a stimulant that raises your heart rate and body temperature, which can bring on a flush. Try gradually cutting back on coffee by blending regular and decaf. Swap your afternoon coffee for herbal teas like peppermint or chamomile.

**Processed sugars and fats**

These can cause spikes in blood sugar, leading to increased body heat and worsening flushes. Try opting for whole foods – vegetables, fruits, and nuts – that nourish your body while keeping blood sugar stable.

**Spicy foods**

Chilli peppers and hot sauces increase body heat, which can exacerbate hot flushes. Try incorporating cooling herbs like sage into your meals. Sage has been shown to help balance hormones and may reduce flushes.

**Hot foods and drinks**

Even hot meals or drinks can raise your core temperature and trigger a flush. Try letting hot beverages or foods cool down before consuming them to help avoid triggering that sudden wave of heat.

Making small changes in your nutrition and lifestyle can also help manage and even reduce hot flushes:

**Hydration**

Staying hydrated throughout the day helps regulate your body's temperature.

*Tip*: carry a water bottle with you and aim for consistent water intake.

**Relaxation**

Breathing exercises, yoga, or mindfulness can calm your nervous system, reducing both stress and hot flush intensity.

*Tip*: take three deep breaths before meals to centre yourself and promote a state of relaxation.

**Cooling techniques**

Keep a small fan or cooling mist handy, and wear light, breathable clothing.

*Tip*: layers can help you adjust quickly to temperature shifts throughout the day.

**Open conversations**

Don't be afraid to talk about your hot flushes with loved ones or colleagues. It can help create a more understanding and supportive environment.

*Tip*: Addressing these changes openly can foster greater empathy and ease the pressure to "push through" alone.

# *Chapter Fifteen*

# Mood Changes and Weight Changes

## 1. Mood changes

"It's a rollercoaster: happy, sad, furious, tearful, blah ... and that can be in the space of one day."

Mood changes are a common experience during menopause, with many women feeling less tolerant and more irritable, or emotionally unpredictable. These fluctuations are directly tied to the hormonal shifts of menopause, especially the decline in oestrogen and progesterone, which play a key role in regulating stress responses, mood stability, and overall emotional well-being. Around 20% of women experience depression at some point during menopause. This highlights the need to prioritise emotional health during this time.

As oestrogen levels drop, the brain's ability to manage stress and regulate emotions becomes compromised. This hormonal shift disrupts the balance of neurotransmitters, such as serotonin and dopamine, which can amplify feelings of anxiety, overwhelm, or emotional instability. The decrease in progesterone, known for its calming effects, further contributes to emotional reactivity and heightened anxiety.

Both oestrogen and progesterone help synthesise and release neurotransmitters like serotonin and gamma-aminobutyric acid (GABA), both of which are essential for mood regulation and stress resilience. When oestrogen levels fall, this process is disrupted, leading to increased neural excitability, which can trigger panic or anxiety symptoms. Additionally, the drop in serotonin production may intensify mood disturbances related to anxiety, increasing feelings of worry, fear, or irritability.

Personally, I'll never forget a moment during my own experience of menopause. I was in a department store, getting my eyebrows waxed – nothing out of the ordinary. Yet, halfway through, I was gripped by such overwhelming anxiety that I couldn't stay. I had to leave with only one eyebrow done. It was as though a simple task had turned into a mountain I couldn't climb. I can laugh at it now, but it was one of the first times I realised just how profoundly these hormonal changes were impacting my emotional state.

## Actionable Tips

**Embrace self-care and mindfulness practice**

Whether it's deep breathing, journaling, yoga, or mindful walking in nature, find practises that help you reconnect with yourself. These activities help lower stress and bring your focus back to the present moment, which can significantly reduce anxiety and mood swings. Experiment with different practises to see what works for you.

**Regular exercise**

Physical movement does more than just strengthen your body; it's also a natural antidepressant. When you exercise, your body releases endorphins, those feel-good chemicals that boost your mood. Aim for at least thirty minutes of moderate activity several times a week. It could be anything from walking and dancing to cycling or strength training. The key is to move your body in a way that feels enjoyable and helps lift your spirits.

**Food is fuel for both your body and your mind**

Pay attention to what you're eating. Nutrient-rich foods like leafy greens, berries, fatty fish, and nuts can have a positive effect on your brain chemistry. Avoid foods that tend to trigger inflammation or worsen mood swings, like processed sugars, refined carbs, and too much caffeine.

**Sleep hygiene**

Sleep disturbances are often a by-product of menopause, but poor sleep can worsen mood swings and anxiety. Create a calming bedtime routine by avoiding screens before bed, dimming the lights, and maybe even indulging in some lavender aromatherapy. Keeping a consistent sleep schedule can help regulate your body's internal clock and improve your overall mood.

**Build your support network**

Surround yourself with people who support and understand you. Whether it's close friends, family members, or a support group for women going through menopause, having someone to talk to can make all the difference. Share your experiences, frustrations, and victories. Emotional connection can act as a buffer against feelings of isolation and mood dips.

**Seek professional support**

Sometimes, mood swings and anxiety become too much for self-care to manage. If you feel that your emotions are getting too overwhelming, don't hesitate to reach out to a healthcare professional. Therapy or counselling can offer additional strategies, and in some cases, hormone replacement therapy (HRT) may be an option worth discussing with your doctor.

Going back to my story about that fateful eyebrow wax appointment, after finding tools and strategies that work for me, I can confidently sit through the entire appointment, both eyebrows done, and leave feeling very proud of myself. It may seem like a small victory, but for me, it's proof that progress is possible, no matter how overwhelming things may seem at the moment.

So, if you're feeling weighed down by mood swings or anxiety, know that even the smallest wins are worth celebrating. Remember, it's not about eliminating every difficult feeling, but learning how to navigate through them with more confidence and resilience.

Take a moment to ask yourself: w*hat small win can you celebrate today?*

## 2. Weight changes

*"Have you noticed changes in your body shape as you've entered your perimenopause?"*

During perimenopause, fluctuations in oestrogen and progesterone often lead to shifts in fat distribution. Typically, premenopausal women store fat in a gynoid pattern – that is, around the hips, thighs, and buttocks. However, as oestrogen levels decline during menopause, this shifts toward an android pattern of fat storage around the abdomen and waist. This change can feel dramatic, as fat begins to accumulate in areas where it wasn't previously stored.

The main culprit behind this shift is visceral fat, which accumulates around internal organs like the liver, pancreas, and intestines. Unlike subcutaneous fat (which sits directly under the skin), visceral fat is metabolically active and releases bioactive substances such as cytokines and adipokines. These compounds can promote chronic, low-grade inflammation and insulin resistance, increasing the risk of developing metabolic conditions like Type 2 diabetes, cardiovascular disease, and hypertension. Postmenopausal women are particularly prone to this increase in visceral fat.

Understanding these hormonal shifts is the first step to supporting weight changes during menopause. Once you're aware of the "why" behind these shifts, you can take targeted steps to manage your body composition in a way that supports both your physical and emotional well-being.

## Actionable Tips

Navigating weight management during menopause requires a more holistic and personalised approach than a simple focus on calorie restriction. Many women find that shifting their perspective away from restrictive diets and towards nourishing the body with balanced, nutrient-rich foods is a far more sustainable path. Restrictive diets can increase stress, prompting the release of cortisol – the hormone that encourages fat storage, particularly around the abdomen. By focusing on whole, natural foods and making sustainable lifestyle adjustments, you can improve your overall health and feel more in control during this transitional time. Here are practical steps to support:

**Emphasise whole foods**

Prioritise nutrient-dense, whole foods such as vegetables, lean proteins, fruits, whole grains, and healthy fats. These foods help regulate blood sugar levels, reducing the likelihood of unhealthy cravings, and provide essential vitamins and minerals that support metabolic health.

**Stay hydrated**

Drinking adequate amounts of water throughout the day is crucial, as dehydration can often be mistaken for hunger. Aim to drink at least eight glasses a day and check the colour of your urine – it should be a light yellow. For variety, try herbal teas or fruit-infused water to stay refreshed.

**Incorporate regular physical activity**

Aim for a balanced mix of cardio, strength training, and flexibility exercises. Regular movement helps maintain your metabolism, preserves muscle mass, and supports bone health, all of which are vital during menopause. Find activities you enjoy – whether it's brisk walking, swimming, or yoga – and aim for thirty minutes most days of the week.

**Mindful eating**

Slow down during meals and take time to truly savour each bite. Pay attention to your hunger and fullness cues to avoid overeating. Try to remove distractions such as phones or television while eating, and take deep breaths before starting your meal to help your body shift into a more relaxed, calm state for optimal digestion

Fuelling your body is about empowering yourself with better nutrition. Taking control of your health isn't about drastic diets or perfection; it's about making consistent, nourishing choices that truly support your body. Each time you opt for nutrient-dense, whole foods, you're feeding not just your physical health but your emotional and mental well-being, too. The beauty of focusing on nutrition is that even small changes, like adding more greens to your plate or drinking an extra glass of water, can create a ripple effect. Over time, these shifts lead to more energy, better digestion, and improved overall health. It's about making choices that work for you and building habits that last.

Remember, you hold the power to transform your health with every meal. Each nourishing choice is a step toward greater vitality and balance. By taking control of your nutrition, you're actively shaping your future health – one bite at a time.

# *Chapter Sixteen*

## Sleep Disruptions

*"Have you found yourself unable to fall asleep or tossing and turning in the early hours of the morning, struggling to drift back into sleep?"*

You're not alone. Sleep disturbances, including insomnia, are common among women transitioning through menopause, affecting up to 60% of women during this phase.

These sleep issues can significantly impact your mood, productivity, and physical health. Hormonal changes, particularly the decline in oestrogen and progesterone, can disrupt the natural sleep-wake cycle. Oestrogen, which plays a role in maintaining healthy sleep, begins to decline, contributing to sleep disturbances. Progesterone, known for its calming effects, also decreases, leading to difficulty relaxing and staying asleep. Additionally, studies have shown that lower oestrogen levels are linked to more frequent awakenings and difficulty falling asleep. Women experiencing severe menopausal symptoms, such as hot flushes or night sweats, are particularly prone to these sleep disruptions, which can interfere with daily functioning. Changes in melatonin production and increased cortisol (the stress hormone) levels also contribute to feelings of restlessness and disrupted sleep patterns.

If sleep disturbances are taking a toll, there are practical steps you can take to foster better sleep. By creating an environment conducive to rest and implementing a few lifestyle adjustments, you can manage menopausal sleep disruptions more effectively.

## Actionable Tips

**Create a sleep-friendly environment**
Keep your bedroom dark, quiet, and cool. Use blackout curtains or eye masks to block out light, white noise machines to mask disruptive sounds, and fans or air conditioning to maintain a comfortable temperature. Choose breathable bedding and sleepwear to reduce discomfort from night sweats.

**Establish a bedtime routine**
Go to bed and wake up at the same time every day to support your body's natural sleep-wake cycle. Incorporate relaxing activities like reading, listening to calming music, taking a warm bath, or meditating before bed. These routines signal to your body that it's time to wind down.

**Relaxation techniques**
Engage in progressive muscle relaxation or deep breathing exercises to calm your mind and reduce tension. Gentle stretches or yoga before bed can relax your muscles and prepare your body for restful sleep.

**Limit screen time**
Avoid blue light exposure from phones, tablets, or computers at least an hour before bed, as it can suppress melatonin

production, the hormone that regulates sleep. Consider using blue-light-blocking glasses if screen use is unavoidable.

**Morning sun exposure**

Getting exposure to natural light in the morning helps regulate your circadian rhythm and can promote better sleep at night. A ten-minute walk outside after waking up can do wonders.

**Be mindful of caffeine**

Caffeine is a stimulant that can interfere with sleep, even if consumed hours earlier. Limit caffeine intake after midday and opt for caffeine-free herbal teas in the evening, such as chamomile or peppermint, to promote relaxation.

**Exercise regularly**

Moderate physical activity during the day can improve sleep quality, but avoid vigorous workouts in the evening, as they can leave you too energised to wind down.

**Consider professional support**

If sleep disturbances persist despite your best efforts, consult a healthcare provider. They can assess your needs and recommend solutions.

Sleep is not a luxury—it's a necessity for your health and happiness. While menopause brings challenges, it also offers an opportunity to reassess and prioritise self-care. With consistent effort and the right strategies, you can cultivate an environment and lifestyle that supports better sleep. Imagine how much more vibrant and energised you'll feel with consistent, restorative rest.

*"Sleep is the single most effective thing we can do to reset our brain and body health each day."*

*-Matthew Walker*

**AC'S STORY**

Menopause hit me hard with severe fatigue and sleep disturbances. I found myself tossing and turning at night, unable to get a restful sleep. During the day, I felt exhausted and struggled to keep up with my work and family responsibilities. This constant state of tiredness was affecting my mood and my ability to enjoy life.

For months, I tried various remedies, from herbal teas to over-the-counter sleep aids, but nothing seemed to work. My frustration grew as I continued to suffer from sleepless nights and weary days.

That's when I found Harmony Health & Menopause and met Julie. She listened to my concerns with empathy and provided me with a comprehensive plan to address my sleep issues and fatigue. Julie helped me understand the connection between hormonal changes and sleep patterns and introduced me to techniques that promote better sleep hygiene.

She recommended a regular sleep schedule, creating a calming bedtime routine, and limiting screen time before bed. Julie also advised me to include foods in my diet that support sleep, such as those rich in magnesium and tryptophan, and to stay hydrated throughout the day.

Additionally, Julie suggested gentle exercises like stretching and deep-breathing exercises to help relax my body and mind before bedtime. These small but effective changes made a world of difference.

With Julie's guidance, my sleep quality improved significantly. I started waking up feeling refreshed and energetic, which positively impacted my mood and daily activities. I could finally enjoy my work and spend quality time with my family without feeling drained.

Julie's knowledge and patient approach were exactly what I needed. Her encouragement to "prioritise rest and self-care" was a game-changer for me. Thanks to Julie, I now have the tools to manage my sleep and energy levels effectively.

# Chapter Seventeen

## Vaginal Dryness

*"Research suggests that up to 40% of postmenopausal women experience some form of vaginal discomfort, with many of these symptoms leading to sexual dysfunction and affecting self-confidence. However, this is not just about physical discomfort; it often affects women on an emotional level, impacting their relationships and overall sense of well-being."*

Changes to vaginal and urinary health are primarily due to declining oestrogen levels. These hormonal shifts can lead to vaginal dryness, a common and often distressing symptom that affects both physical comfort, emotional well-being, and day to day life. They also include a variety of symptoms related to the vulva, vagina, and lower urinary tract, commonly referred to as **genitourinary syndrome of menopause (GSM),**

Here are some of the most common vaginal symptoms experienced during menopause:

**Vulvovaginal dryness**

This results in a lack of lubrication in the vaginal walls, leading to discomfort, itching, and a sensation of dryness, often exacerbated during sexual intercourse.

**Pain during intercourse (dyspareunia)**

Vaginal dryness makes sexual activity uncomfortable, and, in many cases, painful. It can lead to a decrease in libido and avoidance of intimacy, which can strain relationships.

**Painful urination (dysuria)**

Women often feel a burning sensation while urinating, which is due to the thinning of the vaginal and urinary tract tissues.

**Increased urgency or frequency to urinate**

As the bladder and urethral tissues thin due to a decline in oestrogen, women may experience a frequent or urgent need to urinate.

**Higher risk of recurrent urinary tract infections (UTIs)**

Oestrogen plays a protective role in the urinary tract. Without enough oestrogen, the urethra becomes more vulnerable to bacteria, leading to an increased likelihood of UTIs.

**Greater susceptibility to infections like vaginitis and bacterial vaginosis (BV)**

The protective environment of the vagina changes during menopause, making it more susceptible to infections as its pH levels rise.

**Recurrent vaginal yeast infections (candidiasis)**
The disruption of the vaginal microbiome during menopause can also lead to recurrent thrush, which manifests as itching, irritation, and a thick discharge.

The decrease in oestrogen levels is the primary cause of vaginal dryness during menopause, and affects several key aspects of vaginal health:

**Thinning of vaginal tissues**
Oestrogen helps maintain the thickness of the vaginal lining by supporting collagen production. As oestrogen levels fall, this lining becomes thinner and more prone to damage, which can lead to irritation, burning, and pain.

**Loss of natural lubrication**
Without adequate oestrogen, the glands in the vaginal walls produce less natural lubrication, making sexual intercourse uncomfortable or painful.

**Increased vaginal pH**
The vaginal microbiome is the community of beneficial bacteria that protect the vagina from infections. The vagina is normally rich in Lactobacilli, a type of bacteria that helps maintain an acidic pH (3.6-4.5) in the vagina, which is essential for preventing harmful bacteria from growing. As oestrogen levels fall, the population of Lactobacilli decreases, and the vaginal pH becomes less acidic. This change creates a more hospitable environment for harmful bacteria and yeast, increasing the risk of infections such as bacterial vaginosis and thrush.

**Changes in elasticity**

Oestrogen supports the production of elastin and collagen in the vaginal tissues, which allows the vagina to stretch and accommodate sexual activity. As oestrogen decreases, these tissues lose their elasticity, leading to discomfort during intercourse or other physical activities.

These conditions are not only uncomfortable but can also affect your mental health, contributing to feelings of embarrassment, frustration, or a diminished sense of femininity. However, it is essential to understand that these symptoms are not simply a "side effect" of menopause but part of a broader change in your body's physiology. Understanding the underlying causes – primarily oestrogen loss – can help you seek the right treatments and solutions to manage your symptoms effectively.

## Actionable Tips

Managing vaginal dryness and associated symptoms during menopause requires both lifestyle changes and treatments that support vaginal health. Below are effective strategies to help alleviate these symptoms and promote overall vaginal well-being.

**Enhance vaginal moisture and elasticity**

Vaginal lubricants are essential for reducing discomfort during intercourse. Opt for natural, water-based lubricants like YES or INTO THE WYLDE. Ensure you consume nutrients that support skin and tissue health, including Vitamin C, Zinc, Vitamin A, and Vitamin E. These vitamins are essential for collagen production and tissue repair. Consider sea buckthorn oil, rich in omega-7 fatty acids, polyphenols, and beta-carotene. It is renowned for its ability to support mucous membranes, including vaginal tissues and can an provide essential nourishment to help maintain hydration and elasticity. Maintain stable blood sugar levels through a balanced diet rich in protein, healthy fats, and complex carbohydrates.

**Maintain a healthy vaginal microbiome**

Increase the presence of good bacteria like Lactobacilli by consuming fermented foods such as yogurt, kefir, sauerkraut, or kimchi. Additionally, probiotic supplements specifically designed for vaginal health can help restore balance. Consulting a nutritional therapist can ensure you get the correct supplement for your needs. Steer clear of vaginal washes, soaps, or sprays that disrupt the natural vaginal pH balance. Use plain water for cleaning and avoid douching, which can strip the vagina of healthy bacteria. Choose breathable clothing, like cotton underwear. Avoid synthetic fabrics that trap moisture, leading to irritation. Also, avoid using strong detergents and fabric softeners on undergarments. A diet rich in prebiotic foods (like garlic, onions, and bananas) supports the growth of beneficial bacteria in the gut and vaginal microbiome.

Above all, don't be embarrassed. Don't suffer. Don't hesitate to seek professional guidance from your GP and healthcare providers, explore natural remedies, and connect with others who are navigating the same path. However, the main thing is to be kind to yourself and reach out for the help you deserve; you don't have to suffer in silence.

# *Chapter Eighteen*

## Finding Clarity: Menopause Brain Fog

*"Have you ever walked into a room and completely forgotten why you went in there? Or found yourself searching for a word that seems to have vanished into thin air? If this sounds familiar, I'm with you."*

These "brain fog" moments can catch us off guard during menopause, leaving us feeling scattered and frustrated. But here's the truth – your body is adapting to the hormonal shifts, and while these moments can be confusing, they don't define who you are, and they won't last forever.

I'll never forget the first time it happened to me. I was standing in the kitchen, completely blank on why I was even there. But as I learned more about the changes happening inside my body, I realised this wasn't a sign of anything wrong. My brain was adjusting to new rhythms, and what I needed most was patience and self-compassion. Menopause doesn't diminish who we are – it simply asks us to adapt, to be present, and to explore new ways of caring for ourselves.

**Brain Fog**

*The cognitive challenges of:*

- Confusion
- Forgetfulness
- Losing your train of thought
- A sense of mental haziness, struggling to recall words, names, or numbers

Brain fog often accompanies other menopause symptoms such as sleep disturbances, fatigue, and hot flushes. Hormonal fluctuations, inflammation, chronic stress, poor nutrition, and dehydration can all contribute to these feelings of mental fuzziness.

Hormonal changes, especially the decline of oestrogen, play a significant role in these cognitive fluctuations. Oestrogen is essential for brain functions such as memory, focus, and executive functioning, particularly in areas like the hippocampus and prefrontal cortex. When oestrogen levels begin to fluctuate during perimenopause, it can result in temporary difficulties with learning, memory, and overall mental sharpness.

## Brain-derived neurotrophic factor (BDNF)

Hormonal changes during menopause significantly influence the production of Brain-Derived Neurotrophic Factor (BDNF), a protein vital for brain health. BDNF supports the growth, survival, and function of neurons, and plays a central role in synaptic plasticity—the brain's ability to adapt, form new connections, and maintain critical cognitive functions like memory and learning.

Oestrogen helps regulate BDNF levels, but its decline during menopause can result in reduced BDNF production. This decrease may contribute to cognitive challenges such as memory lapses, difficulty concentrating, and heightened sensitivity to stress and depression. You can actively support healthy BDNF levels through targeted nutrition and lifestyle strategies, such as:

**Butyrate**

Recent research highlights the significant role of the gut microbiome in influencing brain functions through the "gut-brain axis," a bidirectional communication system connecting the gut and brain via neural, hormonal, and immune pathways. Butyrate, a short-chain fatty acid (SCFA) produced in the large intestine during the fermentation of prebiotic fibres by gut bacteria, plays a vital role in this process. Butyrate supports brain health by enhancing levels of BDNF and promoting neurogenesis in the hippocampus, both of which are crucial for neuronal development and synaptic plasticity. It also provides energy to colon cells and can influence brain function by crossing the blood-brain barrier. To naturally boost butyrate production, incorporate prebiotic-rich, high-fibre foods into your diet, such as oats, apples, garlic, onions, bananas, berries, and asparagus. These foods support a healthy gut microbiome, enhance butyrate production, and promote overall brain and gut health.

**Curcumin**

(Found in turmeric) offers antioxidant and anti-inflammatory benefits that promote brain health and protect against cognitive decline.

**Magnesium**
Supports BDNF synthesis and cognitive well-being. Green leafy veg, nuts, seeds.

**Niacin (vitamin B3)**
Contributes to BDNF production and cellular energy, supporting overall brain function. Chicken, salmon, legumes, brown rice.

**Exercise**
Hippocampal BDNF increases in response to exercise.

## Taking control of cognitive health

As well as these tips to boost BDNF, there are other impactful ways to take back control of your cognitive health and help regain mental clarity. Let's explore additional steps you can take today to further support your brain, enhance focus, and feel more like yourself again.

## Actionable Tips

**Stay hydrated**
Proper hydration is essential for optimal brain function. Drink plenty of water throughout the day to keep your body and mind functioning at their best.

**Eat a nutrient-rich diet**
Focus on fibre-rich, whole foods, including fruits, vegetables, lean proteins, and healthy fats. Omega-3 fatty acids, in particular, are beneficial for brain health. Fatty fish, flaxseeds, and walnuts are excellent sources of Omega-3s.

**Prioritise sleep**

Quality rest is critical for cognitive clarity and brain function. Create a restful bedtime routine and ensure you're getting enough sleep each night.

**Exercise regularly**

Physical activity not only improves your overall health but also supports brain function. Engage in a physical activity you enjoy, as it can boost your mood, alleviate stress, and enhance overall well-being, all of which contribute to improved cognition. Aim for at least 30 minutes of moderate exercise most days of the week.

**Limit sugar and processed foods**

Reducing sugar and processed foods in your diet can help stabilise energy levels and improve mental clarity.

**Practise self-care and stress reduction**

The brain is an energy-intensive organ, relying on healthy, functioning neurons to support cognitive processes. It requires time for rest, recovery, and rejuvenation, free from constant stimulation or prolonged activation of the stress response.

Incorporating relaxation techniques can help manage stress, improve mental clarity, and support cognitive function. Practices to calm and support the brain include:

**Mindfulness and meditation**

Engaging in mindfulness or meditation practices can reduce stress, enhance focus, and create a sense of calm for the brain.

**Yoga**

This integrative mind-body practice supports mental clarity, improves focus, and boosts overall cognitive performance.

## Keep the brain engaged

**Brain-stimulating activities**

Engaging in cognitive games, puzzles, or challenges helps stimulate the brain, fostering mental agility and cognitive flexibility.

**Memory training**

Regularly practising memory exercises can sharpen the mind and maintain cognitive function, countering some of the effects of menopause-related brain fog.

Remember, if you find that cognitive function is severely impacting your daily life, it's essential to seek advice from your GP. This will help rule out any other underlying conditions and ensure you're receiving the right support.

# Chapter Nineteen

## Skin and Hair Changes

### 1. Skin

*Imagine that one day, you catch yourself in the mirror and notice your skin looking a bit different. Maybe it's a little drier or less firm than you remember. I've been there, staring at my reflection, thinking everything had just dropped! My skin had lost its plumpness, and there were lines that looked as if they'd been drawn on overnight!*

Menopause brings profound shifts with skin and hair. As oestrogen levels drop, the effects show up in ways we can see and feel. Oestrogen is like a guardian of our skin, keeping it hydrated, firm, and resilient. When it declines, our skin can become thinner, drier, and more prone to lines or sagging. The drop in collagen and natural oils only adds to that feeling of "drooping", affecting our skin's radiance and firmness.

But here's the empowering part: while we can't stop these shifts, we can support our skin with some simple, effective steps. Let's explore ways to care for your skin so it feels strong, healthy, and loved through this journey.

Falling oestrogen levels affect your skin in the following ways:

**Blood flow and nutrient delivery**

Oestrogen supports blood flow through the skin's capillaries, ensuring cells receive vital nutrients and oxygen. With declining oestrogen, blood flow decreases, slowing down nutrient delivery and cell turnover. This results in thinner skin, a dull complexion, and a reduced ability to combat oxidative stress, leaving the skin vulnerable to damage.

**Moisture balance**

Oestrogen helps maintain the skin's moisture balance by promoting the production of ceramides, hyaluronic acid, and sebum. When oestrogen levels drop, the skin's moisture barrier weakens, leading to dryness, flakiness, and heightened sensitivity. Strengthening your skin's barrier helps to maintain hydration and counteract age-related changes. Key strategies include healthy fats – Omega-3 fatty acids, found in fish, like salmon and mackerel – which play an essential role in reducing inflammation and supporting the skin's structure and function, and good hydration: drink plenty of water and use gentle, hydrating skincare products to lock in moisture.

**Collagen support**

Collagen, the protein responsible for skin structure and elasticity, declines significantly after menopause. With less oestrogen, collagen levels drop, causing the skin to thin and lose its elasticity, leading to wrinkles and sagging.

**Advanced glycation end products (AGEs) and skin ageing**

These are harmful compounds formed when proteins or fats combine with sugars in the body. This process negatively impacts skin health, especially during menopause, by damaging collagen. AGEs reduce collagen's flexibility and increase its susceptibility to wear and tear, contributing to wrinkles, sagging, and overall loss of elasticity. Menopausal women should be cautious of factors that accelerate AGE formation, such as UV exposure, smoking, and diets high in sugar and fried foods. Since menopause already affects collagen production and skin hydration, these external factors can intensify skin ageing. To minimise AGEs in your dietary intake, look at your cooking methods: favour steaming or poaching over frying or grilling, and choose healthier snacks - swap crisps and processed snacks for nutrient-dense options like nuts and seeds.

**Free radicals and skin health**

Free radicals, or reactive oxygen species (ROS), are by-products of the body's natural metabolic processes. While essential for energy production, free radicals can cause oxidative stress when produced in excess. The skin, being the body's largest organ, is particularly vulnerable to oxidative damage, which can be exacerbated by environmental factors like pollution, UV rays, and chemicals in cosmetics. Excessive free radicals can break down collagen and elastin fibres, accelerating the ageing process and contributing to wrinkles, sagging, and inflammation. Oxidative stress can also trigger inflammatory skin conditions such as acne, eczema, and psoriasis. Minimising the use of synthetic detergents, makeup, and other harsh products that can strip the skin's natural oils is a positive step.

Antioxidants are crucial in neutralising free radicals and protecting the skin from oxidative damage. Harness antioxidant support through lycopene, which is found in tomatoes. It helps support collagen synthesis and overall skin health. Other key antioxidants include:

**Vitamin C:** powerful antioxidant that regenerates vitamin E, supports collagen production, and protects against UV-induced skin damage. Found in citrus fruits (oranges, strawberries, kiwi), bell peppers, broccoli, and tomatoes.

**Vitamin E:** protects cell membranes from oxidative stress and plays a key role in maintaining skin elasticity and resilience. Present in nuts, seeds (almonds, sunflower seeds), spinach, avocado, and olive oil,

**Zinc:** important for skin repair, zinc can be found in shellfish (oysters, crab), beef, chicken, beans, and whole grains.

**Protein:** incorporate lean protein sources like fish, chicken, turkey, tofu, beans, and lentils to support skin repair and renewal.

## Gut-skin axis and skin health

The connection between gut health and skin health, known as the gut-skin axis, plays a significant role in skin health. The gut microbiota influences inflammation and immune function, which in turn affects the skin. Probiotics, which help regulate inflammation and oxidative stress, can support both gut and skin health. Key strategies for improving gut health include:

**Fibre** helps maintain a healthy digestive system, which can directly impact skin clarity. Include fibre-rich foods like whole grains (oats, quinoa), vegetables (broccoli, carrots), fruits (apples, berries), and legumes (lentils, chickpeas).

**Probiotics** support gut flora balance, reducing inflammation and improving digestion. You can find probiotics in fermented foods like yogurt, kefir, sauerkraut, kimchi, and miso.

**Prebiotics** feed the beneficial bacteria in your gut, encouraging a balanced microbiome. Prebiotic-rich foods include garlic, onions, leeks, asparagus, bananas, and Jerusalem artichokes.

## 2. Hair

*"Hair loss during perimenopause and menopause is not just a physical symptom, it often deeply affects emotional well-being. For many women, their hair is tied to their sense of identity and self-esteem. Experiencing hair thinning or loss during an already emotionally turbulent time can lead to stress, anxiety, and even depression. This emotional impact can create a cycle, where stress exacerbates hormonal imbalances, leading to further hair shedding."*

You won't be surprised to learn that hair loss or thinning is driven by our old friends, hormones, and the complex changes they undergo during menopause.

Oestrogen plays an essential role in prolonging the anagen (growth) phase of the hair cycle. This means that higher oestrogen levels promote hair growth by stimulating the production of growth factors that nourish hair follicles. During menopause, as oestrogen levels decrease, many women notice their hair growth slows down, thins or sheds.

Another hormone, testosterone, and its more potent derivative dihydrotestosterone (DHT) may also contribute to hair loss. While these "androgens" are present in both men and women, they become more dominant when oestrogen declines, leading to a condition called androgenic alopecia. This is characterised by thinning hair around the temples or the crown of the head. Women can become more sensitive to these male hormones, which can shrink hair follicles, slow hair growth, and eventually cause hair to shed more rapidly than it regrows.

Additionally, the vasodilatory effects of oestrogen help support blood circulation to the scalp, ensuring that hair follicles receive the necessary nutrients and oxygen to maintain healthy hair growth. As oestrogen decreases, reduced blood flow to the scalp may result in weakened follicles, making them more prone to damage and hair loss.

Beyond hormones, other factors such as genetics, stress, and even nutritional deficiencies can contribute to hair loss during menopause. Telogen effluvium is a condition characterised by a significant increase in daily hair shedding. This occurs when a larger proportion of hairs transition from the active growth phase (anagen) into the resting and shedding phase (telogen). Typically, around 10% of scalp hair is in the telogen phase, but in telogen effluvium, this percentage can rise to 30% or more. The onset is often sudden and may occur about three months following a triggering event. Some common triggers include childbirth and severe trauma or illness. These events can disturb the balance of the hair cycle, leading to a noticeable and temporary increase in shedding.

The thinning of hair can also be exacerbated by physical changes related to ageing, such as a decrease in scalp elasticity and collagen production, both of which play crucial roles in maintaining a healthy environment for hair growth.

As we age, the melanocytes in our hair follicles – the cells responsible for producing pigment – naturally slow down and reduce melanin production, causing hair to turn grey. For some women, letting their grey hair shine can feel empowering, symbolising confidence, wisdom, and individuality. Grey hair holds its own unique beauty, reflecting the strength and experience you've gained over the years. For others, colouring their hair brings joy, boosts self-confidence, and becomes an important act of self-care. A trip to the hairdresser can offer more than a new look; a chance to relax, recharge, and reconnect with yourself.

What truly matters is how *you* feel. Whether you go natural or choose to colour, celebrate yourself and the beauty of this stage in your journey. You are strong, vibrant, and enough just as you are.

## Actionable Tips

Supporting your hair during this time involves taking a holistic approach and finding naturopathic support for hair health. Effective strategies include:

> **Ensure adequate protein intake**
> Hair is made primarily of keratin, a protein. Make sure your diet includes plenty of protein-rich foods like fish, chicken, lentils, beans, and tofu to support hair growth.

**Include biotin (vitamin B7)**

B7's functions in protein synthesis and more specifically, in keratin production, explains its contribution to healthy nail and hair growth. Foods found to have high amounts of biotin include nuts, legumes, whole grains, rice, and egg yolk.

**Include zinc-rich foods**

Crucial for hair tissue repair and growth. Foods like pumpkin seeds, oats, chickpeas, lentils, and mushrooms are excellent sources of zinc.

**Iron-rich foods**

Iron deficiencies can lead to hair thinning. Incorporate iron-rich foods such as leafy greens, grass-fed beef, lamb, and dried apricots into your meals to support healthy hair follicles.

**Get enough vitamin D**

Helps regulate the cells responsible for hair growth. Make sure to get enough sunlight or consider foods like fortified dairy, eggs, and oily fish, or take supplements if needed.

**Healthy fats**

Omega-3 fatty acids, found in oily fish, nuts, seeds, and avocado, help maintain scalp health and provide essential nutrients for hair.

**Balance blood sugar levels**

Imbalances can affect hormone regulation. Including protein with your meals, along with foods that support blood sugar stability, like chromium-rich vegetables (e.g. broccoli), can make a difference.

**Avoid pro-inflammatory foods**

Reduce processed foods, sugar, and alcohol, as they can trigger inflammation, which may worsen hair loss, particularly if you have autoimmune conditions.

**Look after gut health**

Support gut health by including prebiotic and probiotic foods. Prebiotics such as garlic, onions, and bananas feed healthy bacteria, while probiotics like yogurt, kefir, and sauerkraut help maintain a healthy microbiome, which can influence overall health, including hair health.

The key takeaway is that every woman's hair journey through menopause is unique. Whether you're embracing your natural grey or colouring your hair to feel more like yourself, the most important thing is to focus on what brings you joy and confidence.

Finding hairstyles that make you feel confident or exploring new looks can help boost self-esteem. And remember, if you're finding this experience overwhelming, seeking advice from a dermatologist or trichologist can provide personalised support. Empower yourself with self-care, self-compassion, and the understanding that beauty is not tied to age or hair colour – it's tied to how you nurture yourself from the inside out.

## 3. Facial Hair

*"Is it just me, or do those rogue chin hairs seem to have superpowers? You'll swear they weren't there in the evening, and by morning, they've grown long enough to braid."*

We've talked about the changes to hair on the scalp, but we can't finish without a word on our small but mighty nemesis—our little friends, the chin hairs. These unexpected guests often make their debut during menopause, demanding attention and reminding us of the complex hormonal changes our bodies are navigating.

The increase in facial hair growth during menopause, also known as hirsutism, is a result of hormonal changes. Oestrogen levels drop significantly, while testosterone levels decline more slowly, leading to a higher ratio of active testosterone in the body. Oestrogen, which usually keeps hair finer, softer, and lighter, loses its influence, allowing testosterone's effects to become more apparent. This hormonal shift often leads to the development of coarse, darker hairs, particularly on the chin, jawline, and upper lip.

As visceral fat increases—a common occurrence during menopause—it lowers levels of sex hormone-binding globulin (SHBG). Reduced SHBG levels result in higher amounts of free testosterone circulating in the body, which can further contribute to the development of facial hair. Other factors like insulin resistance and hyperinsulinemia, which are more prevalent post-menopause, can also amplify testosterone levels. While overall androgen levels remain within premenopausal ranges, the imbalance between oestrogen and testosterone can result in these noticeable changes.

Beyond facial hair, testosterone can make the skin oilier and more acne-prone, adding to the challenges of managing these changes. But there's good news: these shifts are manageable with the right strategies.

## Actionable tips for managing facial hair

**Start with a professional assessment**
If you're experiencing excessive facial hair growth, don't hesitate to reach out to your GP. They can help assess the situation and explore possible causes. A dermatologist can also provide guidance on safe and effective treatment options tailored to your needs, ensuring you feel supported every step of the way.

**Choose the right removal method**
From waxing and threading to dermaplaning or tweezing, explore the options that work for your skin and lifestyle.

**Support hormones with nutrition**
As we have seen, menopause-related hormonal changes, combined with elevated insulin resistance and inflammation, can exacerbate androgen levels, which are often at the root of unwanted hair growth. The good news is that, with thoughtful dietary choices, it's possible to support hormonal balance and address these underlying factors effectively:

- **Prioritise complex carbohydrates:** Replace refined carbohydrates like white bread, sugary snacks, and pasta with whole grains, legumes, and fibre-rich vegetables. These stabilise blood sugar levels, reducing insulin spikes that can trigger increased androgen production.
- **Incorporate protein and healthy fats:** Balanced meals with quality proteins (like lean meats, eggs, or legumes) and healthy fats (like avocado, nuts, or olive oil) help stabilise glucose levels and support hormone regulation.
- **Include anti-inflammatory foods:** Add omega-3-rich

foods such as salmon, flaxseeds, and walnuts to combat inflammation, which can exacerbate hormonal imbalances.

- **Boost micronutrients:** Leafy greens, cruciferous vegetables, and colourful fruits provide essential vitamins, magnesium, and antioxidants to support hormone metabolism and reduce oxidative stress.
- **Stay hydrated:** Adequate hydration supports liver function, which is crucial for processing and eliminating excess hormones like androgens.

The appearance of facial hair can be challenging, but it's important to remember that you're not alone on this journey. These changes reflect your body's incredible complexity and resilience. While they may feel frustrating, they are manageable with the right care, attention, and support, all while embracing self-compassion.

*"And the beauty of a woman, with passing years only grows."*

*Audrey Hepburn*

# *Chapter Twenty*

## Joint Pain

*Have you noticed joint pain creeping into your daily life as you approach or move through menopause?*

For many women, joint pain is a new and unexpected challenge that can disrupt daily routines – something as simple as getting out of bed in the morning can feel like a struggle. You might find yourself wondering why your knees are stiff after sitting for too long or why your hands ache after holding a pen or cup of tea for just a few minutes. Suddenly, activities that used to bring joy – like gardening, walking, or even playing with your children or grandchildren – can feel daunting. I remember speaking with a friend who shared her frustration about her favourite yoga class becoming more difficult as her body changed. She used to love the stretches and poses, but now she was feeling stiffness in her hips and knees that made it hard to fully participate.

But what exactly is causing such joint pain, and what can you do to ease it?

Joint pain, often referred to as "arthralgia", is a common issue during perimenopause and menopause. This discomfort primarily stems from hormonal fluctuations, particularly the decline in oestrogen levels. Oestrogen plays a crucial role in maintaining joint and connective tissue health by preserving collagen and promoting anti-inflammatory responses in the body. When oestrogen levels begin to drop, joint health may be affected in several ways:

**Collagen breakdown**
Oestrogen helps maintain the strength and elasticity of collagen, which is a vital component of ligaments, tendons, and joints. As oestrogen declines, collagen production slows down, leading to weakened connective tissues and increased joint stiffness.

**Increased inflammation**
Oestrogen has anti-inflammatory properties. Without it, the body's inflammatory responses may become overactive, causing swelling and pain in the joints.

**Decreased flexibility**
Oestrogen supports ligament relaxation, allowing for smooth joint movement. Lower levels can make your joints feel stiff, increasing your risk of injury.

**Compromised mucous membranes**
Oestrogen helps maintain the integrity of mucous membranes, which lubricate and cushion joints. Reduced oestrogen levels can lead to discomfort as this protective cushioning decreases.For many women, these changes make everyday tasks more challenging and

can even reduce motivation to stay active, which is crucial for overall health and hormone regulation.

**Frozen shoulder**

A common condition that affects women during menopause is frozen shoulder, also known as adhesive capsulitis. This painful and debilitating condition causes inflammation and thickening of the connective tissues surrounding the shoulder joint, leading to stiffness and a limited range of motion. While it may present as sudden severe shoulder pain, it can also develop gradually with insidious pain and a progressive loss of motion in the shoulder joint.

Frozen shoulder typically progresses through three distinct stages. In the freezing stage, lasting 6 weeks to 9 months, pain intensifies, and shoulder mobility decreases. During the frozen stage, which lasts 4 to 6 months, the pain may subside, but stiffness persists, making daily activities, such as dressing or reaching, difficult. The final stage, known as the thawing stage, can take 6 months to 2 years, during which joint movement gradually returns to normal or near normal. Symptoms often disrupt sleep and make daily tasks challenging.

While it is not definitively proven that menopause directly causes frozen shoulder, it is most commonly experienced by women between the ages of 40 and 60, and women are four times more likely to develop this condition than men. The timing of its onset often coincides with menopause, suggesting a possible link between declining oestrogen levels and the condition. Additionally, other menopause-related factors, such as poor sleep, fatigue, and depression, may exacerbate joint issues.

If you suspect frozen shoulder, consulting a healthcare provider early can help manage symptoms and prevent further progression.

With proper treatment, recovery can be more manageable, ensuring a smoother and less disruptive journey to regaining shoulder mobility.

## Actionable Tips

If you're experiencing joint pain, here are some holistic strategies to help manage and ease discomfort during menopause:

**Focus on collagen support**
Increase your intake of Vitamin C-rich foods, such as citrus fruits, kiwi, and bell peppers, to support collagen production. Collagen supplements may also be helpful.

**Adopt an anti-inflammatory diet**
Emphasise foods that fight inflammation, like leafy greens, fatty fish (rich in Omega-3s), and whole grains. Herbal teas, such as rosehip, combined with Vitamin C and zinc, can further support joint health.

**Incorporate turmeric and ginger**
Turmeric contains curcumin, and ginger contains gingerols—both are powerful compounds with strong anti-inflammatory properties which can help reduce inflammation and support joints. Add turmeric and ginger to your soups, stews, teas, or juices to enhance their flavour and gain their health benefits.

**Strengthen your gut health**
Nourish your gut with prebiotic and probiotic foods to maintain a healthy microbiome, which can have a positive impact on inflammation. Include fibre-rich foods like bananas, garlic, and asparagus alongside fermented foods like yogurt and sauerkraut.

**Maintain regular exercise**

Gentle exercise, such as walking, swimming, or yoga, can keep your joints flexible and reduce pain. Aim for thirty minutes a day, focusing on low-impact movements that don't strain your joints.

**Eat enough protein**

1.0-1.2g per kg of body weight per day supports muscle mass and joint integrity.

**Manage stress**

Chronic stress can worsen joint pain by increasing inflammation. Incorporate stress-reduction techniques like deep breathing, mindfulness, or meditation to keep your mind and body balanced.

**Seek professional help**

If joint pain is persistent or severe, consult with a healthcare provider to discuss personalised treatment options, such as physical therapy or hormone therapy, which can be tailored to your needs.

# *Chapter Twenty-One*

## Migraines and Headaches

Many women experience an increase in the frequency and intensity of migraines and headaches during perimenopause and menopause due to fluctuating hormone levels, particularly oestrogen and progesterone, as well as non-hormonal factors, such as food sensitivities, stress, and nutritional deficiencies. Likewise, migraines often become more common or severe during perimenopause, since the changes that occur can affect blood vessel dynamics, neural excitability, and brain function. These headaches can be debilitating, affecting daily activities and reducing overall quality of life. Understanding their underlying causes and triggers during this transitional phase is essential for effective management and relief.

### Oestrogen's role:

#### Vasodilation

Oestrogen promotes blood vessel dilation, which can affect

vascular tone and trigger migraines due to increased blood flow and pressure changes in the brain.

**Glutaminergic activity and excitable brain cells**

Oestrogen facilitates the activity of glutamate, a neurotransmitter influencing neural excitability. Increased glutaminergic activity can make brain cells more excitable. When oestrogen levels rise without sufficient progesterone to counterbalance, brain cells may become overly excitable. This can trigger migraines.

**Nitric oxide production**

Oestrogen stimulates nitric oxide production, a molecule that dilates blood vessels. While nitric oxide has beneficial effects, sudden drops in oestrogen – such as those occurring before menstruation – can disrupt nitric oxide balance and trigger migraines.

## Progesterone's role:

Progesterone typically counterbalances some of the excitatory effects of oestrogen by promoting neural stability. However, fluctuations or declines in progesterone levels during perimenopause can lead to:

**Reduced GABA activity**

Progesterone helps modulate GABA, a neurotransmitter that has calming effects on the brain. Lower progesterone levels reduce GABA activity, increasing neural excitability and susceptibility to migraines.

**Heightened susceptibility**

Without adequate progesterone to counterbalance oestrogen, hormonal shifts during menopause can contribute to a higher frequency and intensity of migraines.

## Actionable Tips

**Dietary changes**
Reducing foods high in histamine and tyramine, such as aged cheeses, cured meats, fermented foods, and alcoholic beverages, may be beneficial.

**Relaxation techniques**
Stress is a well-known migraine trigger. Incorporating techniques like deep breathing, meditation, yoga, progressive muscle relaxation, or guided imagery, can manage stress and so potentially lower the occurrence of migraines.

**Stable blood sugar levels**
Blood sugar fluctuations can provoke migraines. Avoid skipping meals and incorporate protein-rich foods like lean meats, fish, eggs, dairy, nuts, seeds, and legumes into your meals and snacks. Choose complex carbohydrates such as whole grains, fruits, and vegetables to maintain steady energy levels and prevent rapid changes in blood sugar.

**Alcohol intake**
In particular, red wine, beer, and some spirits can trigger migraines in certain individuals. Reducing alcohol consumption or abstaining altogether may help reduce their frequency.

**Rest and quality sleep**
Aim for 7-9 hours of quality sleep per night, after establishing a calming bedtime routine and creating an ideal sleep environment. Limiting screen time before bed and engaging in relaxation techniques before sleep can help.

# *Chapter Twenty-Two*

## Increased Allergies

*"I'm a chef who has always loved tomatoes, but I suddenly found myself developing an intolerance to them during perimenopause. Whenever I ate them, I would break out in hives. It was incredibly frustrating – how could something I'd enjoyed for years now cause such discomfort? After Julie helped me focus on improving my gut health, things slowly started to shift. Over time, I've been able to reintroduce tomatoes into my meals without any issues."*

This story is a reminder of how your body's needs can change during menopause, but, with the right support, you can regain balance. If you've experienced something similar, rest assured that these changes in allergies and sensitivities are common during menopause. But why does this happen, and what can you do about it?

During perimenopause and menopause, many women experience an increase in symptoms associated with histamine intolerance – such as migraines, itching, hives, and even food sensitivities. Histamine is a natural chemical in the body that plays a role in immune responses and digestion. It's usually broken down by enzymes like diamine oxidase (DAO) in the gut and histamine N-methyltransferase (HNMT) in the nervous system. However, when your body's ability to break down histamine is compromised, symptoms of intolerance can emerge.

Hormonal fluctuations, particularly the decrease in oestrogen levels, play a significant role in this. Oestrogen stimulates mast cells to release more histamine while simultaneously reducing the activity of DAO, the enzyme that breaks it down. This can create a vicious cycle: as histamine levels rise, they can, in turn, stimulate even more oestrogen production, exacerbating the issue. Additionally, non-hormonal factors like diet, stress, and gut health also play important roles in how well your body manages histamine. Foods high in histamine – like red wine, cheese, and processed meats – may trigger more pronounced symptoms, while poor gut health can further reduce the body's ability to break down histamine effectively. Addressing both the hormonal and non-hormonal contributors to histamine sensitivity is key to managing symptoms.

## Actionable Tips

## Dietary adjustments:

**Avoid histamine-rich foods**
Rather than eliminating everything, begin with a few common triggers and see how your body responds. Start by reducing your intake of high-histamine foods such as aged cheeses, red wine, cured meats, vinegar, and fermented products like sauerkraut.

**Limit alcohol and coffee**
Try reducing or eliminating them from your diet to see if your symptoms improve.

## Supporting Gut Health:

### Microbiome nourishment

Since a healthy gut is key for effective histamine breakdown, incorporate probiotics from sources like yogurt, kefir, or sauerkraut, and eat prebiotic-rich foods like garlic, onions, and leeks to nourish your gut flora.

### Fibre-rich foods

Fibre is essential for promoting healthy digestion and detoxification. Whole grains, fruits, vegetables, legumes, and seeds can help move waste through your system, supporting regular elimination and reducing histamine build-up.

## Increase Antioxidant Intake:

### Vitamin C

A natural antihistamine, Vitamin C can help reduce histamine levels. Include foods rich in Vitamin C such as oranges, strawberries, bell peppers, and broccoli

### Cruciferous vegetables

Broccoli, kale, and cauliflower support liver detoxification, helping your body process excess oestrogen and histamine.

## Environmental Adjustments:

### Reduce exposure to environmental toxins

Consider switching to natural cleaning and skincare products and opt for organic produce when possible. This reduces the toxic load on your body, giving your liver more capacity to break down histamine effectively.

# *Chapter Twenty-Three*

## Digestive Symptoms

*Have you found that your digestion is suddenly unpredictable, or that foods you used to enjoy now cause bloating, discomfort, or other issues? Could your hormonal shifts be affecting your gut?*

Menopause brings about many changes in your body, and one of the most common areas affected is digestion. You might notice that your digestion is less predictable, or certain foods that once were a pleasure may now cause bloating, discomfort, or even digestive distress. Let's explore how hormonal shifts during menopause influence your digestive health and what you can do to find relief.

### How menopause affects digestion

Hormonal fluctuations, particularly the decline in oestrogen and progesterone, are key drivers of many digestive issues. These hormones regulate the body's fluid balance, digestion, and gut motility (the movement of food through the intestines). When these hormones decrease during menopause, the balance in your digestive system is disrupted, leading to various uncomfortable symptoms.

- **Oestrogen:** This hormone supports a healthy gut microbiome (the beneficial bacteria in your gut) and helps maintain the smooth movement of food through your digestive system. As oestrogen drops, fluid retention increases, leading to bloating and constipation. This imbalance can also cause an overgrowth of gas-producing bacteria, worsening digestive discomfort. Furthermore, decreased oestrogen levels can increase cortisol, the stress hormone, which can further slow digestion and contribute to these symptoms.

- **Progesterone:** Known for its role in maintaining fluid balance, progesterone also helps the muscles in your gut relax, promoting regular bowel movements. When progesterone levels fall, digestion can slow down, causing constipation and making it harder for your body to move waste through the intestines efficiently.

## Common digestive symptoms include:

**Bloating:** with reduced oestrogen, fluid retention becomes more common, leading to bloating. Hormonal changes also cause an imbalance in the gut microbiome, which can increase gas production and make bloating worse.

**Constipation:** Slower digestion caused by reduced progesterone and oestrogen levels can lead to harder stools and a feeling of incomplete evacuation. This slowed process may result in the reabsorption of hormones, such as oestrogen, as they remain exposed to gut bacteria for longer periods. This can elevate hormone levels, contributing to imbalances that exacerbate menopausal symptoms. Additionally, constipation-related bloating and discomfort may amplify other symptoms like mood swings, poor sleep, and fatigue. Chronic constipation can also increase systemic inflammation, further intensifying menopausal challenges.

**Diarrhoea:** Some women experience diarrhoea due to increased gut motility triggered by hormonal shifts or stress.

**Heartburn and acid reflux:** as oestrogen levels decline, the lower oesophageal sphincter weakens, allowing stomach acid to rise into the oesophagus more easily, causing heartburn and discomfort after meals.

**Fat malabsorption:** oestrogen plays a key role in bile production, which helps digest fats. With lower oestrogen levels, bile production may decrease, leading to difficulty digesting high-fat meals and causing discomfort after eating.

## The role of the gut-brain axis in digestive health during menopause

The relationship between hormones and digestive health extends beyond the digestive tract; it also involves the gut-brain axis, a bidirectional communication system that connects the gut and the brain. This system allows signals from your digestive system to influence your mental well-being and vice versa, creating a dynamic interplay between your physical and emotional health.

One of the main ways menopause affects the gut-brain axis is through the impact of hormonal changes on stress and anxiety levels. Many women experience heightened stress and anxiety during menopause due to fluctuating hormones which, in turn, can affect the gut. Stress activates the sympathetic nervous system, disrupting normal motility and leading to symptoms such as bloating, abdominal discomfort, and changes in bowel habits. In some cases, stress can also exacerbate existing conditions like irritable bowel syndrome (IBS), which is already sensitive to stress and hormonal fluctuations.

## The gut microbiome: a foundation for wellness

The gut microbiome is made up of a diverse community of trillions of microorganisms, including bacteria, fungi, and viruses, which live in your digestive tract. These microbes play a crucial role in your digestion, immune system, and overall health. They help absorb nutrients, produce essential compounds, and maintain balance in the body.

Emerging research shows that there is a strong connection between menopause and the gut microbiome, highlighting how hormonal fluctuations can significantly change the balance of gut bacteria. These shifts can not only worsen digestive symptoms but also play a role in other issues like inflammation, which further complicates overall health during menopause.

The imbalance in gut bacteria can also have a profound effect on the production of neurotransmitters like serotonin. Since approximately 90% of serotonin is produced in the gut, any disruption in this balance can influence mood, mental clarity, and emotional health. This connection means that disturbances in gut health during menopause can directly impact your mental well-being, creating a vicious cycle of digestive discomfort and emotional distress.

## Tying it all together

The gut-brain axis and the gut microbiome are deeply connected to digestive health, particularly during menopause. Hormonal fluctuations not only affect digestion but can also influence your relationship with food and overall well-being. You might notice that foods you once enjoyed now cause discomfort, or that the stress and anxiety accompanying menopause exacerbate digestive issues. These disruptions can feel overwhelming. However, by understanding the complex interplay between hormonal changes, gut health, and stress, you can take meaningful steps to regain balance. Supporting your gut during menopause is not just about improving digestion; it's about enhancing both your emotional and physical health.

Below, you'll find practical strategies designed to nourish your gut and help you build a strong foundation for long-term well-being.

## Actionable tips to support gut health

**Increase dietary fibre**
Fibre is essential for promoting healthy digestion, especially during menopause. Incorporate fibre-rich foods like fruits, vegetables, legumes, and whole grains to help maintain regular bowel movements and prevent constipation. See the 30-day challenge below.

**Stay hydrated**
Proper hydration is vital for keeping things moving in your

digestive system. Drinking enough water each day helps soften stools and prevents constipation, allowing for more comfortable digestion. Aim for at least eight glasses of water a day to keep things moving.

**Avoid processed foods**

Processed foods, high in unhealthy fats and sugars, can exacerbate bloating and discomfort. Opt for whole, natural foods to reduce digestive issues and improve your overall gut health.

**Exercise regularly**

Physical activity stimulates bowel function and helps prevent constipation. Aim for at least thirty minutes of moderate exercise daily, such as walking or swimming to promote healthy digestion.

**Consider probiotics**

Probiotics are live bacteria that, when consumed in adequate amounts, promote a balanced gut microbiome, improve digestion, support immune function, and enhance overall health. Supporting your gut microbiome with probiotic-rich foods like yogurt, kefir, and fermented vegetables can ease digestive discomfort and improve gut health. For specific health concerns, consult a healthcare professional to ensure the type and dosage of probiotics meet your individual needs.

**Add prebiotics to your diet**

Prebiotics are non-digestible food components that nourish beneficial gut bacteria like *Bifidobacteria* and *Lactobacilli*, essential for a balanced microbiome. A diverse gut microbiome supports optimal digestion, nutrient absorption, and overall well-being. Foods rich in prebiotics include garlic, onions, leeks, artichokes, bananas, chicory and legumes.

**Consume bitter foods**

These stimulate digestive juices and promote optimal digestion by enhancing the secretion of stomach acid and bile. Incorporate foods such as arugula, dandelion greens, radicchio, and endive into your meals to support digestive function. Start your meals with a small salad or appetiser containing bitter greens to stimulate digestion and enhance nutrient absorption.

**Manage stress**

High stress levels can worsen digestive symptoms like bloating and constipation. Incorporate relaxation techniques like meditation, deep breathing, or yoga to reduce stress and support better digestion.

## The 30-plant challenge: nourishing your gut for better digestion

One of the most effective ways to support your gut health is to eat a diverse range of plant foods. Research suggests that consuming 30 different plant foods each week can significantly improve the diversity of your gut microbiome, which plays a crucial role in digestion, nutrient absorption, and overall well-being.

Plant foods include vegetables, fruits, nuts, seeds, herbs, legumes, and whole grains. Each plant type provides different fibres, polyphenols, and prebiotics that feed specific gut bacteria, helping to create a balanced and resilient microbiome. The more variety you include in your diet, the better your gut bacteria can thrive, supporting digestion and reducing bloating, inflammation, and sluggish bowel movements.

## Examples of plant-based foods for the 30-plant challenge

Here are some easy-to-find plant foods you can include in your weekly meals to boost gut health and digestion:

- **Vegetables** - Spinach, Kale, Carrots, Peppers (red, yellow, green), Courgette, Broccoli, Cauliflower, Onion, Garlic, Cabbage (red, green, savoy), Beetroot, Mushrooms, Leeks

- **Fruits** - Blueberries, Strawberries, Apples, Pomegranate, Bananas, Oranges, Kiwi, Mango, Figs, Avocado

- **Nuts** - Almonds, Walnuts, Cashews, Pistachios, Brazil nuts, Pecans

- **Seeds** - Chia seeds, Flaxseeds, Pumpkin seeds, Sunflower seeds, Sesame seeds, Hemp seeds

- **Herbs** - Basil, Coriander, Parsley, Mint, Thyme, Rosemary, Oregano, Fennel

- **Legumes** - Chickpeas, Lentils (red, green, black), Black beans, Kidney beans, Butter beans, Cannellini beans, Pinto beans, Edamame beans, Mung bean

- **Whole Grains** - Quinoa, Brown rice, Whole oats, Barley, Bulgur wheat, Buckwheat, Wholegrain pasta, Spelt

If 30 sounds like a big number, don't worry—you're probably already eating more plants than you think! It's not about overhauling your diet overnight but finding simple ways to increase variety in the meals you already love. Here are some easy ways to get started:

## Simple ways to increase your plant variety

**Supercharge your salads**
Mix in spinach, rocket, kale, or watercress for extra nutrients. Add shredded carrots, cucumber, radishes, or roasted peppers. Top with a sprinkle of nuts, seeds, or pomegranate for crunch and extra flavour.

**Boost your breakfast**
Swap plain porridge or yoghurt for a gut-loving bowl by adding flaxseeds, chia seeds, walnuts, and a mix of berries. If you enjoy smoothies, experiment with different greens, herbs, and nut butters.

**Embrace beans and legumes**
Chickpeas, lentils, and black beans are excellent for gut health. Add them to soups, salads, or stir-fries, or blend them into dips like hummus. Instead of using just one type of bean in a dish, mix two or three varieties for extra diversity.

**Upgrade your soups and stews**
Homemade soups and stews are a fantastic way to incorporate more plants. Throw in lentils, courgettes, leeks, or sweet potatoes, and use fresh herbs like parsley, coriander, or thyme for an extra gut-friendly boost.

**Experiment with herbs and spices**
Fresh and dried herbs not only enhance flavour but also support digestion. Try mint, basil, fennel, or turmeric to give your meals a gut-friendly boost.

By gradually introducing more plant-based foods into your daily routine, you'll be nourishing your gut, improving digestion, and supporting long-term health. This isn't about perfection—it's about consistency and variety. Challenge yourself to try new plant foods each week, and before you know it, you'll be effortlessly reaching 30 different plants and feeling the digestive benefits.

*Tip: Keep a simple checklist of the plant foods you eat each week to track your progress and discover new favourites!*

## Final thoughts

Remember, each woman's experience with menopause is unique, and digestive symptoms can vary widely. It's important to listen to your body, take action to support your gut, and seek professional advice if symptoms persist.

**CN's Story**
I thankfully discovered Harmony Health & Menopause and met Julie who has helped change my life for the better. Talking through my feelings and symptoms was the best thing I did and the start of a new lifestyle. Julie discussed my eating and exercise routine pre and post menopause and came up with a plan. I was introduced to plant based and multi vitamin foods and a good exercise routine which included cycling which is my personal downtime where I can enjoy the outdoor space and have time for me.

# *Chapter Twenty-Four*

## Dizziness & Vertigo

*"I remember the first time it happened to me – it felt like the world was tilting under my feet. I was sitting at my computer, when suddenly, the room started to spin uncontrollably. It felt as if the ground was shifting under me, and I had to grip the edge of the desk to steady myself. As I sat there, my heart raced, and a wave of anxiety washed over me. It was as though I had lost control of my own body, and that feeling of vulnerability was terrifying."*

This one episode affected me in more than just that moment – it shook my confidence. I began worrying that it might happen again at any time. That fear grew over the following weeks, and soon I found myself avoiding everyday activities like going for a walk or even shopping. The anxiety surrounding these unpredictable episodes became overwhelming.

Experiences like these can feel incredibly disorientating, frightening and isolating, especially when you can't immediately pinpoint the cause. However, what many women don't realise is that these episodes are far more common than you might think. As oestrogen levels begin to fluctuate and ultimately decline, these hormonal changes can directly influence the vestibular system – the part of the inner ear responsible for maintaining our sense of balance. When this system is disrupted, it can lead to sensations of dizziness, spinning, or even vertigo. The imbalance, the sudden vertigo, the moments where the world feels off-kilter – all of these can be traced back to the hormonal changes occurring during this transitional time. For some women, too, menopause may exacerbate or even trigger underlying vestibular conditions like Ménière's disease. This condition, characterised by episodes of vertigo, hearing loss, and tinnitus, can be worsened by the hormonal fluctuations that occur during this time.

I encourage you to seek medical advice to rule out any other conditions but understanding that these vestibular symptoms may be linked to menopause offers a sense of validation. You're not imagining it, and you're not alone. I do understand the frustration of not having immediate answers – I underwent many tests without finding the cause for quite some time, and it wasn't until I was diagnosed with early menopause and started hormone replacement therapy (HRT) that I began to improve.

## Actionable Tips

Managing dizziness and vertigo during menopause may feel overwhelming, but there are ways to support your vestibular health. Here are some strategies to help manage these symptoms:

**Seek professional guidance for postural exercises**

Working with a healthcare professional or physical therapist can provide you with tailored postural exercises to strengthen your vestibular system. Vestibular rehabilitation therapy is particularly beneficial in managing dizziness and improving balance.

**Stay hydrated**

Drinking enough water is essential for your overall health and can reduce the intensity of dizziness and vertigo. Dehydration can worsen these symptoms, so aim for at least eight glasses of water a day.

**Balance exercises**

Gentle exercises such as yoga, tai chi, or simple balance drills can improve stability and coordination. Such activities not only support your physical balance but also promote mental clarity and reduce anxiety, which can help manage vestibular symptoms.

**Monitor and adjust your diet**

Certain foods and drinks can worsen dizziness and vertigo. Be mindful of caffeine, alcohol, and high-sodium foods, which can disrupt fluid balance and blood pressure. Focus on a nutrient-rich diet full of whole foods, lean proteins, and healthy fats to help you feel more balanced.

**Manage stress and anxiety**

Stress can aggravate vestibular symptoms, so incorporate relaxation techniques such as deep breathing, meditation, or mindfulness. Regular exercise and sufficient sleep will also help you maintain emotional balance and improve overall well-being.

## Regaining balance and confidence

Every now and again, I still experience small bouts of dizziness, and I've noticed they often coincide with periods of stress. For me, the best way to cope is to lie still in bed, relax my body, and practise meditation or self-Reiki. This helps me feel grounded. I also do balance exercises that my GP recommended, which help recalibrate me when I feel off-balance. This approach works for me, but the key is to find something that resonates with you.

Embrace self-compassion and allow yourself to take small, manageable steps to ease your symptoms. I know it can feel overwhelming, but with the right support and some lifestyle adjustments, relief is within reach. You deserve to live a vibrant, fulfilling life, even through menopause, and I truly believe you can get there. Take it one step at a time and know that I'm right here with you on this journey.

# Chapter Twenty-Five

## Energy and Fatigue

*"Almost everything will work again if you unplug it for a few minutes, including you."*

*Anne Lamont*

Many women find themselves facing unexpected fatigue during menopause, wondering where their vitality went. The main culprit? Hormonal changes again – especially the drop in oestrogen – impact everything from sleep quality to daily stamina.

Oestrogen plays a key role in maintaining energy levels by supporting mitochondrial function, the "powerhouses" of your cells that produce energy, in the form of ATP, the body's main energy molecule. Oestrogen helps create new mitochondria and enhances their efficiency, maximising energy production. However, as oestrogen levels decline during perimenopause and menopause, mitochondrial function can become less efficient, leading to reduced energy output and feelings of fatigue. This slowdown in metabolism can make it harder for your body to convert food into energy, contributing to a persistent sense of tiredness and possibly weight gain. Additionally, shifts in thyroid function during menopause can further impact energy levels, as thyroid hormones also regulate metabolism.

Menopausal fatigue isn't just about feeling tired or being sleepy; many women describe it as an overwhelming sense of physical and mental exhaustion, where even simple tasks feel monumental. You might feel like you're running on empty, with little reserve for daily responsibilities like work, family, and personal commitments. This type of fatigue can affect mood, productivity, and your overall quality of life, sometimes even contributing to feelings of anxiety or depression.

In some cases, the lack of energy is not just a result of lower mitochondrial efficiency, but also poor sleep quality. The hormonal changes associated with menopause can disrupt sleep patterns, leading to insomnia, frequent awakenings during the night, or early morning waking. As a result, you may not get the restful sleep your body needs to recover, exacerbating the feelings of fatigue.

**Energy production through nutrition**

Eating a nutrient-rich diet is essential for supporting energy production. Focus on whole grains, lean proteins, fruits, vegetables, and healthy fats, as they contain vital nutrients – such as vitamins and antioxidants – that improve mitochondrial function and energy levels.

**Magnesium** also plays a vital role in energy production by activating ATP. In fact, most ATP in your cells exists as magnesium-

ATP complexes, which are essential for biological activity and energy metabolism. This is found in foods like almonds, leafy greens, and seeds.

**Iron** is another cornerstone of energy production, as around two-thirds of the body's iron is found in haemoglobin. This protein in red blood cells binds oxygen in its ferrous form (Fe2+), allowing haemoglobin to transport up to four oxygen molecules per molecule. This enables the blood to carry 50-70 times more oxygen than plasma alone, ensuring tissues receive the oxygen needed for energy and metabolic processes. Without sufficient iron, oxygen delivery is compromised, leading to fatigue, reduced physical performance. Iron is found in spinach, red meat, and lentils.

**Antioxidants**

Berries, oranges, broccoli, and carrots protect against oxidative stress which can deplete energy reserves.

**Coenzyme Q10 (CoQ10)** is found in fatty fish, organic meats, and whole grains. CoQ10 improves mitochondrial function and boosts energy efficiency.

**Alpha-lipoic acid (ALA)** is a naturally occurring compound which is both water and fat soluble and acts as a powerful antioxidant as well as playing a crucial role in energy metabolism. It enhances mitochondrial energy production by supporting the citric acid cycle and increasing glucose uptake into cells. Additionally, as a potent antioxidant, ALA protects mitochondrial structures. It is found in foods such as red meat, organ meats, spinach, broccoli, beets, and carrots.

By prioritising a balanced diet rich in these nutrients, you can optimise your body's energy production, reduce fatigue, and support overall vitality. Start small by adding one iron-rich food or a magnesium-dense snack into your daily routine to feel the difference in your energy levels!

## Other actionable tips to boost energy:

**Regular physical activity**
Incorporating consistent exercise into your routine is a great way to boost energy. Aerobic activities combined with strength training and flexibility exercises improve mitochondrial function, enhance stamina, and support overall metabolic health.

**Stress management**
High stress levels can drain your energy. Mindfulness meditation, yoga, and deep breathing exercises can reduce stress and restore your mental and physical energy.

**Prioritise sleep**
Adequate sleep is crucial to recharging your body, so aim for 7-9 hours of quality rest every night. Establish a calming bedtime routine and limit screen time and caffeine intake before bed to improve sleep quality.

**Adrenal support**
The adrenal glands regulate stress responses and can become fatigued during menopause. Set personal boundaries, practise self-care, and learn to say no when necessary to avoid adrenal fatigue and maintain balanced energy levels.

One of the most empowering things you can do is listen to your body and rest when it calls for it. Many women going through menopause are balancing multiple responsibilities – family, work, and sometimes caring for ageing parents. This often leads to placing themselves last on the list for care at a time when rest should be their top priority. Rest is not a luxury, it's essential for your body to recharge and recover, so you can maintain the energy needed to navigate both your own life and the needs of those who rely on you.

# *Chapter Twenty-Six*

## Loss of Libido

*Libido reflects your natural desire for sexual connection and intimacy, which can ebb and flow throughout life due to various factors.*

Loss of libido, or low sex drive, is a deeply personal and often misunderstood concern that many women face, especially during menopause. However, when your desire for sex feels persistently diminished—far from what feels normal or fulfilling for you—it can ripple into your emotional well-being, relationships, and overall quality of life. It's important to acknowledge that this is a common experience and not something you are navigating alone.

Studies show that low sexual desire is the most frequently reported sexual health concern among women, representing 64% of all sexual concerns in one major study. While occasional changes in libido are natural, when the decrease becomes severe and causes significant distress, it may indicate a condition known as hypoactive sexual desire disorder (HSDD).

HSDD is more than just a lowered sex drive—it's an ongoing, distressing struggle with motivation and interest in sexual activity which has persisted for more than 6 months. The International Society for the Study of Women's Sexual Health defines HSDD as:

- **A lack of spontaneous desire,** such as sexual thoughts or fantasies.

- **A reduced or absent response to erotic cues or stimulation,** making it difficult to maintain interest or enjoyment during sexual activity.

- **Avoidance of intimacy,** not due to physical pain or discomfort, but rooted in diminished desire.

What makes HSDD particularly challenging is the emotional toll it takes. Feelings of frustration, sadness, guilt, or even loss of self can arise, affecting not only your sense of identity but also the emotional and physical intimacy you share with your partner.

## How menopause affects libido

Menopause often brings changes in sexual desire and function, resulting in a loss of libido for many women. These changes can stem from declining levels of oestrogen and testosterone, leading to physical discomfort, such as vulvovaginal dryness, discomfort, and even dyspareunia (painful intercourse). This discomfort can further reduce sexual desire, creating a cycle that affects intimacy and connection.

A diminished libido during menopause can also affect emotional well-being and self-confidence. Sexual intimacy is not just a physical act – it plays a crucial role in emotional bonding between partners. When sexual desire decreases, it can cause feelings of frustration, sadness, and disconnection. Additionally, changes in libido can affect self-esteem and body image, intensifying emotional and psychological challenges.

I understand that these changes can be difficult and even isolating at times. With the right information and support, you can explore ways to maintain a fulfilling and intimate relationship, both with your partner and yourself. Let's delve into some of the primary reasons for decreased libido and potential solutions that may help improve sexual well-being.

## Factors contributing to loss of libido:

### Oestrogen decline

Oestrogen plays a vital role in vaginal lubrication, tissue elasticity, and blood flow to the genital area. As oestrogen levels drop during menopause, many women experience vaginal dryness, discomfort, and thinning of the vaginal walls, making sexual activity uncomfortable or even painful. These physical changes can naturally lead to reduced sexual desire and arousal.

### Testosterone decline

Though often associated with male sexual function, testosterone is also produced in small amounts by women, particularly in the ovaries and adrenal glands. It plays a significant role in libido, sexual arousal, and sensitivity to stimuli. A decline in testosterone during menopause can further reduce sexual desire and responsiveness.

**Psychological factors**

Emotional stress, relationship concerns, body image issues, and mood disturbances such as anxiety and depression can all contribute to diminished libido. These psychological factors often create additional barriers to sexual desire, further complicating the physical changes of menopause.

## Actionable Tips

**Open communication**

Engage in honest and supportive conversations with your partner about how you feel. Open communication helps strengthen intimacy and can help address issues that may be affecting your sexual desire. Sharing your thoughts and feelings allows you both to work together to find ways to reconnect emotionally and physically.

**Vulvovaginal care**

Consider using lubricants and moisturisers specifically designed for menopausal women to alleviate vaginal dryness and discomfort. In some cases, vaginal oestrogen therapy or other medical treatments may be recommended by a healthcare provider to improve vaginal health and make intercourse more comfortable.

**Stress management**

Reducing stress can help address psychological barriers to libido. Incorporating relaxation techniques such as mindfulness meditation, yoga, deep breathing exercises, or other forms of stress relief can enhance your emotional well-being and help restore sexual desire.

**Healthy lifestyle habits**

Maintaining a balanced diet, exercising regularly, getting sufficient sleep, and moderating alcohol and smoking can all help support hormonal balance and enhance libido. Eating nutrient-rich foods can also contribute to overall well-being, positively impacting sexual desire and energy levels.

**Professional help**

If lifestyle changes and self-care measures aren't enough, consider seeking advice from healthcare providers, such as a gynaecologist or sex therapist who specialises in menopausal sexual health. They can offer personalised guidance, assess any underlying conditions, and suggest treatments to improve sexual satisfaction and intimacy.

It's essential to approach this with compassion for yourself. Your body is transitioning, and with that comes the need for patience and understanding. Just as your body has adapted through different stages of life, it will find a new balance in time. Be kind to yourself as you explore what works best for your unique situation, whether that's communicating openly with your partner, seeking medical advice, or incorporating lifestyle changes that help you feel more comfortable and in tune with your body.

Most importantly, remember that your worth and your ability to experience connection go beyond these changes. You are deserving of intimacy, love, and care. By taking small, manageable steps – whether it's trying new methods of self-care, reaching out for support, or simply giving yourself permission to rest and reflect – you can reclaim the joy of intimacy on your terms.

# *Chapter Twenty-Seven*

## Oral Changes

*Could hormonal changes during menopause be the reason behind your aching gums, increased sensitivity, or unexpected dental issues?*

Menopause changes many things about our bodies, and oral health is no exception. It's a topic that isn't often discussed, but it's one that deserves our attention because the health of your mouth is deeply connected to your overall well-being.

Just like your gut and vagina, your mouth has its own microbiome: a community of bacteria that play a crucial role in maintaining optimal health. When this delicate balance is disrupted, it can lead to inflammation, infections, and other oral health issues.

I know exactly how menopause can affect your oral health—because I've been there. A little over a year ago, I was diagnosed with periodontal disease. The news came as a shock to me; I had always considered myself someone who took good care of their teeth. I'd noticed that my gums ached when I was run down, and every Christmas (when stress levels skyrocketed), I seemed to get toothache, but I dismissed it as part of the season.

Since that diagnosis, I've been on a year-long journey to improve my oral health, and I can finally say I'm finally starting to see real progress. I've had the privilege of working with the best dentist and hygienists I've ever met, and they've educated me on many aspects of oral health. I now follow a detailed daily oral care routine, and while it takes commitment, it's paying off and my gums are now much healthier.

This chapter is my opportunity to share what I've learned—because if you're navigating menopause and noticing changes in your oral health, you're not alone. And trust me, there's so much you can do to protect your smile and feel good about it again.

## Menopause and oral health: understanding the impact

The oral mucosa and salivary glands contain oestrogen receptors, suggesting that fluctuations in oestrogen levels during menopause can directly affect oral health. Postmenopausal women often report oral discomfort, with increased risks of periodontal disease, xerostomia (dry mouth), burning mouth syndrome, altered taste perception, atrophic gingivitis and weakened jawbones. These issues arise due to the thinning and atrophy of the oral mucosal epithelium, which becomes more susceptible to mechanical injuries, infections, and changes in pain tolerance.

## Periodontal disease in menopausal women

Periodontal disease is a progressive inflammatory condition that can lead to tooth loss. It develops due to the accumulation of dental plaque, bacterial dysbiosis, the formation of periodontal pockets, and subsequent tissue destruction, including alveolar bone loss. Menopausal women are particularly susceptible to this condition, as declining oestrogen levels exacerbate inflammation and weaken the periodontium. Research suggests a strong association between menopause and periodontitis, with oxidative stress and reduced antioxidant defences playing significant roles in disease progression.

## Salivary glands and oral health

Dryness of the mouth or xerostomia is one of the most common symptoms reported by women in the menopausal period. Salivary glands are hormone-dependent, and menopause-induced hormonal changes can alter saliva secretion and consistency. Reduced saliva production affects the oral cavity by increasing the risk of infections, dental caries, and periodontal disease.

As women transition through menopause, the hormonal changes that occur can significantly impact the health of your mouth. Lower levels of oestrogen can alter the oral microbiome, making your gums and teeth more susceptible to inflammation and infections. Just as I learned through my own journey with periodontal disease, these changes can be unexpected and challenging—but with the right knowledge and care, they're absolutely manageable.

## Actionable Tips

### Talk to your dentist and hygienist

The first and most crucial step is to partner with dental professionals. Regular check-ups and cleanings are vital. They can monitor changes in your oral health, provide targeted treatments, and recommend products or techniques tailored to your unique needs. Don't hesitate to discuss any symptoms like dry mouth, gum sensitivity or discomfort when brushing

### Build your oral health arsenal

I'm not a dentist or hygienist, but maintaining a routine of brushing twice daily, flossing, using interdental brushes, and incorporating a water flosser has been a game-changer for me. In fact, I've got all my tools lined up on a specially designated shelf—it's like a mini dental clinic in my bathroom! This routine has worked for me, but we're all unique, and our oral health needs differ. By speaking to your dentist or hygienist, you can create your own personalised arsenal of tools and techniques to keep your smile in top shape.

### Hydrate and moisturise

Stay hydrated by drinking plenty of water throughout the day to support saliva production and keep your mouth moist.

### Be aware of hormonal changes

Hormonal shifts during menopause can impact gum health and saliva production. Monitor your symptoms and share these observations with your dentist. They can help address hormone-related issues with targeted strategies.

**Stay consistent**

Consistency is key. Even small daily habits, like thorough brushing and regular hydration, add up over time to protect your teeth and gums during menopause.

**Your smile is worth it**

My advice to you? If you have any concerns about your oral health as you enter perimenopause, don't wait—speak to your dentist. It's never too early or too late to take steps toward protecting your smile and overall health. Taking care of your oral health is an act of self-care that benefits your entire well-being. You deserve to feel confident, comfortable, and empowered every time you smile.

# *Part Three*

## Menopause Vitality: A Guide to Nutrition and Lifestyle

# *Chapter Twenty-Eight*

# Nurturing Your Body Through Menopause: Macronutrients

*"Let food be thy medicine and medicine be thy food."*

*Hippocrates*

I remember a time in my own menopause journey when I felt like everything was slipping through my fingers: my body, my emotions, and my energy. They were all out of balance, with days when even the smallest of tasks felt overwhelming, and I just wanted to feel steady again, like myself again. I came to realise that while I couldn't control everything that was happening to my body, I *could* control how I nourished it. Food became more than just fuel it became a way to care for myself, to rebuild strength from within. It wasn't an overnight solution, but it was a starting point, a small, intentional shift that reminded me of my own resilience.

As the earlier chapters have shown us, the power of food cannot be underestimated. Every nutrient you consume plays a part in supporting your hormones, lifting your mood, and keeping your body strong. It's a powerful tool you can use to thrive, even during the most challenging parts of this transition. By making intentional, informed choices, you can create a foundation of health that carries you not just through menopause, but well beyond it. This isn't about a rigid diet or giving up the foods you love – it's about finding ways to nourish your body and mind with intention and care.

All the nutrients highlighted in the next few chapters have a role to play, whether it's helping to balance your hormones, protect your bones, or boost your energy. Think of these as the building blocks your body needs to thrive. With this knowledge, you'll be able to make choices that feel good in the moment and set you up for long-term health and vitality.

## Macronutrients

These are the proteins, fats and carbohydrates that form the cornerstone of our diet.

### 1. Protein

Proteins are essential molecules made up of amino acids that perform vital functions in the body. These amino acids are classified as essential: they must be obtained through diet (e.g., leucine, lysine) and non-essential: produced naturally by the body (e.g., alanine, glutamine).

Protein is essential during menopause to:

**Preserve muscle mass:** declining oestrogen levels can accelerate muscle loss, impacting strength and metabolism. Sarcopenia, the natural age-related loss of muscle mass and function, leads to a 3–8% decline in lean muscle every decade after the age of 30. This condition affects around 30% of individuals over 60 and over 50% of those aged 80 and above. Adequate protein intake plays a vital role in addressing sarcopenia by helping to preserve muscle mass, support physical strength, and maintain overall health.

**Regulate hormones:** amino acids support the production of hormones like insulin and thyroid hormones, which are crucial for metabolic and energy balance.

**Support tissue repair:** protein aids in tissue growth and repair, particularly important as oestrogen levels decline.

**Balance blood sugar:** protein slows sugar release into the bloodstream, keeping energy steady and helping you feel fuller for longer.

Good sources of protein can be animal-based, such as chicken, turkey, eggs, salmon, mackerel, lean beef, and Greek yogurt. Or plant-based, like lentils, chickpeas, quinoa, tofu, tempeh, chia seeds, and almonds. Menopausal women should aim for 1g-1.2g of protein per kg of body weight daily, distributed throughout your meals and snacks to support muscle repair and hormone balance.

| Typical Portions of Protein | |
|---|---|
| Chicken Breast (100g): | 30g per serving |
| Salmon Fillet (100g) | 22g |
| 2 Boiled Eggs | 14g |
| Cooked Lentils (1 cup) | 12g |
| Greek Yogurt (120g) | 7g |
| Edamame (0.5 cup) | 8g |
| Almonds (1oz) | 6g |
| Cottage Cheese (0.5 cup) | 14g |
| Chickpeas (1 cup) | 15g |
| Tofu (1 cup) | 10g |
| Quinoa (1 cup) | 8g |
| Black Beans (1 cup) | 15g |
| Tempeh (1 cup) | 10g |

## 2. Carbohydrates

These are your body's energy source, its primary fuel, which is especially important during menopause when energy levels and blood sugar balance can fluctuate.

**Energy stabilisation**
Complex carbohydrates, such as those found in whole grains, vegetables, and legumes, release glucose slowly, preventing energy crashes and supporting steady energy throughout the day.

**Digestive support**
Fibre from carbohydrates aids digestion, promotes regular bowel movements, and supports the detoxification of excess hormones like oestrogen.

**Blood sugar regulation**
Low-GI carbohydrates help maintain consistent blood sugar levels, reducing fatigue, irritability, and mood swings.

**Nutrient delivery**

Carbohydrates are rich in essential vitamins, minerals, and antioxidants that promote overall health.

The glycaemic index (GI) measures how quickly foods raise blood sugar levels. During menopause, prioritising low-GI foods helps maintain steady energy, reduces mood swings, and prevents fatigue. Low GI foods include whole grains (quinoa, oats, barley), legumes (lentils, chickpeas) and non-starchy vegetables (broccoli, leafy greens). High GI Foods include sugary cereals, white bread and rice and processed snacks.

| Tips for Incorporating Carbohydrates | |
|---|---|
| Focus on Whole Grains | Include brown rice, quinoa, and oats for sustained energy and fibre. |
| Load Up on Vegetables | Make leafy greens, cruciferous vegetables, and colourful options like sweet potatoes a dietary staple. |
| Choose Low-GI Foods | Stabilise energy and hormones by swapping refined carbs for whole grains and legumes. |
| Increase Fruits | Enjoy berries, apples, and pears for antioxidants, fibre, and a natural energy boost. |

## 3. Fibre

Fibre is your menopausal superhero. It's a plant-based carbohydrate that your body doesn't fully digest. Instead, it passes through your digestive system, providing benefits along the way. Fibre helps regulate digestion, manage blood sugar, and eliminate excess hormones like oestrogen, supporting hormonal balance during menopause.

There are two types of fibre: **soluble**, which dissolves in water, forming a gel-like substance in your gut and slows digestion, stabilises blood sugar, and lowers cholesterol. Examples include oats, flaxseeds, broccoli, and apples. And **insoluble** fibre that adds bulk to stools, promoting regular bowel movements and helps prevent constipation (a common menopausal issue). Whole grains, lentils, spinach, and almonds are high in insoluble fibre.

Fibre is essential during menopause for:

**Hormonal regulation:** fibre helps eliminate excess oestrogen from the body, reducing symptoms like bloating and mood swings.

**Blood sugar control:** by slowing the release of glucose into the bloodstream, fibre helps maintain stable energy levels and reduces cravings.

**Weight management:** high-fibre foods promote satiety, helping you feel fuller for longer and making it easier to manage weight.

**Heart health:** soluble fibre supports cardiovascular health by lowering cholesterol levels, a critical factor as heart disease risk increases post-menopause.

**Digestive support:** fibre feeds beneficial gut bacteria, promoting a healthy microbiome and reducing bloating and digestive discomfort.

Women are encouraged to aim to take in 30g of fibre daily. Here's how you can achieve it:

| | |
|---|---|
| ½ avocado | 7g fibre |
| 2 tbsp chia seeds | 10g |
| 1 cup broccoli | 5g |
| 1 pear | 5.5g |
| ½ cup cooked lentils | 8g |
| 1 apple with skin | 4g |
| 1 slice whole-grain bread | 3g |

Practical tips for increasing fibre include:

**Starting your day right:** add chia seeds to smoothies or oatmeal for a fibre-packed breakfast.

**Making vegetables the star:** fill half your plate with colourful vegetables like broccoli, spinach, or sweet potatoes.

**Snack smart:** choose fibre-rich snacks like carrots and hummus or a handful of nuts.

**Hydrate well:** drink plenty of water to help fibre move through your digestive system smoothly.

**Go gradually:** increase fibre intake slowly to avoid digestive discomfort.

## 4. Fats: essential building blocks for hormonal health

Fats are a vital component of a healthy diet, especially during menopause. They serve as building blocks for hormone production, support cellular function, and aid in reducing inflammation—

all crucial for managing menopausal symptoms. Among these, omega-3 and omega-6 fatty acids, often called "essential fats," stand out because the body cannot produce them on its own and must obtain them from food.

Not all fats are created equal. Healthy fats like omega-3s and unsaturated fats promote hormone production, heart health, and brain function, while excessive consumption of saturated and trans fats can lead to inflammation and other health issues. By focusing on the right sources, you can harness the benefits of fats to support your body's needs during menopause.

## Healthy fats are essential for:

**Hormone production:** cholesterol serves as a building block for hormones like oestrogen, progesterone, and testosterone. Adequate fat intake ensures the body has the resources needed to maintain hormonal equilibrium.

**Nutrient absorption:** fats enable the absorption of fat-soluble vitamins like A, D, E, and K, which are vital for bone health, immunity, and vision.

**Cellular function:** healthy fats maintain the integrity of cell membranes, aiding communication and fluidity across the body.

**Cardiovascular support:** fats from avocados, olive oil, and fatty fish can reduce cholesterol and inflammation, protecting against heart disease, which becomes a greater risk post-menopause.

**Cognitive and emotional health:** Omega-3 fatty acids, especially DHA, support brain health and emotional stability, helping reduce mood swings and memory challenges.

**Inflammation control:** Omega-3s form anti-inflammatory compounds, which can ease joint pain and other menopause-related symptoms.

## The balancing act: omega-3 and omega-6

Omega-3 and omega-6 fatty acids are essential nutrients that play key roles in overall health, influencing cellular function, hormonal balance, and inflammation regulation. Omega-3 fatty acids, including eicosapentaenoic acid (EPA) and docosahexaenoic acid (DHA), are primarily found in oily fish such as salmon, mackerel, and sardines, as well as plant-based sources like flaxseeds, chia seeds, and walnuts.

These fats deliver a wide range of health benefits, including anti-inflammatory, vasodilating, and anticoagulant effects that support brain health, cardiovascular function, and the management of inflammation-related conditions. EPA and DHA, derived from marine sources, are particularly crucial for brain function, eye health, and maintaining cell membrane integrity. While the body can convert alpha-linolenic acid (ALA) from plant-based foods into EPA and DHA, this conversion process is relatively inefficient. Therefore, obtaining EPA and DHA directly from dietary sources is highly recommended for maintaining optimal well-being.

Omega-6 fatty acids, such as linoleic acid (LA), are found in seed oils (e.g., sunflower and corn oil), nuts, and seeds. These fats are vital for immune responses, cellular function, and growth. However, excessive omega-6 intake—common in modern diets due to the widespread use of processed foods and seed oils—can contribute to inflammation.

A healthy ratio of omega-6 to omega-3 is typically around 4:1, but many Western diets skew heavily toward omega-6, with ratios as high as 20:1 or more. To restore balance, focus on increasing omega-3 intake through foods like fatty fish, flaxseeds, and walnuts while reducing omega-6-heavy processed foods and seed oil consumption.

By incorporating omega-3-rich foods and moderating omega-6 intake, you can effectively help to reduce inflammation, support hormonal health, and promote overall well-being.

| **Practical Strategies for Incorporating Healthy Fats** | |
|---|---|
| Include Omega-3 fatty acids | Add fatty fish, flaxseeds, chia seeds, or walnuts to your weekly meals. Use fish oil or algae-based supplements if dietary intake is insufficient. Always seek the help of a Nutritionist to determine the right supplement for you. |
| Prioritise Unsaturated Fats | Focus on avocados, olive oil, almonds, and seeds to support hormone production and heart health. |
| Reduce Saturated and Trans Fats | Minimise intake of fried and processed foods, replacing them with whole, nutrient-dense options. |

By understanding the role of fats, carbohydrates, proteins, and fibre during menopause, you can empower yourself to make intentional, informed choices that nurture your body. These essential macronutrients work together to support energy levels, stabilise mood, and promote overall well-being during this transformative stage of life. Remember, even the smallest changes can have a profound impact. Swapping refined carbohydrates for whole grains, incorporating more healthy fats, ensuring an adequate intake of quality protein, or adding fibre-rich foods to your meals can all contribute to better health and vitality.

*"Every time you eat is an opportunity to nourish your body."*

*-Unknown*

# *Chapter Twenty-Nine*

## Micronutrients and Menopause (1): Vital Vitamins

*"A wise man ought to realise that health is his most valuable possession."*

*Hippocrates*

Micronutrients are those small but mighty vitamins, minerals, and other essential compounds, the unsung heroes that support your body every single day. They're not just silent supporters in the background; they're actively involved in almost every process your body undertakes. From producing hormones to boosting immunity, supporting bone health, regulating energy levels, and even lifting your mood. Micronutrients are indispensable.

Vitamins are organic compounds that the body needs in small quantities to support normal metabolic functions.

## 1. Vitamin A

Fat-soluble Vitamin A is essential for vision, skin health, immune function and cellular growth. It exists in two forms: retinol, sourced from animal-based foods, such as liver, eggs, fortified dairy, and fish liver oils; carotenoids, which are plant-derived compounds that the body converts into Vitamin A. These are sourced from carrots, sweet potatoes, spinach, kale, and red peppers. Aim to include a mix of animal-based and plant-based sources for a balanced Vitamin A intake. Foods rich in beta-carotene (e.g., colourful fruits and vegetables) also provide powerful antioxidant benefits:

**Skin health and cellular renewal**
Menopausal hormonal changes often lead to skin dryness and a loss of elasticity. Vitamin A promotes skin cell regeneration, helping to combat these effects and maintain a healthy, hydrated complexion. Retinoids, derived from Vitamin A, are frequently used in skincare to improve skin turnover and reduce signs of ageing.

**Immune function**
Vitamin A supports the health of mucous membranes in the respiratory and digestive systems, which serve as the body's first line of defence against infections. Since menopause can weaken the immune system, maintaining adequate Vitamin A levels is crucial for strengthening immunity.

**Eye health**
Essential for retinal function, Vitamin A supports healthy vision, particularly in low-light conditions. As menopause can exacerbate age-related eye concerns, Vitamin A contributes to long-term eye health.

## 2. B Vitamins

B Vitamins are water-soluble nutrients that play a critical role in energy production, brain function, and stress regulation. This group includes thiamine (B1), riboflavin (B2), niacin (B3), pantothenic acid (B5), pyridoxine (B6), biotin (B7), folate (B9), and cobalamin (B12):

**Energy metabolism**
B Vitamins aid in breaking down carbohydrates, fats, and proteins to produce cellular energy. This function helps counteract menopause-related fatigue and supports sustained energy levels throughout the day.

**Cognitive and neurological health**
Hormonal shifts during menopause can lead to brain fog, mood swings, and memory lapses. Vitamins B6, B12, and folate play key roles in neurotransmitter synthesis, promoting mental clarity and emotional stability.

**Stress management**
B Vitamins, particularly B5, help regulate cortisol production by supporting adrenal gland function. Adequate intake can ease the physical and emotional stress that often accompanies menopause.

**Cardiovascular support**
B6, folate, and B12 help lower homocysteine levels, a marker linked to cardiovascular risk. By supporting heart health, they help mitigate the inflammation and oxidative stress that rise during menopause.

## 3. Vitamin C

Vitamin C is well-known for its immune-boosting properties, but its importance during menopause extends far beyond that. This water-soluble vitamin is critical for collagen production, maintaining energy levels and combating oxidative stress. Menopause often brings heightened stress, which depletes Vitamin C levels in the adrenal glands. As the body uses Vitamin C to manage stress-related hormones, maintaining adequate intake is crucial for overall hormonal balance.

**Collagen production**

Vitamin C aids in the production of collagen, a protein essential for skin elasticity, joint health, and bone strength. This is particularly vital as declining oestrogen levels can weaken these structures.

**Antioxidant and anti-inflammatory effects**

Vitamin C neutralises free radicals and reduces oxidative stress, alleviating menopausal symptoms like joint pain, skin ageing, and inflammation.

**Immune function**

Hormonal fluctuations during menopause may weaken immune defences. Vitamin C helps bolster immunity, protecting against infections and promoting overall resilience.

**Energy production**

By supporting the production of carnitine, Vitamin C aids in transporting fatty acids to mitochondria for energy, helping combat menopausal fatigue.

**Enhanced iron absorption**
Vitamin C improves the absorption of non-haem iron from plant-based foods, essential for preventing anaemia and supporting energy levels.

## 4. Vitamin D

Known as the "sunlight vitamin", Vitamin D is actually a hormone essential for several bodily functions. It plays a vital role in maintaining bone health by aiding calcium absorption in the intestines, which is critical for preserving bone density and strength. The body naturally synthesises Vitamin D when the skin is exposed to sunlight, though it can also be obtained from dietary sources.

**Bone health**
As oestrogen levels decline, the risk of bone loss and fractures increases. Vitamin D enhances calcium absorption and regulates its levels via the parathyroid hormone. Women deficient in Vitamin D have up to a 77% higher risk of fractures, particularly hip fractures, making adequate intake essential during menopause.

**Immune support**
Vitamin D activates T cells that help fight infections and modulate immune responses. This function is especially valuable during menopause when immunity may weaken.

**Blood sugar regulation**
Deficiencies in Vitamin D are linked to insulin resistance and inflammation, particularly in the context of hormonal imbalances. Maintaining optimal Vitamin D levels helps improve metabolic health.

### Mental health

Low Vitamin D levels are associated with a higher risk of depression, highlighting its importance for emotional balance during menopause. Adequate levels can support a more stable mood and overall mental well-being.

There are three main sources of Vitamin D: dietary, such as fatty fish (e.g. salmon, mackerel), fortified dairy products, egg yolks, and fortified plant milks); sun exposure: aim for 15–20 minutes of sun exposure a few times a week, taking care to balance sun safety with Vitamin D synthesis, and supplements. If sun exposure or dietary intake is insufficient, consider supplements. Always consult your healthcare provider for appropriate dosage and monitoring.

## 5. Vitamin E

A fat-soluble vitamin renowned for its potent antioxidant properties, which protect cells from oxidative stress. The various forms of Vitamin E include alpha-tocopherol, the most biologically active in the body. Vitamin E supports immune function, skin health, and cellular protection – key areas affected by oxidative stress and hormonal shifts during menopause.

### Antioxidant protection

Menopause increases oxidative stress, accelerating ageing and contributing to skin dryness and inflammation. Vitamin E helps neutralise free radicals, reducing cellular damage.

### Skin and hair health

Declining oestrogen levels often result in skin dryness, thinning, and loss of elasticity. Vitamin E aids hydration, repairs skin cells, and may improve the appearance of fine lines and wrinkles. It also supports scalp health and reduces hair loss linked to hormonal changes.

**Cardiovascular support**

Vitamin E protects blood vessels from oxidative damage and improves circulation, reducing the risk of cardiovascular complications associated with menopause.

**Immune function**

By enhancing immune cell activity, Vitamin E supports the body's defences, which may weaken during menopause.

## 6. Vitamin K

Vitamin K is a fat-soluble vitamin available in two primary forms: **Vitamin K1 (Phylloquinone**), found in green leafy vegetables like spinach and kale and **Vitamin K2 (Menaquinone),** in fermented foods and animal products, synthesised by gut bacteria.

Vitamin K plays a pivotal role in bone mineralisation, supporting bone density and preventing arterial calcification, which becomes increasingly important during menopause.

**Calcium regulation**

Vitamin K2 directs calcium to bones and teeth while preventing it from accumulating in soft tissues and arteries. This helps protect against arterial calcification and supports bone strength.

**Bone health**

Research shows Vitamin K improves vertebral bone density, reducing the risk of fractures in postmenopausal women with osteoporosis. It ensures calcium is effectively utilised within bones.

**Micronutrient synergy**

Vitamin K works closely with Vitamin D, calcium, and magnesium to enhance calcium absorption and utilisation, providing a multi-faceted approach to bone health during menopause.

| Vitamin-Rich Foods – Cheat Sheet 1 | | |
|---|---|---|
| Vitamin A | Liver, eggs, fortified dairy, and fish liver oils; carrots, sweet potatoes, spinach, kale, and red peppers. | To boost Vitamin A intake, pair colourful vegetables like carrots, sweet potatoes, or spinach with healthy fats, such as olive oil, avocado, or nuts. Vitamin A is fat-soluble, so combining it with fats enhances its absorption in the body. |
| B Vitamins | Whole grains such as brown rice, quinoa and oats; lean meats and organic meats, like chicken, turkey, liver; legumes including lentils, chickpeas, and beans; and leafy greens such as spinach, kale, and dark greens. | A variety of these ensures an optimal balance of all B Vitamins. They work synergistically to support energy and metabolism. |
| Vitamin C | Red peppers, kiwi, strawberries, broccoli, and oranges. | Since it is sensitive to heat, consume foods like raw peppers or lightly steamed broccoli to retain full nutrient value. |
| Vitamin D | Fatty fish (e.g. salmon, mackerel), fortified dairy products, egg yolks, and fortified plant milks | Pairing Vitamin D-rich foods like oily fish or fortified plant milks with healthy fats (e.g. Olive oil, avocado) to maximise absorption. |

| | | |
|---|---|---|
| Vitamin E | Nuts and seeds, such as almonds, sunflower seeds, and hazelnuts; leafy greens, like spinach, Swiss chard, and broccoli; vegetable oils including cold-pressed sunflower oil, safflower oil and avocados | Snack on sunflower seeds or almonds and pair Vitamin E-rich foods with healthy fats (e.g., avocado, nut butter) for improved absorption. |
| Vitamin K | Fermented foods like natto and sauerkraut; grass-fed animal products such as meat, dairy and egg yolks; and there is evidence to suggest cheeses like gouda and brie provide a reduced risk of heart disease linked to menaquinone intake. | Including leafy greens like spinach or kale with healthy fats (e.g. olive oil, avocado) to optimise absorption of Vitamin K. For added benefits, combine these with fermented foods for both nutritional and probiotic support. |

# *Chapter Thirty*

## Micronutrients and Menopause (2): Mighty Minerals

Minerals are inorganic elements that the body requires in varying amounts to perform essential functions and maintain overall health.

### 1. Calcium

Calcium is a crucial structural component of bones and teeth, making them strong and dense. Approximately 99% of the body's calcium is stored in bones and teeth, while the remaining 1% plays critical roles in muscle function, nerve transmission, blood clotting, and hormone secretion.

**Bone density**

During menopause, declining oestrogen levels lead to a reduction in bone density, increasing the risk of osteoporosis and fractures. Ensuring adequate calcium intake, especially when combined with vitamin D, is essential for preserving bone strength.

**Critical bodily functions**

Beyond bone health, calcium is vital for numerous physiological processes, including vascular contraction and dilation, muscle function, nerve transmission, intracellular signalling, digestion, blood clotting, and heart function regulation. The body tightly regulates plasma calcium levels through the actions of two key hormones—parathyroid hormone (PTH) and calcitonin—to prevent disruptions that could affect overall health.

- **Parathyroid Hormone (PTH):** Produced by the parathyroid glands, PTH raises blood calcium levels by releasing calcium from bones, enhancing intestinal absorption, and reducing calcium excretion by the kidneys. This ensures proper nerve, muscle, and bone function.

- **Calcitonin:** Produced by the thyroid gland, calcitonin lowers blood calcium by inhibiting calcium release from bones and increasing calcium excretion through the kidneys. It counterbalances PTH, preventing excess calcium in the blood and maintaining bone integrity.

Ensuring sufficient calcium intake during menopause supports both structural and regulatory functions, contributing to overall health and vitality.

## 2. Magnesium

Magnesium is a critical mineral involved in over 300 biochemical reactions in the body. It supports protein synthesis, nerve and muscle function, blood sugar regulation, and blood pressure maintenance.

Magnesium also plays a pivotal role in DNA and RNA synthesis, stabilising cell membranes, and promoting bone health.

**Bone health**

Aids bone formation by regulating osteoblasts and osteoclasts, the cells responsible for building and breaking down bone tissue. It also ensures optimal parathyroid hormone and vitamin D function, for bone strength.

**Hormonal balance**

Influences neurotransmitters like serotonin, supporting mood regulation and stress response – crucial for hormonal fluctuations.

**Blood sugar regulation**

Improves insulin sensitivity, helping regulate blood sugar levels – a vital function as hormonal changes can disrupt glucose metabolism.

**Thyroid support**

Reduces inflammation and supports healthy thyroid function, which affects metabolism and energy levels.

**Improved sleep**

By relaxing muscles and calming the nervous system, magnesium promotes restful sleep, often disrupted during menopause.

**Energy production**

Supports mitochondrial function, the "powerhouses" of cells, ensuring efficient energy production and combating fatigue.

Consequences of magnesium deficiency include fatigue and low energy, muscle cramps and twitches, sleep disturbances, heightened anxiety or heart palpitations and digestive issues such as constipation.

## 3. Zinc

Zinc is a trace mineral involved in over 300 enzyme reactions, making it vital for immune function, inflammation regulation, and cellular repair.

**Immune boost**
Enhances the activity of immune cells like T cells and B cells, strengthening the body's defences during a time when immune resilience may weaken.

**Inflammation control**
Zinc's anti-inflammatory properties help regulate chronic inflammation, reducing discomfort linked to menopausal symptoms like joint pain.

**Antioxidant defence**
As a potent antioxidant, zinc neutralises free radicals, reducing oxidative stress that accelerates cellular ageing.

**Skin and collagen health**
Promotes collagen synthesis, helping maintain skin elasticity and repair. It alleviates common concerns like dryness and wrinkles associated with declining oestrogen levels.

**Mood and neurotransmitter support**
Helps balance neurotransmitters like serotonin and dopamine, reducing anxiety and mood swings often experienced during menopause.

## 4. Selenium

Selenium is a trace mineral essential for antioxidant protection and thyroid health. It plays a crucial role in neutralising free radicals and maintaining metabolic stability.

**Cellular health**
Acts as an antioxidant, reducing oxidative stress and promoting healthy ageing, and supports collagen production, which maintains skin elasticity and joint health.

**Thyroid function**
Vital for producing thyroid hormones that regulate metabolism and energy levels. Also helps alleviate symptoms like fatigue and weight changes linked to thyroid imbalance.

## 5. Iron

Iron is a mineral critical for oxygen transport via haemoglobin and energy production. Found in two forms: heme (animal-based) and nonheme (plant-based) – iron is essential for preventing fatigue and supporting metabolic health.

**Energy production**
Enables oxygen delivery to cells, reducing fatigue and supporting cellular energy.

**Cognitive function**
Adequate iron ensures optimal oxygen flow to the brain, improving memory and focus.

**Immune health**
Helps produce immune cells, bolstering defences.

**Fatigue prevention**
Prevents anaemia, a common cause of exhaustion and weakness.

## 6. Iodine

Iodine is a trace mineral essential for synthesising thyroid hormones, which regulate metabolism, energy levels, and cognitive health.

**Thyroid regulation**
Ensures proper production of T3 and T4 hormones, stabilising metabolism. Supports hypothyroidism, which can exacerbate menopausal symptoms like fatigue and weight gain.

**Metabolic balance**
Helps maintain stable energy levels and cardiovascular health.

## 7. Potassium

Potassium is a vital mineral essential for maintaining overall health and body function.

**Muscle function**
Supports proper muscle contraction, reducing the risk of cramps and spasms, especially during exercise or in hot conditions when potassium is lost through sweat.

**Fluid balance**
Along with sodium, potassium regulates the body's fluid balance, ensuring optimal hydration.

**Nerve signal transmission**
Critical for transmitting nerve impulses, enabling sensory, motor, and cognitive functions.

## 8. Sodium

Sodium is a key mineral that plays an integral role in maintaining the body's fluid and electrolyte balance.

**Fluid regulation**
Works alongside potassium to balance fluid levels, maintaining proper hydration and preventing dehydration.

**Nerve function**
Assists in nerve signal transmission, enabling effective communication between the brain and muscles.

**Muscle function**
Essential for proper muscle contractions and overall mobility.

Sodium is primarily obtained from sodium chloride (table salt), often added to processed foods for preservation. While sodium is essential for fluid balance, nerve signalling, and muscle contractions, excessive consumption—especially from packaged and processed foods—can contribute to health risks.

## 9. Copper

Copper is essential for multiple physiological processes in the body:

**Red blood cell formation**
Facilitates the absorption and utilisation of iron, aiding in the production of haemoglobin.

**Bone and connective tissue health**
Supports the formation of collagen and elastin, vital for strong bones, skin, and blood vessels.

**Immune function**
Plays a role in maintaining immune defences.

**Co-factor for enzymes**
Acts as a cofactor for several enzymes, enabling metabolic and antioxidant processes.

## 10. Phosphorus

Phosphorus is the second most abundant mineral in the body and serves several essential functions:

**Bone and teeth health**
Combines with calcium to form and strengthen bones and teeth.

**Genetic material**
Essential for the formation of DNA and RNA, which carry genetic instructions.

**Cell membranes**
Forms phospholipids, which are key structural components of cell membranes.

**Energy production**
Plays a critical role in generating ATP (adenosine triphosphate), the primary energy source for cellular processes.

**Muscle function**
Assists in muscle contraction through creatine phosphate.

**pH balance**
Acts as a buffer to maintain the body's acid-base balance, ensuring proper fluid homeostasis.

| Mineral-Rich Foods – Cheat Sheet 2 | | |
|---|---|---|
| Calcium | **Dairy Products:** Milk, yogurt, and cheese offer highly absorbable forms. **Fish with Bones:** Sardines and salmon are rich sources of calcium and healthy fats.<br>**Leafy Greens:** Kale, broccoli, and bok choy.<br>**Nuts and Seeds:** Almonds, chia seeds, and sesame seeds.<br>**Tahini:** A sesame seed paste. | Combine calcium-rich foods with vitamin D sources, such as fatty fish or fortified dairy, to enhance absorption. Try adding chia seeds to yogurt or sprinkling sesame seeds on salads for an extra calcium boost. |
| Magnesium | **Nuts and Seeds:** Almonds, cashews, peanuts, and pumpkin seeds.<br>**Leafy Greens**: Spinach, kale, and Swiss chard.<br>**Whole Grains:** Quinoa, oats, and brown rice provide magnesium alongside fibre and other nutrients.<br>**Legumes:** Beans, lentils, and chickpeas also support gut health.<br>**Fatty Fish:** Salmon & mackerel. Avocados. | Incorporate magnesium-rich snacks like almonds or add spinach and quinoa to meals for a healthy magnesium boost. Pair magnesium-rich foods with vitamin D for enhanced benefits, particularly for bone health. |
| Zinc | **Oysters:** Highest natural source of zinc.<br>**Red Meat:** Beef and lamb<br>**Legumes:** Chickpeas, lentils, and beans provide plant-based zinc.<br>**Seeds and Nuts:** Pumpkin seeds and cashews are nutrient-dense options. | Increase zinc intake during illness using zinc lozenges to shorten the duration of symptoms.<br>Consult a healthcare provider for dosage recommendations |

| | | |
|---|---|---|
| Selenium | **Brazil Nuts**<br>**Seafood:** tuna and shrimp.<br>**Sunflower Seeds**<br>**Whole Grains:** brown rice. | Just one to two Brazil nuts a day can meet your selenium needs. |
| Iron | **Heme Sources:** Lean meats, chicken, turkey, and fish.<br>**Nonheme Sources:** Lentils, spinach, kale, and beans. | Pair plant-based iron sources with Vitamin C-rich foods, like citrus fruits or tomatoes, to enhance absorption. |
| Iodine | **Seaweed:** Easily added to soup and salads.<br>**Iodised Salt:** Convenient option for daily iodine intake.<br>**Dairy:** Milk, cheese, and yogurt provide iodine and calcium.<br>**Eggs** | Include seaweed in your meals or cook with iodised salt to support thyroid function and metabolism. |
| Potassium | **Fruits:** bananas, kiwi, apricots, guava.<br>**Veg:** avocado, beetroot, spinach, courgettes, mushrooms, endives, potatoes.<br>**Nuts and Seeds:** almond, sunflower seeds. | More than 90% of potassium is absorbed from the diet. Olive oil can increase the absorption. |
| Phosphorus | **Meat and poultry**<br>**Legumes:** beans, lentils.<br>**Nuts:** especially cashews and Brazil nuts. | Be Aware: Phosphorus is present in many processed fast foods, soda and packages snacks. |
| Copper | **Shellfish, Organ Meats,**<br>**Nuts and Seeds**<br>**Mushrooms**<br>**Whole grain products:** wheat-bran cereals.<br>**Legumes:** beans and lentils. | Nuts and seeds -particularly almonds, cashew and sesames seeds- are good sources of copper. |

# *Chapter Thirty-One*

# Lesser-Known Essential Nutrients

## 1. Choline

Choline is a water-soluble nutrient essential for brain health, serving as a precursor for acetylcholine, a neurotransmitter crucial for memory, learning, and mood regulation:

**Cognitive function**
Choline supports acetylcholine production, aiding memory, learning, and mental clarity.

**Memory enhancement**
Boosts acetylcholine levels, improving memory retention and recall during menopause.

**Mood regulation**
Supports anxiety by modulating the parasympathetic nervous system and counteracting adrenaline effects.

## 2. Inositol

A glucose-like compound that acts as a secondary messenger in cellular functions, supporting insulin sensitivity, neurotransmitter production, and hormonal balance:

**Improved insulin sensitivity**
Regulates blood sugar and reduces the risk of metabolic syndrome.

**Neurotransmitter regulation**
Enhances serotonin production, alleviating anxiety and emotional instability.

## 3. Coenzyme Q10 (CoQ10)

Coenzyme Q10 (CoQ10) is a fat-soluble, vitamin-like compound that supports cellular energy production and acts as a powerful antioxidant:

**Antioxidant protection**
Reduces oxidative stress and slows cellular ageing.

**Energy boost**
Fuels ATP production, enhancing overall energy levels and combating fatigue.

**Heart health**
Supports energy production in cardiac cells, reducing menopause-related cardiovascular risks.

**Skin and brain support**

Promotes collagen production for youthful skin and helps protect against cognitive decline.

**Gum health**

Diseased gum tissues have significantly lower levels of CoQ10 compared to healthy gums. Research shows that daily supplementation with CoQ10, combined with standard periodontal care, can lead to notable improvements in periodontal disease.

## 4. Phytoestrogens

Phytoestrogens are plant-based compounds that share structural similarities with oestrogen, allowing them to interact with oestrogen receptors in the body. These interactions enable phytoestrogens to either mimic or moderate oestrogen's effects, making them a valuable ally during menopause when natural oestrogen levels begin to decline.

They belong to four principal categories: flavonoids, phenolic acids, lignans, and stilbenes. Although they do not contain actual oestrogen, their structural similarity enables them to act as Selective Estrogen Receptor Modulators (SERMs). This means they can mimic oestrogen in some tissues while blocking its effects in others, offering a natural means to support hormonal balance without overstimulation.

Incorporating a variety of phytoestrogen-rich foods into your diet is a natural and effective way to support hormone health.

| Lesser-Known Essential Nutrients – Cheat Sheet 3 | |
|---|---|
| Choline | Lecithin (soy, seeds, eggs). Organ meats (liver). Poultry and fish (chicken, turkey, salmon). Nuts, dairy, and cruciferous vegetables (almonds, broccoli). |
| Inositol | Fruits, beans, grains, and nuts. Supplementation may be necessary for therapeutic benefits. Consult a healthcare provider for tailored advice. |
| Coenzyme Q10 (CoQ10) | Organic meats (liver, kidney, heart). Fatty fish (salmon, mackerel). Poultry and beef. Vegetables (spinach, broccoli). Nuts and seeds (peanuts, sesame seeds). |
| Phytoestrogens | **Lignans:** Found in flaxseeds, sesame seeds, whole grains, nuts, fruits, and vegetables. Flaxseeds are particularly rich, offering an easy addition to smoothies, yoghurts, or salads.<br>**Isoflavones:** Present in soy-based products such as tofu, tempeh, and soy milk, as well as lentils, chickpeas, and red clover.<br>**Coumestans:** Found in legumes like split peas, pinto beans, mung bean sprouts, alfalfa sprouts, and red clover. |

Incorporating these foods into your diet is a simple yet powerful way to nurture your hormonal health. Remember, there's no perfect formula—your journey is as unique as you are. Embrace variety and balance in your choices, and if you ever feel unsure or have specific concerns, reaching out to a trusted healthcare professional can provide the personalised support and reassurance you deserve. You're not alone, and every step you take towards nourishing yourself is a step towards greater vitality and well-being.

# *Chapter Thirty-Two*

## Superfoods and Super Thoughts: Mindful Nutrition in Menopause

"*Take care of your body. It's the only place you have to live in.*"

*Jim Rohn*

You may be wondering about mindful nutrition – surely nutrition and eating are naturally mindful processes You eat the food, and the food gets digested, right?

Well, not quite. Mindful nutrition goes beyond simply eating food – it's about *how* we eat, the state we're in when we eat, and the attention we give to the act of nourishing our bodies. In today's fast-paced world, where meals are often rushed or eaten on autopilot, mindfulness can feel like a foreign concept. However, it plays a critical role in how effectively we digest, absorb, and utilise nutrients.

When we eat in a hurry, under stress, or while distracted, our body shifts into "fight or flight" mode, a state that's designed to help us escape danger, not digest a meal. In this state, our digestive system takes a back seat, reducing its efficiency. Chewing gets skipped, enzymes and stomach acid production can slow down, and the entire process of nutrient absorption becomes compromised. Low stomach acid can impair protein digestion and the absorption of key minerals. It also reduces the production of intrinsic factor, a glycoprotein produced by the stomach lining-that is essential for Vitamin B12 absorption. Intrinsic factor binds to B12 allowing it to be absorbed in the Small Intestine. Without adequate intrinsic factor B12 uptake becomes significantly impaired. On the other hand, when we approach eating mindfully – calm, present, and aware – we engage our parasympathetic nervous system, also known as the "rest and digest" mode. This state allows our body to fully break down food, absorb its nutrients, and send those nutrients to where they're needed most.

Mindful eating bridges the gap between what you eat and how your body benefits from it.

**Are You Eating Mindlessly or Mindfully?**

Take a moment to reflect on your eating habits:

□ I eat on the run or while multitasking

□ I scroll through your phone or watch TV during meals?

□ I sit at a table, pause, and savour each bite?

If your routine aligns with the first two habits, you might be practising mindless eating – consuming food without thought or intention. This can lead to overeating, poor food choices, and reduced nutrient absorption. Mindful eating, on the other hand, is about slowing down, paying attention to your body's hunger and fullness cues, and truly appreciating your meal.

## A guide to practising mindful eating

To help you cultivate the art of mindful eating, here's a step-by-step approach to bring presence and awareness to every meal:

- **Listen to your body:** let your natural hunger and fullness cues – not the clock – guide your eating. This helps prevent overeating and promotes better digestion.

- **Engage your senses:** as you begin eating, focus on the colours, textures, and aromas of your food. Take time to savour each bite, allowing your senses to fully appreciate the meal.

- **Start with a bitter salad:** a small salad of bitter greens like arugula or radicchio can stimulate stomach acid production, enhancing your digestion for the rest of the meal.

- **Pause for three deep breaths:** before your first bite, take three deep breaths. This simple ritual helps shift your body from stress to relaxation mode, setting the stage for better digestion.

- **Chew slowly and thoroughly:** remember, your stomach doesn't have teeth! Chew each bite fully to break down your food and support optimal digestion. This also gives your brain time to recognise when you're full.

- **Take breaks between bites:** put your utensils down between bites and check in with how you're feeling. Are you still hungry, or are you satisfied? This helps prevent overeating.

- **Eliminate distractions:** turn off the TV, put down your phone, and focus entirely on your meal. By being present, you can enjoy your food more and support better digestion.

- **Create a dedicated eating space:** whenever possible, sit down at a table for your meals. A calm, intentional space fosters mindful eating and makes the experience more satisfying.

- **End with gratitude:** reflect on how your meal nourished your body. A moment of gratitude strengthens your connection with food and reinforces a positive mindset.

The saying "we are what we eat" holds truth, but let's take it further: we are also what we absorb. It's not just about eating healthy foods but about giving your body the best chance to break down and absorb those nutrients.

## Superfoods

Superfoods play a vital role in promoting hormonal balance and overall well-being during menopause. Packed with vitamins, minerals, and antioxidants, these foods help detoxify the liver, regulate hormone levels, and combat oxidative stress – key factors in reducing menopause symptoms. Incorporating these nutrient-dense foods into your daily routine can empower you to nourish your body from within and feel more in control of your health:

**Cruciferous vegetables** (broccoli, kale, Brussels sprouts) support liver detoxification in that they contain Indole-3-carbinol (I3C), which aids the liver in breaking down oestrogen into less harmful forms, reducing oestrogen-related health risks. They are also important for hormone metabolism by helping balance oestrogen levels by promoting beneficial metabolic pathways. Roast them, steam them, or toss into soups and salads for easy, delicious meals.

**Berries** (blueberries, strawberries, raspberries) are rich in antioxidants. They combat oxidative stress and reduce inflammation, which can alleviate joint pain and stiffness. They also offer hormonal support by helping the body manage hormonal fluctuations by reducing cellular stress. Add berries to smoothies, oats, or enjoy as a snack for a burst of flavour and health benefits.

**Leafy greens** (spinach, Swiss chard, kale) are all nutrient dense. They provide magnesium, calcium, iron and fibre – essential for hormone production and overall vitality. Blend them into green smoothies, sauté with garlic, or add to soups and stews for an easy nutrient boost.

**Garlic** has an active compound called allicin, which helps reduce inflammation, supports liver detoxification, and processes excess hormones. It also aids heart health by supporting cholesterol-management and blood pressure regulation, protecting against menopause-related cardiovascular risks. Garlic enhances immune resilience, which can be impacted by hormonal changes. Incorporate it into stir-fries, soups, or roasted vegetables for a flavourful, health-boosting addition.

**Turmeric's** active compound, curcumin, is renowned for its potent anti-inflammatory and antioxidant effects. These properties can help support menopausal symptoms like joint pain, stiffness, and inflammation, particularly beneficial for women with arthritis or other age-related discomforts. Curcumin also aids liver function, which is essential for hormone metabolism. A healthy liver helps detoxify excess hormones, promoting better hormonal balance. Add turmeric to soups, curries, or golden milk lattes. These small but consistent dietary changes can offer long-term support for hormonal health.

**Cinnamon** enhances insulin sensitivity, helping stabilise blood sugar levels. This is particularly important during menopause when metabolic changes can increase the risk of insulin resistance and Type 2 diabetes. By preventing blood sugar spikes and crashes, cinnamon can help stabilise mood and energy levels, reducing feelings of fatigue and irritability. Sprinkle cinnamon over overnight oats, blend it into smoothies, or add it to baked goods for both flavour and metabolic benefits.

**Ginger** is celebrated for its ability to reduce inflammation, making it a powerful tool for managing joint pain, muscle aches, and stiffness. It also supports digestion, helping to ease bloating, nausea, and indigestion – common issues during menopause. A healthy digestive system contributes to overall comfort and well-being. Use fresh ginger in stir-fries, soups, or teas, or add powdered ginger to smoothies and baked treats for a warming, health-boosting kick.

By incorporating these nutrient-rich superfoods into your meals, you can take meaningful steps to nurture your hormonal health and overall well-being. With a little creativity in the kitchen, your food becomes a powerful ally in helping you thrive during menopause.

You don't need to transform your diet overnight. Start small—perhaps with a vibrant, nutrient-packed breakfast or by adding an extra portion of colourful vegetables to your plate. Every mindful choice you make strengthens your body, supports your journey, and honours the incredible resilience within you.

Remember, the care you show yourself today is an investment in your future well-being. This is your time to prioritise self-care, embrace the power of nourishing foods, and rediscover your vitality—one intentional meal at a time.

**Food as Self-Care: a case study**

I once spoke to a woman who had spent years caring for everyone else: her children, partner, and parents. When menopause hit, her body demanded attention she hadn't been giving it. She told me, "I realised I had nothing left to give because I had spent so long putting myself last."

She decided to make her meals a form of self-care, preparing nourishing food for herself as if she were caring for a dear friend. She sat down to eat with no distractions, just herself and her plate. Over time, she noticed not only better digestion and more energy but also a sense of peace and connection with her body.

"It wasn't just about the food," she explained. "It was about saying, 'I matter too.'"

Her experience shows that food is more than fuel; it's a way to care for yourself deeply. In a world that demands so much from us, how often do we stop to nourish ourselves with the same love and attention we give to others? Could your next meal be a moment of self-care?

# Chapter Thirty-Three

## Strong Foundations: Bone Health

*"Menopause is a time to rediscover yourself. And what better way to embrace this time than with a strong heart and bones that can carry you through life with strength and resilience?"*

We've come full circle here, back to our old friend oestrogen, which is crucial for maintaining bone health. It supports osteoblasts (the cells responsible for building bone) and regulates osteoclasts (the cells that break down bone tissue). When oestrogen levels drop, this balance is disrupted, causing bone formation to slow and bone breakdown to accelerate. Oestrogen also plays a vital role in the body's ability to absorb calcium from the diet and helps retain calcium within the bones. However, when oestrogen levels fall during menopause, calcium absorption becomes less efficient, and the body begins extracting calcium from the bones to support other critical functions. This depletion exacerbates bone mineral density (BMD) loss.

Research indicates that BMD in areas such as the lumbar spine and hip can decrease by up to 20% in perimenopausal and postmenopausal women compared to premenopausal levels. The first decade post-menopause is a particularly critical window, with women losing up to 10% of their total BMD during this time. Nearly half of all lifetime bone loss occurs in these years, significantly increasing the risk of osteoporosis – a condition characterised by fragile, brittle bones. By the age of eighty, approximately one in four women will develop osteoporosis, highlighting the importance of proactive bone health management.

## Understanding bone health

Osteoporosis, or "porous bones," is a condition marked by reduced bone mass and structural deterioration of bone tissue, resulting in increased fragility and a higher risk of fractures. Although it often presents without symptoms, fractures linked to osteoporosis can be both debilitating and expensive to manage.

Bones are made up of a collagen matrix strengthened by essential minerals such as calcium. Bone health relies on a balance between osteoblasts, which create new bone, and osteoclasts, which break down old bone. Oestrogen plays a key role in maintaining this balance by stimulating osteoblasts and supporting bone remodelling. When this balance is disrupted, bone mass declines, and this can lead to osteoporosis. This condition increases the risk of fractures, particularly in the hip and spine, which can cause pain, disability, and even severe health consequences.

Globally, the condition affects 1 in 3 women over fifty with a total of around 21.2% of the female population experiencing it. In the UK, osteoporosis-related fractures account for over 240,000 incidents annually, costing approximately £1.7 billion. During menopause, women can lose up to 20% of their bone mass, primarily in the hips and spine, significantly increasing fracture risk. Differentiating between osteopenia and osteoporosis is crucial for understanding the progression of bone health issues:

| Osteoporosis | Osteopenia |
|---|---|
| Represents an advanced stage of bone weakening, characterised by compromised structural integrity and heightened fracture risk.<br><br>Hormonal imbalances, particularly the decline in oestrogen and progesterone levels during menopause, significantly contribute to accelerated bone loss, exacerbating the risk of developing osteoporosis. | Serves as an early warning sign, indicating a stage of decreased bone density that precedes osteoporosis.<br><br>Recognising osteopenia underscores the importance of implementing proactive measures to prevent further deterioration of bone density and reduce the risk of progression to osteoporosis. |

## Importance of bone density scans

Bone density scans are essential for evaluating bone health, particularly in individuals at risk of osteoporosis or osteopenia. Typically performed using X-rays or CT technology, these scans measure bone mineral content and density, providing valuable insights into bone strength. The most common method, a DEXA (Dual-Energy X-ray Absorptiometry) scan, is a quick, non-invasive procedure that uses low-dose X-rays to measure Bone Mineral Density (BMD). This test provides detailed information about bone strength and helps identify early signs of bone loss.

BMD is evaluated using a T-score, which compares an individual's BMD to that of a healthy young adult. The categories are as follows:

- **Normal BMD: T-score greater than -1.0**
- **Osteopenia: T-score between -1.0 and -2.5**
- **Osteoporosis: T-score less than -2.5**

The World Health Organisation (WHO) defines osteoporosis as a T-score of ≤ -2.5, with osteopenia characterised by T-scores between -1.0 and -2.5. Recognising these distinctions is essential for early intervention and implementing preventative measures to reduce the risk of fractures and other complications associated with low bone density.

## Nutrition and lifestyle for bone health

Bone health requires a combination of nutrients beyond just calcium. Here are some (familiar!) essentials:

**Calcium** is essential for building and maintaining strong bones as it forms the structural foundation of bone architecture. It plays a critical role in the mineralisation process, where calcium combines with phosphate to create hydroxyapatite crystals, which give bones their hardness and strength. This mineralisation is vital for supporting the skeletal framework, enabling bones to withstand daily stresses and reducing the risk of fractures. Sources include dairy products, sardines (with bones), leafy green vegetables (kale, spinach), broccoli, chia seeds, and figs. However, to be absorbed in the intestines, calcium must be in its ionised form. This absorption process depends heavily on the secretion of gastric acid, which is often reduced in up to 40% of postmenopausal women.

To help boost your gastric acid levels and improve calcium absorption, try incorporating these steps into your routine:

- Take deep, calming breaths before meals: Pause to take three slow, deep breaths before eating. This activates the parasympathetic nervous system, helping your body focus on digestion.

- Chew your food thoroughly: Proper chewing not only aids in breaking down food into smaller, more digestible pieces but also stimulates the production of gastric acid, supporting efficient digestion.

- Start with a bitter salad: Include a small salad with bitter greens like radish, rocket, or dandelion greens before your main meal. These naturally stimulate gastric acid production, preparing your stomach for better nutrient absorption.

**Magnesium** supports bone health by aiding in vitamin D activation, converting it to its active form, and regulating the release of parathyroid hormone (PTH) and calcitonin, both essential for maintaining calcium balance and bone strength. Good dietary sources of magnesium include nuts, seeds, whole grains, and leafy greens.

**Vitamin D** plays a vital role in calcium absorption in the intestines and directly supports bone turnover, with insufficient levels linked to bone loss and fractures. As we age, vitamin D levels decline due to reduced sun exposure, dietary intake, and absorption efficiency. Additionally, vitamin D enhances muscle function, balance, and strength by improving calcium uptake in muscle cells and aiding muscle contraction, thereby reducing the risk of falls.

When combined with calcium, vitamin D provides greater benefits for bone health than either nutrient alone. Key sources include sunlight exposure, fatty fish, and egg yolks.

**Vitamin K** serves as a cofactor in enzymatic processes that convert glutamate residues into gamma-carboxyglutamate residues in vitamin K-dependent proteins. This activation is essential for proteins like calbindin and osteocalcin, which are involved in calcium uptake and bone mineralisation. Proper activation of these proteins ensures calcium and other minerals are deposited in the bones, enhancing bone strength and structure. This regulates calcium use, directing it to bones instead of arteries. Found in leafy greens and fermented foods.

**Proteins** are essential for bone health, providing structural support and actively contributing to bone metabolism and mineralisation. They are vital for producing collagen, a key component of the bone matrix that regulates bone mass and provides the framework for minerals like calcium to bind. Collagen-rich foods, such as bone broth and gelatine, supply the amino acids necessary for collagen synthesis. Maintaining an adequate protein intake through lean meats, poultry, fish, dairy products, legumes, nuts, tofu, and tempeh supports collagen production, promotes bone strength, and enhances overall bone health.

**Copper** plays a vital role in bone metabolism by supporting enzymes like lysyl oxidase, which help integrate collagen and elastin into the organic framework of bones, contributing to their strength and structure. Rich dietary sources include liver, oysters, mushrooms, cashew nuts, sunflower seeds.

**Boron** is essential for the growth and maintenance of healthy bones, aiding in the activation of vitamin D into its active form, 1,25-(OH)2D3, which is crucial for calcium absorption and bone formation. By activating oestrogen, boron also enhances the body's ability to utilise this hormone for bone health, providing additional benefits to bone density and maintenance. Fruit and vegetables are the primary sources of boron.

**Zinc** is crucial for producing metalloenzymes involved in forming the bone matrix. It also inhibits the formation of osteoclast-like cells (which break down bone) and promotes the programmed cell death of mature osteoclasts, supporting overall bone health and maintenance. Rich sources include oysters, beef, pumpkin seeds, chickpeas, and lentils.

A bone-healthy diet includes: **phytonutrient-rich foods** such as berries and leafy greens that provide antioxidants to combat bone-damaging oxidative stress; **Omega-3 fatty acids**, found in fatty fish, flaxseeds, and walnuts, which reduce bone resorption; and **whole foods:** whole grains, legumes, nuts, and seeds. On the other hand, it's best to avoid excess caffeine and alcohol as these can weaken bones by reducing calcium absorption; soda/fizzy drinks, because phosphoric acid may leach calcium from bones; and processed foods that are often lacking in the nutrients necessary for bone health.

## Building bone strength with exercise

Along with diet, weight-bearing exercise is an essential component of maintaining bone health, especially during menopause. As hormonal changes accelerate bone density loss, these exercises stimulate your bones and muscles to work against gravity, strengthening them in the process. Regular practise reduces the risk of osteoporosis and fractures, helping you remain active, resilient, and independent as you age. These exercises target the bones most prone to weakness, such as those in the legs, hips, and spine. By placing stress on the skeletal system, they encourage the formation of new bone tissue, slowing down the loss of bone density that naturally occurs during menopause.

Simple and effective weight-bearing activities include:

**Walking** is one of the easiest, most accessible forms of weight-bearing exercise. It strengthens bones in the legs, hips, and spine, and can seamlessly fit into your daily life, whether it's a brisk walk in the park or a stroll through your neighbourhood.

**Jogging or running:** For those seeking a higher-impact option, jogging or running provides more intense stimulation for bone growth. Focus on gradual progression to avoid injury and ensure your joints stay protected.

**Dancing** is a joyful and effective way to improve bone health. Styles like salsa, ballroom, or even freestyle dancing, engage multiple muscle groups while targeting the hips, legs, and lower body. Plus, it's a mood booster!

**Stair climbing** is a straightforward yet powerful way to strengthen bones in the lower body and back. Take the stairs at home or work or use a stair-climbing machine at the gym to intensify your efforts.

**Strength training:** Resistance exercises with free weights, machines, or resistance bands help build bone density. Moves like squats, lunges, and deadlifts target large muscle groups and encourage bone-building activity.

**Yoga and pilates:** While not traditional weight-bearing exercises, yoga and Pilates strengthen muscles that support bones and enhance balance and posture. Poses such as plank, warrior, and downward dog can contribute to overall bone health and prevent falls.

**Julie's Story**

The timing of menopause significantly impacts long-term bone health. Research highlights that women who experience early menopause face a higher risk of fractures and osteoporosis later in life. This makes supporting bone health early on even more essential.

I know this well, as I went through menopause early, and maintaining strong bones is something I continue to prioritise. Luckily, I've always enjoyed weight training far more than cardio. My attempt at running a half marathon is proof enough! My husband, Craig, and friends, Heather and Arlene, joined me on my first training day for motivation. Heather and Craig took off like gazelles, while Arlene and I exchanged looks of mutual understanding—running was not for us. We walked the rest of the way and left the half-marathon completion to Heather while we happily played the role of her cheer squad.

What this taught me is that finding an activity you enjoy makes all the difference. Taking steps to strengthen your bones doesn't have to feel like a chore—it can be fun and empowering, setting the stage for a healthier, stronger future.

# *Chapter Thirty-Four*

## The Heart of the Matter: Cardiovascular Health

*"Are you ready to give your heart the attention it deserves during menopause?"*

As you journey through menopause, prioritising your heart health becomes more essential than ever. Did you know that, after menopause, a woman's risk of cardiovascular disease (CVD) increases dramatically, even exceeding that of men? Shockingly, CVD is responsible for 55% of postmenopausal deaths among women, compared to 43% in men. This makes heart health one of the most important areas for women to focus on during perimenopause, menopause, and beyond.

Oestrogen – as you might expect by now – plays a vital role in maintaining heart health in women, offering multiple layers of protection. It promotes the health and flexibility of blood vessels, manages cholesterol levels, and reduces inflammation in the cardiovascular system. Pre-menopausal women benefit greatly from oestrogen's heart-protective effects, which help keep the risk of heart disease lower compared to men.

## Cholesterol: understanding its role in health

One of oestrogen's key roles is its impact on cholesterol, which often gets a bad reputation for its association with heart disease. However, cholesterol plays essential functions in the body. It is a type of lipid—a substance that doesn't dissolve in water—that is crucial for overall health. Found in every cell of the body, cholesterol helps build and maintain cell membranes, supports the production of hormones like oestrogen and testosterone, aids in the creation of vitamin D, and assists the liver in producing bile for digesting fats.

Despite its importance, excessive cholesterol is a key factor in the development of plaque formation in arteries, which can lead to cardiovascular issues. Cholesterol cannot travel through the bloodstream alone due to its fat composition. Instead, it binds with proteins to form lipoproteins, which transport cholesterol and other fats throughout the body.

There are three main types of cholesterol-carrying lipoproteins, each with a distinct role:

**High-density lipoproteins (HDL):** Often referred to as "good cholesterol," these play a crucial role in maintaining cardiovascular health. HDL removes excess cholesterol from peripheral tissues and transports it to the liver for excretion through bile—a process known as reverse cholesterol transport. Since the liver is the only organ capable of disposing of cholesterol, HDL's role is essential in preventing cholesterol from accumulating in the bloodstream and arterial walls. This removal process helps to reduce the formation of plaque, which can narrow or block arteries, leading to conditions such as atherosclerosis. By supporting this cholesterol clearance and reducing inflammation in blood vessels, HDL lowers the risk of cardiovascular events.

**Low-density lipoproteins (LDL):** Often referred to as "bad cholesterol," LDL carries cholesterol from the liver to cells for functions like cell membrane repair and hormone production. However, elevated LDL levels can lead to cholesterol accumulation in arteries, increasing the risk of cardiovascular events such as strokes and heart attacks.

**Very-low-density lipoproteins (VLDL):** VLDL transports triglycerides, a major energy source, throughout the body. Triglycerides are either used immediately for energy or stored as fat for future use. Consuming excessive carbohydrates and sugars can increase triglyceride production in the liver, resulting in higher VLDL levels. As VLDL particles deliver triglycerides to cells, they break down into LDL particles, which can accumulate in artery walls, forming plaque over time. This process narrows or blocks arteries, significantly raising the risk of heart attacks, strokes, and other cardiovascular diseases.

## Apolipoproteins and cardiovascular health

Apolipoproteins are the protein components of lipoproteins that enable the efficient transport and metabolism of lipids throughout the body. They play a critical role in lipid homeostasis and cardiovascular health. There are two primary apolipoproteins associated with cholesterol regulation:

**Apolipoprotein A (ApoA)** is primarily associated with high-density lipoproteins (HDL), often referred to as "good cholesterol." It facilitates the removal of excess cholesterol from peripheral tissues and transports it to the liver for excretion via bile. Higher levels of ApoA are associated with a reduced risk of cardiovascular disease due to its role in cholesterol clearance.

**Apolipoprotein B (ApoB)** is the main protein component of low-density lipoproteins (LDL) and very-low-density lipoproteins (VLDL), which carry cholesterol and triglycerides through the bloodstream. It acts as a structural component of these particles, allowing them to function effectively. ApoB is directly linked to LDL particles, which deliver cholesterol to arterial walls. Elevated ApoB levels indicate a higher number of LDL particles, increasing the risk of atherosclerosis and cardiovascular events.

## ApoB: the key to understanding your cardiovascular risk

ApoB levels provide a more accurate measure of cardiovascular risk than LDL cholesterol alone as they reflect the number of cholesterol-carrying particles in the bloodstream. High ApoB levels indicate an increased risk of atherosclerosis and cardiovascular disease, making it a valuable marker for assessing individual cardiovascular health.

## What can raise LDL cholesterol?

- **Genetics:** Some individuals inherit genetic traits from their parents that lead to excessively high cholesterol levels, a condition known as familial hypercholesterolemia.

- **Diet:** A diet high in trans fats—commonly found in fried and processed foods—can significantly raise LDL cholesterol levels. Trans fats, also known as "partially hydrogenated oils," are used in baked goods like pastries, pizza dough, pie crusts, cookies, and crackers.

- **Lifestyle:** Lack of physical activity, smoking, and excessive alcohol consumption are lifestyle factors that contribute to elevated LDL cholesterol levels.

## Understanding the role of inflammation

While cholesterol plays a role in plaque formation, arteriosclerosis (the thickening and loss of elasticity in arterial walls) often begins with oxidative damage to the vascular endothelium. This damage triggers inflammation, causing LDL to deposit in the affected areas, where it becomes oxidised and attracts immune cells. This process leads to cholesterol build-up and plaque formation, which is the body's way of stabilising damaged blood vessels.

Rather than cholesterol itself being the root cause, this process highlights deeper metabolic issues such as insulin resistance, elevated insulin levels, or high triglycerides. Addressing these underlying factors and reducing oxidative stress is crucial for improving cardiovascular health and preventing disease progression.

## Oestrogen and cardiovascular health

Oestrogen plays a crucial role in maintaining healthy cholesterol levels and overall cardiovascular health. Research indicates that oestrogen accounts for approximately 30% of the cardiovascular advantage observed in pre-menopausal women. However, during menopause, as oestrogen levels decline, this protective effect diminishes, triggering physiological changes that increase the risk of heart disease.

## How hormonal changes affect the heart

- **Adverse Changes in Cholesterol Levels:** As oestrogen declines, LDL ("bad cholesterol") levels often rise, while HDL ("good cholesterol") levels may decrease. This imbalance heightens the risk of plaque build-up in arteries, leading to atherosclerosis.

- **Reduced Vasodilation:** Oestrogen promotes vasodilation (the widening of blood vessels) by stimulating nitric oxide production, which relaxes and dilates blood vessels. With lower oestrogen levels, blood vessels become stiffer, reducing blood flow efficiency, and increasing strain on the heart.

These hormonal changes, coupled with shifts in body composition and fat distribution during menopause, contribute to a higher risk of cardiovascular issues such as heart attacks and strokes. However, adopting heart-healthy foods and lifestyle changes can empower you to maintain a strong, resilient heart through this stage of life. Menopause brings many changes, but by making intentional, informed decisions, you can protect your heart and thrive.

## Nutrition for a healthy heart

## Fibre: Your heart's best friend

Fibre, particularly soluble fibre, is the heart's best friend. It plays a powerful role in supporting cardiovascular health. Soluble fibre binds to cholesterol in the digestive system, helping to eliminate it from the body and reducing "bad" LDL cholesterol levels. By incorporating fibre-rich foods into your diet, you can effectively reduce cardiovascular risks while nourishing your body.

The top fibre sources for a healthy heart are: whole grains including oats, barley, and quinoa for their cholesterol-lowering benefits and added nutrients; fruits such as apples, berries; and oranges; and vegetables like broccoli, carrots, and Brussels sprouts.

## Antioxidants: cellular protection

Antioxidants are crucial for heart health, as they boost cardiovascular resilience by protecting cells from damage caused by oxidative stress – a key contributor to heart disease. Foods rich in antioxidants, such as berries, nuts, and cruciferous veg, strengthen your body's defences and help maintain cardiovascular function during menopause.

## Omega-3 fatty acids: anti-inflammatory support

Omega-3 fatty acids are essential for heart health due to their anti-inflammatory properties. These fats – found in fatty fish, such as salmon, mackerel, and sardines (rich in EPA and DHA), and plant sources like flaxseeds and walnuts (rich in ALA) – help reduce inflammation, improve blood vessel function, and lower the risk of cardiovascular issues. The overall effect on blood lipids for marine omega-3 EPA and DHA seems to be protective due to overall improvements in LDL particle size and density as well as reductions in VLDL, TGs, and increases in HDL. Regularly including Omega-3s in your diet can provide metabolic benefits, making them particularly valuable during menopause.

## Magnesium: your heart's hidden ally

Magnesium is the unsung hero of cardiovascular wellness. It supports heart health by helping regulate blood vessel function, heart rhythm, and blood pressure. A magnesium deficiency can increase risks like hypertension and diabetes, which become more prevalent during menopause. Foods like leafy greens, seeds, nuts, and avocados are excellent sources to incorporate into your diet, supporting both heart function and metabolic balance.

## Avoid trans fats

Trans fats are harmful to cardiovascular health as they increase LDL cholesterol levels and contribute to arterial plaque build-up. To limit trans fats:

- Avoid baked goods like pastries, cookies, and crackers made with shortening or partially hydrogenated oils.
- Limit commercially fried foods and fast food.

## Lifestyle strategies for heart health

## Increase physical activity

Regular physical activity is key to maintaining cardiovascular health. Both aerobic and strength-training exercises are beneficial. Research shows that the amount of exercise matters more than the type. Aim for at least 150 minutes of moderate exercise weekly, such as:

- Walking
- Swimming
- Strength training

Consistency is key. Choose activities you enjoy and commit to at least 30 minutes daily.

## Try to stop smoking

Smoking significantly increases cardiovascular risk by lowering HDL cholesterol and raising triglyceride levels. If you smoke, seek support from a healthcare professional. Evidence suggests that you're more likely to quit successfully with expert guidance.

Your heart health is a pillar of long-term vitality. Whether you're exploring hormone replacement therapy (HRT) with your GP or taking a natural approach, your heart's well-being is central to your menopausal care. Heart health is not something to delay. By prioritising it now, you're building a foundation for a strong, healthy heart that will serve you well through menopause and beyond. Remember, with the right knowledge, you hold the power to make meaningful changes that protect your heart and strengthen your future. Let your heart guide you toward a healthier, stronger you.

*Once a day, sit quietly and place your hand over your heart. Send it love and allow yourself to feel the love your heart has for you. It has been beating for you since you were born. Your heart is love. All is well, and you are safe."*

*-Louise Hay*

# Chapter Thirty-Five

## Mastering Metabolic Menopause: Taking Control of Blood Sugar

*Have you ever felt irritable or "hangry" when you don't eat regularly? Do you find yourself needing a mid-afternoon snack just to get through the rest of the day?*

"Hangry" feelings or energy crashes often come down to your blood sugar levels. During menopause, managing blood sugar becomes even more important as it's closely tied to how we feel and function each day. Blood sugar, or glucose, is your body's primary energy source. It fuels your cells and supports vital functions like mood regulation, energy, cognitive clarity, and overall well-being.

Your body thrives when it achieves a stable state called homeostasis, regulating essential chemicals like glucose in your bloodstream. Glucose is your body's primary energy source, fuelling your cells for vital functions such as mood regulation, focus, and overall well-being. However, when glucose levels rise too high, it can damage blood vessels and nerves. To maintain balance, your body relies on an intricate system to keep blood sugar within a healthy range. Two key hormones work together to regulate blood sugar:

**Insulin**: Produced by beta cells in the pancreas, insulin lowers blood sugar after meals by moving glucose from your bloodstream into your cells for energy. Excess glucose is stored as glycogen in the liver and muscles.

**Glucagon:** Secreted by alpha cells in the pancreas, glucagon acts when blood sugar drops between meals or during exercise. It triggers the liver to release stored glucose (glycogenolysis) and stimulates the production of glucose from non-carbohydrate sources (gluconeogenesis).

But when blood sugar isn't balanced, it can strain your adrenal glands, exacerbating hormonal imbalances and potentially causing:

- Energy highs and lows
- Abdominal fat gain
- Sugar or carbohydrate cravings
- Dependence on stimulants like caffeine
- Mood swings
- Trouble concentrating
- Feeling faint

A common example of this is the mid-afternoon energy slump, which often stems from consuming high-sugar foods for lunch. Meals high in quickly absorbed carbohydrates cause blood sugar levels to spike rapidly, prompting an overproduction of insulin to clear the glucose. This leads to a blood sugar crash, leaving you fatigued and craving more sugary foods, perpetuating a "rollercoaster" of highs and lows. Over time, this cycle strains the metabolic system and increases the risk of insulin resistance, type 2 diabetes, and weight gain.

When blood sugar drops, cortisol—a stress hormone essential for maintaining energy balance—is triggered. Cortisol works to raise blood sugar by stimulating gluconeogenesis (the production of glucose from non-carbohydrate sources), reducing insulin sensitivity, and breaking down muscle protein. Chronic stress exacerbates this process, keeping cortisol levels persistently elevated and further disrupting normal blood sugar regulation. This ongoing strain creates a cycle of sharp highs and lows, intensifying the 'blood sugar rollercoaster' and leading to persistent fatigue and intense cravings.

The type of carbohydrates you choose plays a crucial role. Fibre-rich options like whole grains and vegetables release energy gradually, supporting gut health and preventing sharp blood sugar swings. In contrast, refined carbs and sugary foods cause rapid spikes and steep drops, which fuel the cycle of highs and lows. Adding protein and healthy fats to meals helps stabilise blood sugar, reduces cravings, and promotes satiety.

**Assessing Your Blood Sugar Balance**

□ Do you experience energy highs and lows through the day?
□ Do you struggle to lose abdominal fat?
□ Do you crave sugar or carb-heavy foods?
□ Do you rely on caffeine or sugar for energy?
□ Do you feel "hangry" when you're hungry?

*If you've ticked the boxes, blood sugar imbalance could be at play.*

Snacks can help maintain blood sugar levels, especially during the mid-afternoon slump. Choose balanced snacks that contain protein and healthy fats to ensure steady energy levels:

**Balanced Snacks for Blood Sugar Control**

- Carrot sticks, cherry tomatoes, or sliced red peppers with hummus
- One hard-boiled egg
- One oatcake with unsweetened nut butter
- A small pot of Greek yoghurt with chia seeds and blueberries
- Sliced apple with 1 tbsp unsweetened nut butter
- 5-6 almonds or 4-5 Brazil nuts with half an avocado
- Homemade energy bites like Seed and Nut Power Balls or Dark Chocolate Nut Delight *(See snack recipes)*

**DA's Story**

At the beginning of my menopausal journey, I started experiencing erratic blood sugar levels, leading to energy crashes, mood swings, and weight gain. My typical day was a rollercoaster of highs and lows, with cravings for sugary snacks. I struggled to find a balance on my own. My energy levels were unpredictable, and I was constantly tired, which impacted my work and family life. I didn't feel like myself and was desperate. A friend recommended Harmony Health & Menopause, where I met Julie. From our first conversation, I felt hopeful. Julie took the time to understand my symptoms, lifestyle, and eating habits. She explained how hormonal changes during menopause could affect blood sugar balance and provided me with practical advice tailored to my needs.

Julie introduced me to a balanced diet rich in fibre, protein, and healthy fats, which helped stabilise my blood sugar levels. She also recommended regular exercise, like walking at lunchtime and yoga, which was easy to incorporate into my routine and greatly improved my energy levels.
With Julie's support, I learned to manage my cravings and maintain a steady energy level throughout the day. The personalised plan she developed for me was easy to follow and I now feel more in control, my mood has stabilised, and I've regained my confidence and zest for life. I have a better work/life balance which benefits myself and my family. I have more energy to enjoy activities at night and at the weekend such as cycling and walking – and from someone who most nights was in bed the same time as the children, this is a huge positive shift!!

## What is metabolic menopause?

As we age, maintaining metabolic health becomes crucial for long-term vitality. Yet menopause introduces hormonal shifts that make stable blood sugar levels harder to sustain. The term "**metabolic menopause**" refers to the physiological and metabolic changes women experience during this transition, primarily driven by declines in oestrogen and progesterone. It can lead to:

**Increased insulin resistance:** Even women with no prior metabolic concerns may experience rising fasting glucose and insulin levels during perimenopause. Insulin resistance occurs when cells become less responsive to insulin, leaving glucose in the bloodstream instead of being utilised for energy. This not only affects energy levels but also raises the risk of obesity and of Type 2 diabetes, in which the pancreas struggles to keep up, resulting in chronically high blood sugar levels. This form of diabetes often develops in midlife but is increasingly seen in younger adults.

Insulin resistance doesn't just affect blood sugar. It disrupts hormonal systems, including sex and thyroid hormones, leading to broader health impacts. Excess sugar in the bloodstream can damage nerves, blood vessels, and increase abdominal fat – common challenges during menopause.

**Abdominal fat accumulation:** Before menopause, oestrogen directs fat storage to the hips and thighs (gluteo-femoral fat), which is metabolically protective. Post-menopause, fat distribution shifts to the abdominal area, resulting in **visceral fat.** Unlike subcutaneous fat, visceral fat surrounds internal organs and contributes to inflammation, insulin resistance, and cardiovascular risks.

**Loss of muscle mass:** Muscle mass naturally declines with age, but menopause accelerates this loss due to hormonal changes. Since muscle burns more calories than fat, this reduction lowers your basal metabolic rate (BMR), slowing metabolism and making weight management more difficult.

**Lipid and fat metabolism shifts:** Menopause alters how your body processes and stores fats. Common changes include increased levels of triglycerides and LDL cholesterol (the "bad" cholesterol), along with reduced HDL cholesterol (the "good" cholesterol). These shifts heighten the risk of cardiovascular disease.

**Cardiovascular concerns:** The risk of heart disease rises sharply post-menopause, driven by changes in lipid profiles and fat distribution.

### Sleep disruption

Blood sugar imbalance also impacts sleep. Elevated glucose before bed or drops during the night can cause disruptions. Your body may release adrenaline to restore balance, waking you up and affecting your overall rest.

## Liver health and metabolic menopause

Menopause also affects liver health, increasing the risk of Non-Alcoholic Fatty Liver Disease (NAFLD). This condition, characterised by fat build-up in the liver, ranges from simple steatosis (fat accumulation without inflammation) to Non-Alcoholic Steatohepatitis (NASH), which includes liver inflammation and damage. If left unmanaged, NAFLD can progress to more severe liver conditions. Menopause increases NAFLD risk due to:

### Oestrogen decline

Oestrogen plays a protective role in lipid metabolism. Its reduction promotes liver fat storage.

### Insulin resistance

Increased glucose and insulin levels stimulate fat production in the liver.

### Adipokine imbalances

hormonal disruptions in leptin and adiponectin promote inflammation and further fat storage in the liver.

### Gut microbiota dysbiosis

imbalanced gut bacteria allow harmful substances to enter the liver, triggering inflammation.

Processing alcohol adds strain to the liver, so that chronic alcohol consumption can impair liver function and detoxification pathways. If you notice that alcohol triggers hot flushes, consider alternating alcoholic drinks with sparkling water or diluting wine with water to make spritzers.

## Strategies for supporting metabolic health

While metabolic menopause can feel overwhelming, it's important to remember that you're not powerless in this process. With informed choices and proactive steps, you can manage these changes and safeguard your health. There are several proactive steps you can take now:

Prioritise balanced nutrition by:

- Eating complex, low-glycaemic index (GI) carbohydrates.
- Eating protein-rich food
- Eating healthy fats
- Aiming for 5-6 portions of fresh vegetables per day
- Optimising blood sugar balance
- Drinking sufficient water
- Reducing alcohol intake

Considering a Mediterranean diet (MD)which emphasises a variety of plant-based foods, such as vegetables, fruits, legumes, nuts, whole grains, and extra-virgin olive oil as the primary source of fat. Known for its high levels of unsaturated fats and rich bioactive compounds with antioxidant and anti-inflammatory properties, the MD has been shown to lower the risk of cardiovascular disease and metabolic syndrome. Additionally, postmenopausal women who follow the MD report milder menopausal symptoms, improved psychological health, and lower BMI.

There are also several lifestyle modifications you can begin to make:

**Prioritise sleep:** Quality sleep is essential for insulin sensitivity and metabolic balance. Poor sleep increases insulin resistance and raises blood sugar levels. Establishing a consistent sleep schedule and practicing good sleep hygiene are key to optimising metabolic health.

**Manage stress:** Chronic stress elevates cortisol, which can lead to insulin resistance and high blood sugar. Stress-reduction techniques like deep breathing, meditation, yoga, and mindfulness help reduce cortisol levels and support hormonal balance.

**Maintain regular physical activity**

- **Strength training:** builds muscle mass, increases metabolic rate, and improves insulin sensitivity.

- **Aerobic exercise:** walking, swimming, and cycling enhance cardiovascular health and glucose metabolism. Aim for at least 150 minutes per week.

- **Movement after meals:** even a 10–15-minute walk after eating can lower post-meal blood sugar spikes.

| Your Guide to Balanced Nutrition – Cheat Sheet 4 | |
|---|---|
| Complex Carbohydrates (Low GI foods) | Non-starchy vegetables: spinach, kale, tomatoes, carrots, and broccoli.<br>Whole grains: quinoa, barley, bulgur, and whole wheat products.<br>Fruits: raspberries, blackberries, blueberries. |
| Protein | Poultry: chicken, turkey, and duck.<br>Fish: salmon, tuna, trout, and mackerel.<br>Plant-based proteins: tofu, tempeh and legumes such as beans, lentils, chickpeas.<br>Eggs. |
| Healthy Fats | Avocados: rich in monounsaturated fats and fibre<br>Nuts and seeds: almonds, walnuts, chia seeds, flaxseeds, and pumpkin seeds.<br>Olive oil/Extra virgin olive oil.<br>Fatty fish: salmon, sardines, and mackerel. |
| Vegetables | Brussels sprouts, cauliflower, cabbage, broccoli, and kale contain compounds like indole-3-carbinol (I3C) and sulforaphane, which support liver detoxification. |
| Blood sugar regulators | Avoid refined sugars and processed carbohydrates, which cause sharp glucose spikes and crashes.<br>Include soluble fibre (oats, legumes) to slow glucose absorption and insoluble fibre (vegetables, whole grains) for digestive health. |
| Liver health | Antioxidant-rich foods: turmeric, garlic, and green tea protect against oxidative stress.<br>Fibre from vegetables and whole grains to promote detoxification pathways. |
| Mediterranean diet | Fruits, vegetables, nuts, legumes, and olive oil. |
| Good hydration | Drink at least 8 glasses of water a day. |
| Alcohol intake | Consume responsibly – the UK guidelines advise no more than 14 units per week. |

# *Chapter Thirty-Six*

## The Role of Chronic Inflammation

Have you ever wondered if the fatigue, joint discomfort, or mood swings you experience during menopause could be linked to chronic inflammation? While inflammation is a natural response that supports healing after injury or infection, it becomes harmful when prolonged. Chronic inflammation can disrupt hormone balance, drain energy, and increase the risk of age-related conditions such as heart disease, osteoporosis, and cognitive decline.

During menopause, declining oestrogen levels exacerbate chronic inflammation. Oestrogen naturally helps regulate the immune system and dampen inflammatory responses. As oestrogen levels decline, the body becomes more prone to a persistent immune activation, producing an excess of pro-inflammatory proteins, or cytokines, such as IL-1β, IL-6, and TNF-α. These cytokines amplify joint pain, fatigue, and mood swings, while also impairing cognitive function, leaving you feeling sluggish and mentally foggy.

## Oxidative stress: a key driver of inflammation

Oxidative stress occurs when the production of reactive oxygen species (ROS), which you may know of as "free radicals", exceeds the body's capacity to neutralise them using antioxidants. ROS are unstable molecules created as by-products of normal cellular processes, such as energy production in the mitochondria, and external factors like pollution, UV radiation, and smoking. In small amounts, ROS play a role in cell signalling and immune defence. However, when produced in excess, they can damage proteins, lipids, and DNA, accelerating the ageing process and perpetuating chronic inflammation.

## What are antioxidants?

Antioxidants are molecules that neutralise free radicals, preventing oxidative damage and maintaining cellular integrity. The body produces its own antioxidants, known as endogenous antioxidants, including glutathione and superoxide dismutase (SOD). These molecules work by neutralising ROS and converting them into harmless substances like water and oxygen, thereby protecting cells from damage.

In addition to endogenous antioxidants, we rely on dietary sources to bolster our defence system. Foods rich in vitamins, minerals, and bioactive compounds provide exogenous antioxidants that complement the body's natural mechanisms. Key dietary antioxidants include:

Vitamin C: Found in citrus fruits, bell peppers, and strawberries, vitamin C neutralises free radicals and regenerates other antioxidants, like vitamin E.

Vitamin E: Present in nuts, seeds, and avocado, vitamin E protects cell membranes from oxidative damage.

Polyphenols: Compounds in foods like green tea, dark chocolate, and berries that offer strong antioxidant activity.

Selenium: Found in Brazil nuts, fish, and eggs, selenium supports the function of antioxidant enzymes like glutathione peroxidase.

## How chronic inflammation impacts menopausal health

The interplay between oxidative stress and chronic inflammation has far-reaching effects on menopausal symptoms and overall health, including:

- **Joint pain and stiffness:** Inflammation accelerates cartilage breakdown, contributing to joint discomfort and conditions like osteoarthritis.

- **Fatigue and mood swings:** Chronic inflammation impacts energy production and neurotransmitter balance, leading to exhaustion and emotional instability.

- **Cognitive function:** Oxidative stress damages brain cells and disrupts neural communication, contributing to memory problems and brain fog.

- **Bone health:** Inflammation promotes bone resorption, increasing the risk of osteoporosis and fractures.

- **Heart health:** Chronic inflammation damages blood vessels and increases the risk of cardiovascular disease, which becomes a leading concern post-menopause.

## Autoimmunity: when the immune system misfires

Within this chapter on inflammation, its essential to consider autoimmunity as another significant source of chronic inflammation. Autoimmune conditions occur when the immune system, designed to protect the body, mistakenly targets its own healthy cells and tissues. Normally, the immune system defends against harmful invaders like viruses and bacteria by producing antibodies or activating white blood cells (lymphocytes). However, in autoimmune diseases, this protective mechanism malfunctions, leading to persistent immune activation. This can result in tissue damage, disrupted organ function, and a wide range of autoimmune disorders.

## Types of autoimmunity

Autoimmune diseases can be broadly categorised into two types: organ-specific and non-organ-specific:

- **Organ-specific autoimmunity:** The immune response primarily targets a specific organ, leading to its gradual destruction or dysfunction. Examples include:

- **Hashimoto's thyroiditis***:* An autoimmune condition affecting the thyroid gland.

- **Type 1 diabetes***:* The immune system attacks insulin-producing cells in the pancreas.

- **Non-organ-specific autoimmunity:** Immune response targets multiple systems throughout the body. Examples include:

    - **Systemic lupus erythematosus (SLE)**: A chronic inflammatory disease caused by autoantibodies attacking the body's own cells

    - **Rheumatoid arthritis (RA)**: An autoimmune condition targeting the joints and potentially other organs.

Autoimmune conditions like SLE and RA predominantly affect women, and hormonal shifts may exacerbate symptoms. More than 90% of lupus cases and the majority of RA diagnoses occur in women, underscoring the significant impact of hormonal changes on autoimmunity. This unique interplay between hormones, inflammation, and immune response makes understanding these conditions particularly important.

## Systemic Lupus Erythematosus (SLE)

Often referred to simply as *lupus*, SLE is a complex autoimmune condition triggered by a combination of genetic and environmental factors. It occurs when the body's immune system produces autoantibodies that mistakenly attack nuclear and cytoplasmic antigens within healthy cells resulting in widespread inflammation and tissue damage.

## What are the Key Symptoms Associated with SLE?

SLE presents with a wide range of symptoms that can vary greatly from person to person, making it a complex and often challenging condition to manage. Joint and muscle aches and pains, along with extreme fatigue, are the two most commonly reported symptoms. Nearly 90% of lupus patients experiencing fatigue severe enough to significantly impact their quality of life and ability to work.

Other symptoms include:

- Rashes, often in a butterfly shape across the face.
- Light sensitivity, where exposure to sunlight can trigger skin or systemic symptoms.
- Raynaud's phenomenon (discolouration and numbness in the fingers and toes when exposed to cold or stress).
- Hair loss, sometimes in patches or thinning overall.
- Oral or nasal ulcers, which can be painful and persistent.
- Headaches or migraines, which can disrupt daily activities.
- Brain fog, characterised by memory problems and difficulty focusing.
- Anaemia, leading to feelings of weakness and shortness of breath.

These symptoms reflect the systemic nature of lupus, which can affect multiple organs and systems, including the kidneys, heart, and lungs.

## Rheumatoid arthritis (RA)

RA is a chronic autoimmune condition where the immune system mistakenly attacks the lining of the joints, known as the synovium. This leads to inflammation, pain, swelling, and eventually damage to the cartilage and bones within the joint. Over time, RA can cause joint deformities, loss of function, and systemic effects throughout the body.

Common symptoms include:

- Joint pain, stiffness, and swelling, often worse in the morning or after periods of inactivity.

- Fatigue and general sense of malaise.

- Symmetrical joint involvement, meaning it often affects both sides of the body, such as both wrists and knees.

Autoimmunity is more than just a medical term—it's something I've seen up close through my sister-in-law, Jacqueline. Diagnosed with lupus at 17, Jacqueline has never allowed the condition to define her or hold her back. Despite its challenges, she is a dedicated mother to our two nieces, Kelsey and Abbie, and a compassionate Nursery Practitioner, having returned to her studies later in life.

Jacqueline's resilience and determination serve as a constant source of inspiration. Her journey is a powerful reminder of the incredible strength and courage needed to navigate life with an autoimmune condition.

## Supporting health with anti-inflammatory nutrition

The good news? Chronic inflammation can be managed and reduced through the foods you eat. Embracing anti-inflammatory nutrition supports hormone health, restores balance, and boosts energy levels during menopause. Foods naturally rich in essential nutrients and bioactive compounds help lower inflammation. By incorporating these powerful foods into your daily meals, you can promote overall well-being and reduce your risk of inflammation-related health conditions.

| **Examples of Anti-Inflammatory Foods:** | |
|---|---|
| Fruits and Vegetables | Rich in antioxidants – berries, spinach, and kale are excellent choices. |
| Fatty Fish | Salmon, mackerel, and sardines are loaded with Omega-3 fatty acids. |
| Herbs and Spices | Turmeric, ginger, and garlic are natural anti-inflammatory powerhouses. |
| Nuts and Seeds | Flaxseeds, walnuts, and chia seeds provide healthy fats and Omega-3s. |
| Whole Grains | Fibre-rich options like oats, quinoa, and brown rice help reduce inflammation. |
| Healthy Oils | Olive oil and avocado oil offer heart-healthy monounsaturated fats. |

## “Eat the rainbow" for menopausal health

A simple yet powerful way to reduce inflammation and enhance vitality during menopause is by embracing the concept of "eating the rainbow." This approach involves incorporating a variety of colourful fruits and vegetables into your daily meals.

Each vibrant hue represents a unique set of vitamins, minerals, and phytonutrients essential for overall health. By diversifying the colours on your plate, you can ensure your body receives a balanced range of nutrients to support hormonal balance, reduce inflammation, and promote overall well-being.

**The Benefits of Eating the Rainbow**

- Blue/Purple/Black Foods (e.g. aubergines, berries, grapes)
    - *Nutrients:* Flavonoids, polyphenols, anthocyanins
    - *Benefits:* Boost mood, brain health, and memory.
- Red Foods (e.g., tomatoes, pomegranates, red peppers)
    - *Nutrients:* Lycopene, quercetin
    - *Benefits:* Strengthen the immune system and reduce inflammation.
- Orange Foods *(e.g. sweet potatoes, mangoes, oranges)*
    - *Nutrients:* Beta-carotene, carotenoids
    - *Benefits:* Promote glowing skin, healthy vision, and immune function.
- Yellow Foods (e.g. bananas, lemons, pineapples)
    - *Nutrients:* Vitamin C, potassium
    - *Benefits:* Strengthen cellular health and immune defences.
- Green Foods (e.g. broccoli, Brussels sprouts, spinach)
    - *Nutrients:* Isothiocyanates, vitamin K
    - *Benefits:* Support detoxification, protect DNA, and improve cardiovascular health.
- White/Brown Foods (e.g. mushrooms, onions, garlic)
    - *Nutrients:* Probiotics, lignans
    - *Benefits:* Enhance gut health and strengthen immunity.

## Beware of ultra-processed foods

While whole, nutrient-dense foods nourish your body, ultra-processed foods do the opposite. Foods high in refined sugars, unhealthy fats, and artificial additives can disrupt hormonal balance, contribute to inflammation, trigger systemic inflammation, and increase the risk of chronic conditions. Diets high in ultra-processed foods are linked to a 28% increased risk of cardiovascular disease. By minimising ultra-processed foods and choosing whole, nourishing alternatives, you actively reduce inflammation and protect your long-term healing.

Chronic inflammation during menopause can feel overwhelming, affecting not just your body but also your sense of well-being. But this chapter is here to remind you that you are not alone. There is simple yet meaningful steps you can take to support yourself through this transition. Every small change—whether it's adding more vibrant, nutrient-rich foods to your meals or adopting anti-inflammatory habits like prioritising quality sleep, staying hydrated, and reducing processed foods—can help you feel more balanced and in control.

This is your opportunity to care for yourself in a way that feels truly nourishing and compassionate. Food is not just fuel; it's a way to nurture your body, calm inflammation, and build resilience.

As Heather Morgan wisely said:

*"Every time you eat or drink, you are either feeding disease or fighting it."*

With every mindful choice, you are honouring your body's needs and laying the foundation for a healthier, more vibrant future. You deserve that care.

# *Chapter Thirty-Seven*

## The Intricate Dance: The Relationship Between Stress and Hormones

*"Have you ever noticed that when you're stressed, your menopause symptoms seem to worsen? That's no coincidence. Stress is one of the biggest disruptors of hormonal balance."*

Think back to a recent moment when you felt overwhelmed. Maybe it was a day when everything seemed to pile on, or perhaps a sudden situation that left you feeling out of control. What physical or emotional changes did you notice? Did your heart start racing, as though you couldn't quite catch your breath? Did your thoughts scatter, jumping from one worry to the next? Perhaps your shoulders felt tense, your jaw clenched, or your body felt weighed down by fatigue.

These responses aren't just in your mind. They are your body's way of signalling that it's under stress. Your heart might beat faster because your body thinks you need extra energy to escape a threat, even if that "threat" is a work deadline or a difficult conversation. Your scattered thoughts are part of a survival mechanism, scanning for potential danger. And that physical tension? It's your body bracing for action, ready to protect you.

For many, stress manifests differently. Some experience the classic "fight or flight" response, feeling edgy, anxious, or restless. Others, like me, experience the "freeze" response, where even the smallest stressors feel monumental, leaving you immobilised.

Stress means different things to different people and can vary depending on the situation. The first and most generic definition of stress was that proposed by Hans Selye, a pioneering scientist, who extensively studied stress and its effects on the body. He defined stress as: "the nonspecific response of the body to any demand". Selye's research showed that, while stress is a natural and adaptive response, chronic or prolonged stress can harm physical and mental health. His work highlighted the importance of understanding how stress affects the body and emphasised the need for effective stress management to support overall well-being.

## Your journey/my journey: personalising stress relief

Stress has been a constant presence in my life and learning how to manage it has been both a deeply personal and transformative journey. Over the years, I've explored various techniques, but three practices have truly stood out, reshaping how I navigate and cope with stress.

**Reiki** has provided me with a profound sense of calm and grounding, helping me step out of my busy mind and reconnect with my body. It's a practice that offers not only support but also balance and peace, creating a space to recharge and recentre.

**Silent counselling,** guided by the incredible Louise at Maiya's Light, opened the door to releasing deeply held stress and self-doubt I hadn't even realised I was carrying. Louise's compassionate approach made the experience profoundly freeing and transformative, allowing me to process emotions I had long suppressed.

Finally, writing became an unexpected lifeline. Under the expert guidance of my coach, Sarah, I discovered that writing is more than just putting words on a page—it's about uncovering, and processing emotions buried deep within. Writing has given me a safe space to let go, gain clarity, and rediscover my voice, helping me better understand myself in the process.

These three tools have been instrumental in my journey, each offering a unique way to relieve stress and restore balance. I share more about how they've helped me, along with practical tips, at the end of this chapter.

However, stress management isn't one-size-fits-all. My friends Arlene and Heather are perfect examples of this. Arlene finds peace in creating essential oil blends that help her switch off from her busy life. Heather, on the other hand, turns to road cycling, where speed and distance allow her to escape into the rhythm of movement. Personally, cycling would be anything but calming for me – I tried it once, and the stress of ringing the bell and staying balanced was enough to convince me to leave the roads to Heather! The point is this: what works for one person might not work for another. The key is to find what helps you reconnect with yourself. Whether it's through movement, creativity, mindfulness, or connection with loved ones, the goal is the same – to create moments of peace that allow you to recharge and reset. When the three of us come together, our stress seems to melt away. We laugh, share, and simply enjoy each other's company. It's a reminder that sometimes the best stress relief isn't a practice or a tool, it's the people who make you feel safe and supported.

## Understanding stress: what it is and how it affects you

Stress isn't just in your mind; it's also in your body. It affects how you think, feel, and even how your body functions. But the good news is that stress doesn't have to control your life. Let's dive deeper into what's happening behind the scenes in your body and explore actionable ways to manage stress and find your inner calm.

Stress can be short-term (acute) or long-term (chronic). Acute stress helps you react quickly to threats, but chronic stress can harm physical and mental health.

| Acute Stress | Chronic Stress |
|---|---|
| Short-term and triggered by immediate challenges like deadlines or traffic.<br>Activates the "fight or flight" response, increasing heart rate, blood pressure, and stress hormones like adrenaline and cortisol.<br>Once the challenge is over, the body returns to normal. | Long-term and caused by ongoing problems like financial struggles, work pressure, or relationship issues.<br>Leads to constant release of cortisol, which can harm the body over time.<br>Associated with sleep problems, weakened immunity, digestive issues, and mental health conditions like anxiety and depression. |

Your nervous system is like the control centre for your body's stress response. It's responsible for how you react to challenges, whether they're physical, emotional, or psychological. The autonomic nervous system (ANS), which governs involuntary functions like breathing and heart rate, has two key branches:

**Sympathetic Nervous System (SNS):** the "fight or flight" system, activated when you perceive a threat. It releases stress hormones like adrenaline and cortisol, increasing your heart rate, raising blood sugar, and redirecting energy to help you respond to the challenge.

**Parasympathetic Nervous System (PNS)**: the "rest and digest" system helps your body recover after the threat has passed. It slows your heart rate, supports digestion, and promotes relaxation and repair.

When these systems are balanced, your body functions optimally. But chronic stress can tip the balance too far toward the SNS, keeping your body in a constant state of alert. Over time, this wears down your physical and emotional resilience.

## Understanding allostatic load

Allostatic load refers to the cumulative impact of chronic stress and adverse life experiences on the body. When the demands of daily life exceed our ability to cope effectively, the body's stress response systems remain activated for prolonged periods. This repeated exposure to stress without adequate recovery leads to allostatic overload, increasing the risk of long-term health consequences.

First introduced by neuroendocrinologist Bruce McEwen and psychological psychologist Eliot Stellar in 1993, allostatic load describes how the body's ability to adapt to stress—a process known as allostasis—comes at a physiological cost. While short-term stress responses, such as the fight-or-flight reaction, are essential for survival, chronic activation of stress hormones like cortisol and catecholamines can lead to widespread effects on metabolic, cardiovascular, and immune function.

## What is cortisol?

Cortisol is the body's primary stress hormone, produced by the adrenal glands, and it plays a critical role in regulating the body's response to stress. It is essential for survival, enabling us to react to challenges by mobilising energy, enhancing focus, and activating the "fight or flight" response.

Under normal conditions, cortisol follows a natural rhythm throughout the day. Levels peak in the morning to wake you up and gradually decline in the evening to help you unwind and sleep. This morning surge is known as the Cortisol Awakening Response (CAR)—your body's natural "wake-up call." Within the first hour of waking, cortisol levels rise significantly—by as much as 50–60%. This rise is triggered by two key factors:

- **Circadian rhythm:** The hypothalamic–pituitary–adrenal (HPA) axis releases hormones in alignment with your internal body clock.

- **Daylight exposure:** Light activates the suprachiasmatic nucleus in your brain, which stimulates cortisol production.

The CAR is essential for preparing your body for the day ahead. It mobilises energy, primes your heart and muscles for action, and sharpens mental focus, ensuring you feel alert and energised.

However, the CAR is influenced by more than just sleep and light exposure. Chronic stress, anxiety, depression, and even past trauma can alter how this response functions. Understanding your CAR can provide valuable insights into how well your body manages stress and adapts to daily challenges.

## Long-term impacts of elevated cortisol

In short-term (acute) stress, cortisol acts protectively, allowing the body to adapt and recover. However, when stress becomes chronic, cortisol levels remain elevated, shifting its effects from protective to harmful. Chronic stress keeps the body in a heightened state of alert, leading to overproduction of cortisol. This disrupts metabolic processes and strains the adrenal glands. Prolonged cortisol elevation can have wide-ranging health consequences, including:

**Increased abdominal fat:** cortisol encourages fat accumulation around the abdomen, which raises the risk of cardiovascular disease.

**Elevated blood pressure:** persistently high cortisol levels can lead to hypertension, increasing the risk of heart disease.

**Muscle wasting and protein breakdown:** cortisol breaks down proteins, including collagen, leading to muscle loss and weakened connective tissues.

**Bone loss:** chronic stress can demineralise bones, heightening the risk of osteoporosis.

**Immune suppression:** elevated cortisol weakens the immune system, leaving the body more vulnerable to infections.

**Gut health and inflammation:** cortisol increases intestinal permeability ("leaky gut"), allowing toxins and bacteria to enter the bloodstream, potentially triggering inflammation and digestive issues. It also disrupts the gut microbiome, further impairing digestion and overall health.

**Thyroid dysfunction:** chronic stress impacts the thyroid gland, which regulates metabolism. Cortisol can interfere with thyroid hormone conversion, causing fatigue, weight fluctuation, temperature sensitivity, appetite changes. These disruptions can lead to hypothyroidism, hyperthyroidism, or insulin resistance, increasing the risk of metabolic conditions such as diabetes.

## The Hypothalamic-Pituitary-Adrenal (HPA) axis: your body's stress regulator

The HPA axis is a vital neuroendocrine pathway composed of three core structures: the paraventricular nucleus in the hypothalamus, the anterior pituitary gland, and the adrenal gland. This system works together to help the body manage and adapt to stress and is a central regulator of the stress response. When stress is detected, the hypothalamus releases corticotropin-releasing hormone (CRH), which stimulates the pituitary gland to secrete adrenocorticotropic hormone (ACTH). ACTH then triggers the adrenal glands to produce cortisol, alongside the other stress hormones adrenaline and noradrenaline.

**Adrenaline (Epinephrine)**

A hormone that prepares the body for "fight or flight" during stress by increasing heart rate, blood flow to muscles, and energy availability.

**Noradrenaline (Norepinephrine)**
Works alongside adrenaline to manage stress response by constricting blood vessels and maintaining blood pressure.

While this system is crucial for managing acute stress, chronic activation overburdens the HPA axis, leading to "adrenal fatigue" and long-term disruptions in physical and emotional resilience.

## DHEA: the body's stress buffer

Dehydroepiandrosterone (DHEA), often called the "youth hormone," is produced in the adrenal glands and plays a protective role against the harmful effects of prolonged cortisol elevation. While cortisol is a catabolic hormone (i.e. it breaks down tissues and suppresses immune function), DHEA is anabolic (i.e. it promotes tissue repair, immune support, and stress resilience, helping to buffer the body from cortisol's damaging effects and fostering a balanced and resilient stress response).

DHEA also serves as a precursor for oestrogen and testosterone, contributing to hormonal balance, cognitive function, and overall well-being. However, during periods of prolonged stress, cortisol levels can remain high while DHEA production declines, leading to an imbalance that amplifies cortisol's harmful effects and undermines the body's ability to recover.

## Cortisol and hormonal health: the menopause connection

Stress and hormonal health are deeply interconnected, especially during menopause. As oestrogen and progesterone levels fluctuate, the body becomes more sensitive to stress. Chronic stress not only intensifies these hormonal changes but can also worsen menopause symptoms such as hot flushes, fatigue, and mood swings.

Cortisol is produced in the adrenal glands from pregnenolone—a precursor for many hormones, including progesterone. Think of pregnenolone as a key ingredient in the body's biochemical assembly line. Under stress, the body prioritises converting pregnenolone into cortisol to handle perceived threats, rather than into progesterone to support reproductive health. This process, often called "cortisol stealing," occurs because, during stress, the body's focus shifts to survival, temporarily side-lining non-essential functions like reproduction.

While this stress response is a remarkable survival mechanism, it can pose significant challenges during menopause. As ovarian production of oestrogen and progesterone declines, the adrenal glands are meant to step in and compensate. However, if the adrenal glands are already overburdened by chronic stress and excessive cortisol production, they may struggle to meet this demand. The result? Progesterone levels drop even further, amplifying symptoms such as anxiety, poor sleep, and irritability—symptoms that are already heightened during menopause.

There are several strategies we can employ to support healthy cortisol levels and reduce allostatic load. It will come as no surprise that diet plays a significant role in how your body manages and responds to stress. Nutrient-dense foods can help stabilise your mood, support your adrenal glands, and reduce the physical effects of stress. We talked comprehensively about nutrition in earlier chapters (see the "Cheat Sheets"), so just to summarise:

**Stable blood sugar levels** are crucial. Avoid sugary snacks, reduce caffeine intake, and choose regular, balanced meals with high-quality proteins to nourish your stress glands and help reduce stress responses.

**Boost your B vitamin intake** because stress depletes it, especially B5 and B6, which are involved in adrenal hormone synthesis. Eat leafy greens, eggs, mushrooms, lentils, black beans, and chickpeas to support adrenal health and well-being.

**Vitamin C** is highly concentrated in the adrenal glands, and again, is quickly depleted under stress, as it protects the adrenals from free radical damage. Nutritional sources include red peppers, guava, dark leafy greens, kiwi, strawberries, tomatoes, and broccoli.

**Zinc** supports stress resilience and immune function. Good sources include oysters, pumpkin seeds, sunflower seeds, and grass-fed meats.

**Magnesium** is involved in over 300 enzymatic reactions, including those that regulate the stress response. It also aids in muscle relaxation and sleep quality. Include magnesium-rich foods in your diet, like leafy greens, seeds, beans, and dark chocolate.

**Omega-3 fatty acids** found in fatty fish, flaxseeds, and walnuts. Omega-3 fatty acids have anti-inflammatory properties that may help reduce the effects of stress on the body. They support cognitive function, mood stability, and cardiovascular health, especially during times of heightened stress.

## Beyond nutrition

The good news is that, even beyond nutrition, *you* have further power to manage stress and lessen its impact on your hormonal health. There is no one-size-fits-all solution, and that's okay. What matters most is discovering practical strategies that align with your unique needs, integrate naturally into your daily life, and nurture both your body and mind.

Take your time, explore what resonates with you, and trust that every small step is a meaningful act of self-care. When needed, seeking support from healthcare or mental health professionals can be invaluable in reducing stress and safeguarding your long-term well-being.

Let's take a closer look at some simple yet powerful ways to help manage stress and restore balance.

## Mindful movement

**Yoga** combines mindful movement, breathwork, and meditation, making it a holistic approach to stress relief. It stretches tight muscles, releases tension, and encourages relaxation.

**Gentle walking** is one of the simplest yet most effective forms of stress relief. A mindful walk outdoors allows you to connect with nature, clear your head, and release pent-up tension. Pay attention to the rhythm of your steps, the sounds around you, and the feeling of the ground beneath your feet. This brings a meditative quality to your walk.

**Dancing** is a joyful way to move your body while reducing stress. Whether it's a formal dance class or simply moving to your favourite playlist in your living room, dancing releases tension and uplifts your mood.

## Meditation: cultivating inner calm

**Mindfulness** involves focusing on the present moment without judgment. It can be as simple as paying attention to your breath, your surroundings, or the taste of your food. Set aside 5-10 minutes each day to sit quietly and observe your thoughts without trying to change them.

**Meditation** fosters deep relaxation and mental clarity. Regular practice has been shown to lower cortisol levels, improve mood, and enhance overall well-being. Sit comfortably in a quiet space. Focus on your breath or repeat a calming word or mantra, such as "peace" or "calm." Start with just 5 minutes a day and gradually increase the duration.

**Gratitude practice** is a method of reflecting on what you're grateful for shifts your focus away from stressors and toward positive aspects of your life. Try writing down three things you're thankful for each day in a journal.

*"Meditation is not a way of making your mind quiet. It's a way of entering into the quiet that is already there."*

*-Deepak Chopra*

## Breathing techniques

Breathing is something we do every moment, yet we often take it for granted.

| | | |
|---|---|---|
| **Conscious Breathing** | Tuning into your breath and using it as a tool to calm your mind and body. | Sit in a comfortable position with your feet grounded. Inhale deeply through your nose for a count of four, feeling your belly rise. Hold your breath for four counts, then exhale slowly for four counts. Repeat for several minutes. |
| **Box Breathing** | Used by athletes, military personnel, and those in high-stress roles to improve focus and reduce anxiety.<br>Particularly helpful before bed or during moments of heightened stress. | Visualise drawing a square as you breathe.<br>Inhale through your nose for four counts, tracing one side of the square.<br>Hold your breath for four counts, tracing the second side.<br>Exhale through your mouth for four counts, tracing the third side.<br>Hold your breath for four counts, tracing the final side. |
| **4-7-8 Breathing** | The "relaxing breath" that helps activate the parasympathetic nervous system and quiet the mind.<br>Especially helpful for winding down before sleep. | Inhale deeply through your nose for four counts.<br>Hold your breath for seven counts, then exhale slowly and fully through your mouth for eight counts.<br>Repeat for four to six cycles. |

## Holistic therapies

**Reiki** is a gentle and restorative energy healing practice designed to bring balance to both the body and mind. By addressing blocked or stagnant energy, Reiki promotes relaxation, reduces stress, and fosters a sense of inner harmony. Practicing Reiki has been deeply fulfilling for me, and I'm honoured to volunteer with Reiki-Medic Care, a service providing free distance Reiki to NHS staff. It's a privilege to hold space for my clients and witness the transformative, positive effects it can bring to their lives. Below, you'll find GS's inspiring story, which illustrates how Reiki has supported her on her journey.

**Reflexology** involves applying pressure to specific points on the feet or hands that correspond to different areas of the body. This therapy helps activate the parasympathetic nervous system, reduce cortisol levels, and promote overall well-being. My friend Jane, who I met during our studies in Naturopathic Nutrition and who has since become one of my closest friends, is a highly skilled and qualified Reflexologist. Her expertise and insights are truly remarkable, far exceeding my own. I am truly grateful for her valuable contribution below. Thank you, Jane, for sharing your knowledge so beautifully!

**Silent counselling** is a transformative energy release technique that I first experienced under the gentle guidance of Louise at Maiya's Light. By addressing tension stored in the body, Silent Counselling promotes both emotional and physical well-being, revealing just how much unacknowledged stress can affect our overall health and vitality. During our session, Louise's warmth, kindness, and expertise created a safe and deeply personal experience. As a Reiki Master Teacher and a practitioner of various other modalities, she has an incredible ability to make you feel seen, understood, and supported. At the end of this chapter, you'll find some heartfelt words from Louise, where she shares her "why" and the passion behind her incredible work. Her story is a testament to the power of healing and the impact of releasing what no longer serves us.

**Writing:** Under the guidance of my wonderful coach, Sarah, I've come to realise that writing isn't just about putting words on a page—it's a deeply personal process of uncovering emotions and thoughts I'd buried for years. Writing gives voice to what's been unsaid, helps process unresolved feelings, and allows us to release what no longer serves us. It's a path toward clarity, healing, and empowerment.

Through Sarah's writing course, I began to find my voice. On the very first day, when she gave us a prompt and just ten minutes to write a story, I felt paralysed by fear—my mind went blank, and I didn't know where to start. But then I began writing, and, to my surprise, I couldn't stop. It was as though a floodgate had opened, and the words just poured out. That moment was transformative—it marked the start of something entirely new for me. After the course, I continued working with Sarah as my writing coach, and she became so much more than just a mentor. She has been a constant source of encouragement and inspiration, offering guidance and support every step of the way. I feel incredibly fortunate to have her by my side on this journey.

If the idea of writing feels overwhelming, don't worry—there are simple, gentle ways to begin. Start small. Journaling can be a great first step, especially at the end of the day. Try jotting down your thoughts, particularly anything that's been weighing on your mind or keeping you from sleeping. Writing can help process emotions, recognise stress triggers, and bring clarity to your thoughts.

Consider asking yourself:

- What is causing me stress right now, and how can I approach it differently?
- What small victories have I achieved today?
- What brings me peace, and how can I invite more of it into my life?

In the morning, take a moment to write down one or two things you're grateful for. These small steps can help you tap into the therapeutic power of writing, guiding you on a journey of self-discovery and healing.

Sarah has written a truly beautiful and heartfelt piece about how nature and writing have supported her during her menopause journey, which I'm sharing with you below. Her words so perfectly capture the way writing can help us process, reflect, and make sense of emotions that often go unspoken. Let's take a moment to celebrate the power of shared experiences and the strength that comes from opening up about life's transitions. Thank you, Sarah, for your wisdom and inspiration!

## Final thoughts

Chronic stress can take a significant toll on both your body and mind, especially during menopause. But here's the empowering truth: you have the power to regain control. By incorporating practices like mindfulness, regular movement, and prioritising quality sleep, you can restore balance and feel more at ease. And remember, seeking support from healthcare or mental health professionals is a sign of strength—an important step toward nurturing your long-term health.

As Wayne Dyer wisely said:

*"Peace is the result of retraining your mind to process life as it is, rather than as you think it should be."*

Reflect on this quote and consider the power you hold within yourself to create calm and resilience, especially during challenging times. Menopause, with all its changes, may feel overwhelming at moments, but it also offers an opportunity to embrace who you are becoming. By practicing self-compassion, letting go of unrealistic expectations, and accepting the present moment, you can begin to heal from within.

Now, take a deep breath. What would it feel like to stop fighting against the changes and simply allow yourself the peace of being, as you are? You deserve to experience the calm and clarity that comes from embracing this moment, just as it is. And most importantly, you deserve to feel your best.

**GS's Story**

*Julie has such a soothing presence that I felt relaxed right away. At my Reiki session, I was grieving the loss of my father, who I loved very much, yet Julie made me feel quite at ease and supported. I came away from my Reiki appointment with a deeper sense of calm and slept that night better than I had done in a very long time.*

**Silent Counselling by Louise Anderson**

*"Silent Counselling's rapid energy release exercises are designed to help us first let go of stress, worry, self-doubt, and anxiety, providing a foundation for emotional balance and well-being."*

My own past debilitating experience with stress and anxiety, and learning how to overcome it, is what drives me to help others not only to release stress and anxiety but also to understand how to regain control and develop tools to manage it effectively in their lives. I can completely relate to the hormonal changes and the increasing issues like anxiety and self-doubt. I am so grateful to be able to use these techniques for myself as well, allowing me to release these feelings.

Louise Anderson, BA
Maiya's Light
Reiki Master Teacher/Silent Counselling/Crystal Reflexology/
Angel Healing, Meditation/ Mindfulness

**Nature, Writing, and Menopause by Sarah Clayton**

Nature has always been my sanctuary, but during menopause, it has become something more, a guide through the upheaval and uncertainty. Menopause isn't just a physical storm; it's an emotional and psychological reshaping that can leave you questioning who you are. For me, it shattered the identity I'd built, leaving me feeling raw and exposed. For a long time, I didn't know who I was as a writer, or even a human being. But stepping outside, into the woods or beside a restless sea, I found reflections of my own struggles. The trees in autumn don't cling to their leaves, they let go, trusting the cycle to bring something new. Nature reminds me that change, no matter how disorienting, is part of life's rhythm.

Writing is the bridge between my inner turmoil and the steady wisdom of the natural world. When my mind is foggy or restless, putting pen to paper feels like grounding myself, like planting roots in uncertain soil. I write through the sleepless nights, the sudden tears, and the quiet rage that sometimes bubbles up. In those moments, writing isn't just a creative outlet, it is a lifeline. It gives me space to process the losses and rediscover my voice in the chaos. Nature teaches me to see the beauty in transitions, and writing allows me to honour them. Together, they remind me that this wild, unpredictable phase is just another part of the cycle, messy, yes, but also brimming with potential for growth and transformation. Through writing, I've learned to lean into the wildness of menopause, trusting that even in this untamed phase, there's power, renewal, and a new kind of creativity waiting to emerge.

Sarah Clayton MA (HONS), MLitt
Writing Mentor & Creativity Coach
Write Wild Books
https://www.writewildbooks.com

**Reflexology For Menopause by Jane Kerridge**

I first began to have regular reflexology sessions in my late 40's when menopausal symptoms - for me, the most impactful being hot flushes - started to manifest. I found the whole experience of deep relaxation and calm was so positive for my wellbeing. I had monthly treatments, and I noticed such a positive difference in how I experienced my menopause journey. It inspired me to study reflexology myself so that I could help others.

Reflexology is an ancient holistic therapy. Based on the principle that areas of the feet (or hands and even ears) map via the nervous system to corresponding parts of the body, the application of pressure to these reflex points stimulates the movement of energy along the nerve channels, inducing a surge of energy that activates our parasympathetic nervous system, leaving us in a deep state of relaxation and allowing our bodies to balance – it promotes homeostasis in the whole body.

It can support a woman's wellbeing at this important time of transition on many levels. Certain reflex points correspond to key glands involved in hormone regulation - hypothalamus, pituitary, pineal, thyroid and ovaries. By stimulating these points, the aim is to support hormonal balance, potentially with a resultant easing of symptoms. One research study demonstrated that foot reflexology was effective in reducing hot flushes.

Chronic stress (and therefore chronically elevated cortisol levels) can heighten the severity of menopausal symptoms. At this time, the adrenal glands will produce cortisol and adrenaline at the expense of oestrogen and progesterone. Elevated cortisol levels are associated with insulin resistance. Stimulating the reflex points associated with the brain, spinal cord, and nerve bundles can promote calm and balance, thereby countering the stress response.

It is very common to experience disrupted sleep patterns during our menopausal years, which has such a huge impact on our wellbeing, both mentally and physically. By inducing a deeply relaxed state, Reflexology can improve our sleep and alleviate insomnia.

The benefits of reflexology in the menopause further extend to supporting anxiety, fatigue and low mood – even reducing depression in women at this time.

As with many complementary therapies, formal research doesn't always reflect the benefits that we know can happen in practice. It is such an accessible non-invasive therapy with very few contraindications, and is generally safe for all. It should be considered by everyone navigating this often challenging (but ultimately liberating) time.

Jane Kerridge
Bsc(Hons), DipCNM, mBANT, rCNHC, ITEC, mFHT
www.thebalancedhealthclinic.com
Nutritional Therapy | Holistic Massage | Reflexology

# *Chapter Thirty-Eight*

## Self-Care and Stress Resilience: Building Your Toolkit

*"With menopause comes a surge of creativity and energy. It's the perfect time to start a business, write that book, or pursue that long-held dream."*

*Trinny Woodall*

One of the most powerful things you can do for your nervous system during menopause is to create a self-care toolkit – a personalised collection of practices and habits to help you manage stress, find calm, and support your body through this transformative time.

As mentioned in Chapter 5, many women are part of the "sandwich generation" juggling children, aging parents and careers as well as navigating fluctuating hormones. These demands can feel overwhelming, and the instinct to prioritise others can often leave your own needs at the bottom of the list. But here's the truth: self-care isn't a luxury, it's a necessity. Without investing time and energy in yourself, it becomes harder to manage stress, maintain your energy, and respond to life's challenges. You cannot pour from an empty cup.

Self-care is about showing yourself the same love and compassion that you so readily offer to others. It's an act of empowerment, a way to take charge of your health and well-being. As the World Health Organisation reminds us, prioritising self-care during menopause is vital for maintaining overall health.

Your self-care toolkit is a gift you give to yourself, a way to reclaim balance, energy, and joy. It's not about grand gestures or perfection, it's about small, meaningful steps that remind you: *you matter too*. When you dedicate time to self-care, you allow your body to function optimally. Engaging in relaxation practices like deep breathing and mindfulness helps regulate stress hormones such as cortisol, which can worsen menopausal symptoms. The ripple effects of consistent self-care include improved hormone regulation, balanced metabolism, strengthened immunity, and greater emotional well-being.

For me, recognising the power of self-care was transformative. I realised how stress had amplified my symptoms. I was constantly in a heightened state of worry, either about the future or unresolved events from the past. When perimenopause hit, everything I had ignored surfaced all at once. But it was through small, intentional acts of self-care – like mindfulness, nurturing my body, and finding time for relaxation – that I began to regain my balance. If it worked for me, it could work for you too. Start by asking yourself, when did you last prioritise your own self-care?

| **Ten ways to weave self-care into your daily life: Even when time feels limited** | |
|---|---|
| Take Time for Joy | Make space every day for one activity that brings you happiness and calm, whether it's reading, gardening, or simply sitting in quiet reflection. |
| Practice Mindful Moments | Integrate short mindfulness breaks into your day. Deep breathing, meditation, or a short walk can help reset your mind and reduce stress. |
| Move Gently | Find a form of exercise that feels nurturing rather than exhausting. Yoga, Pilates, or even stretching can ease tension while supporting flexibility and strength. |
| Prioritise Sleep | Create a bedtime routine that supports restful sleep. Diminish screen time before bed, set a comfortable environment, and wind down with calming activities like reading or meditation. |
| Nourish Your Body | Eat wisely to support your hormonal health. Include Omega-3-rich foods, essential nutrients, and plenty of water to stay hydrated and balanced. |
| Indulge in Creative Outlets | Whether painting, journaling, or playing an instrument, creativity can soothe the mind and rekindle joy. |
| Bath Bliss | Elevate your bath time with Epsom salts and essential oils like lavender for a calming, spa-like retreat. |
| Connect with Loved Ones | Share your feelings with friends and family. Emotional support and laughter are powerful tools for combating stress and improving mood. |
| Embrace Nature | Spend time outdoors, whether on a quiet walk or an adventurous hike. Nature has a remarkable ability to calm the mind and rejuvenate the soul. |
| Explore Lifelong Learning | Keep your mind sharp by pursuing new hobbies, attending workshops, or diving into topics that inspire you. |

Think about your own go-to stress relievers. Are they working for you, or is it time to try something new? Whether it's reconnecting with an old hobby, discovering a new practice like meditation, or simply carving out quiet time for yourself, know that every small step you take is a step toward balance. Self-care is not a luxury.

*"When you recover or discover something that nourishes your soul and brings joy, care enough about yourself to make room for it in your life."*

*Jean Shinoda Bolen*

**CH's Story of Self Care**

*Julie has an extensive knowledge and was exceptionally easy to talk to and work with. I am now in a better space and enjoy my food, exercise, and family time - Julie's message to me was: 'look after yourself and you'll be able to get through the menopause and enjoy life.'*

## Stress resilience in menopause

I used to think stress was something to avoid at all costs, but now I realise that it's in moments of discomfort where my greatest personal growth has occurred. It wasn't until I started to face those uncomfortable feelings that I could truly move forward. During my menopause journey, it felt as though everything I hadn't wanted to address or deal with came crashing down all at once. It was as if my nervous system had been protecting me throughout my life by keeping certain issues buried. I now see this as a form of self-preservation. After all, our bodies are designed with survival and reproduction in mind. For years, my body seemed to do everything it could to help me navigate life – pushing unresolved trauma and emotions aside, almost as if it was saying, "Not now. Focus on getting through, creating, and caring for others."

But as menopause approached, it felt as though the dam gates finally burst open. With the reproductive window closing, my body seemed to declare, "OK, now it's time to deal with everything that's been stuck for so long – the things that have been holding you back from truly moving forward." It wasn't gradual or gentle; it was more like being thrown into the deep end. And believe me, it was uncomfortable. So many old emotions, fears, and unprocessed experiences surfaced, leaving me feeling overwhelmed at times. Looking back, I now realise how necessary this process was for me. It felt as though, once my body decided reproduction was no longer its main priority, it gave me permission to finally address the things I had buried. It was as though menopause was saying, "You've done enough. Now it's time to focus on you."

I won't sugar-coat it – taking responsibility for your emotional baggage, owning your past experiences, and working through them can be incredibly challenging. But I can say, without a doubt, that it's worth it. Through my journey with the incredible coach, Lorna Dougan, at Mind Positive, I've experienced nothing short of life-changing growth. Each session has peeled back layers, helping me uncover more of my true self. At 56, I can finally say that I'm finding my voice and discovering the real me. While I'm still working through things, the fear I once carried no longer holds me back. Confronting these long-suppressed emotions has empowered me to move forward in ways I never thought possible. I share this because I know how difficult it can be to face what menopause brings, especially when it forces you to confront emotions you've buried for years.

Resilience is the ability to adapt, recover, and bounce back from adversity and difficult experiences. Building stress resilience is about understanding that it's okay to feel uncomfortable – that you can survive it – and recognising that on the other side of discomfort lies growth and healing. Resilience doesn't mean avoiding the hard stuff; it means being willing to face it and trusting in your strength to get through it.

If there's one thing I've learned, it's that building resilience during menopause is a process. It's about embracing the changes, even when they feel overwhelming, and trusting that your body knows what it's doing. Your nervous system has been protecting you for years, and now it's giving you the opportunity to truly heal and evolve. Be patient with yourself, honour your journey, and know that it's never too late to find your inner strength and peace.

As Nayyirah Waheed beautifully expressed:

*"And I said to my body, 'I want to be your friend.' It took a long breath and replied, 'I have been waiting my whole life for this.'"*

# *Part Four*

## Nourishing Recipes for Menopause

# *Recipe Inspirations*

This recipe section provides breakfast, lunch, dinner, and snack ideas that are easy to prepare using ingredients you likely already have in your cupboards. I've been there – I know that when menopause fatigue or brain fog kicks in, the thought of cooking with too many ingredients or following time-consuming recipes can feel completely overwhelming. These simple, nourishing recipes are designed for those days, offering quick and balanced options to keep you energised, satisfied, and feeling your best.

At the same time, I also know there are moments when you may feel more motivated and inspired to spend a little extra time in the kitchen. Cooking can be such a powerful form of self-care, a chance to reconnect with yourself and find joy in creating something nourishing and delicious. Whether you're keeping it simple or feeling ready to experiment, these recipes are here to meet you where you are – helping you take care of your body and rediscover your energy and joy, one meal at a time.

## Why these recipes are beneficial during menopause:

**Diverse nutrients**
Each recipe includes a variety of nutrients crucial for overall health, including bone health, hormonal balance, and heart health.

**Balanced macronutrients**
Recipes offer a mix of proteins, healthy fats, and complex carbohydrates for sustained energy.

**Anti-inflammatory ingredients**
Many recipes incorporate ingredients with anti-inflammatory properties to support overall well-being.

**Support for specific menopausal symptoms**
Ingredients like Omega-3 fatty acids, phytoestrogens, and bone-supportive nutrients address common menopausal challenges.

**Digestive-friendly options**
Including ingredients that aid digestion, such as fibre-rich vegetables and probiotic-rich yogurt.

**Bone health**
Choices like leafy greens and quinoa provide essential nutrients for bone health.

**Gut-friendly options**
Probiotic-rich yogurt and fibre-rich ingredients support gut health, interconnected with hormonal balance.

# BREAKFASTS

## Berry-licious chia pudding

**Ingredients:**

- 1/4 cup of chia seeds
- 1 cup of almond milk
- 1 cup of mixed berries (blueberries, raspberries, strawberries)
- 1 tablespoon of maple syrup or honey
- 1 teaspoon of vanilla extract

**Instructions:**

1. In a bowl, mix chia seeds, almond milk, maple syrup (or honey), and vanilla extract.
2. Stir well and let it sit for 5 minutes.
3. Stir again to break up any clumps.
4. Cover and refrigerate for at least 2 hours or overnight.
5. Top with mixed berries before serving.

**Nutritional Benefits:**

- Chia Seeds: provide Omega-3 fatty acids and fibre, supporting heart health and aiding in digestion.
- Berries: offer antioxidants, fibre, and vitamins, combating oxidative stress and supporting immune health.

## Sweet potato toast with avocado and egg

*A nutrient-packed start to your day.*

**Ingredients**

*Serves 1*

- 1 medium sweet potato, sliced lengthwise into ½-inch slices
- ½ avocado, mashed

- 1 egg, poached or fried
- 1 teaspoon olive oil
- Salt and pepper, to taste

**Instructions**

1. Preheat a toaster or oven to medium-high heat. Toast the sweet potato slices until tender and slightly browned (about 5-7 minutes).
2. Mash the avocado with a pinch of salt and pepper.
3. Spread the avocado onto the sweet potato slices.
4. Top with the poached or fried egg.
5. Drizzle with olive oil if desired and serve warm.

**Nutritional Benefits**

- Sweet Potato: provides complex carbohydrates and fibre for sustained energy, along with beta-carotene (vitamin A) for immune support and skin health.
- Avocado: rich in monounsaturated fats that support hormonal balance, as well as potassium to help regulate blood pressure.
- Egg: source of high-quality protein, choline for brain health, and vitamin D to support bone health and immunity.
- Olive Oil: Adds healthy fats that aid in the absorption of fat-soluble vitamins.

## Greek yoghurt with mixed berries & seeds

**Ingredients**

*Serves 1*

- 1 cup Greek yoghurt (unsweetened)
- Mixed berries: ½ cup (e.g. blueberries, strawberries, raspberries)

- 1 teaspoon chia seeds
- 1 teaspoon pumpkin seeds

**Instructions**

1. Scoop the Greek yoghurt into a bowl.
2. Top with mixed berries of your choice.
3. Sprinkle with chia seeds and pumpkin seeds.
4. Drizzle with honey or maple syrup if you prefer added sweetness.
5. Serve immediately and enjoy!

**Nutritional Benefits**

- Greek Yoghurt: high in protein and probiotics, which support gut health and help with digestion. Also rich in calcium for strong bones.
- Mixed Berries: loaded with antioxidants, fibre, and Vitamins C and K, supporting skin health and reducing inflammation.
- Chia Seeds: a great source of Omega-3 fatty acids and fibre, which help balance hormones and improve digestion.
- Pumpkin Seeds: provide magnesium, zinc, and healthy fats, which can help alleviate stress and support restful sleep.

## Egg omelette with mushrooms

**Ingredients**

*Serves 1*

- 2 large eggs
- ½ cup sliced mushrooms
- ¼ cup spinach
- ¼ onion, finely chopped
- Olive oil 1 teaspoon

**Instructions**

1. Heat olive oil or butter in a non-stick pan over medium heat.
2. Sauté the onion.
3. Add the mushrooms and cook until soft, then toss in the spinach and cook until wilted. Remove the mixture from the pan and set aside.
4. In a bowl, whisk the eggs with salt and pepper.
5. Pour the eggs into the pan, tilting it to spread the mixture evenly.
6. Allow the eggs to set slightly, then add the mushroom and spinach mixture to one side of the omelette.
7. Fold the omelette in half and cook for 1–2 more minutes until the eggs are fully set.
8. Slide onto a plate and serve warm.

**Nutritional Benefits**

- Eggs: packed with protein and essential nutrients like vitamin D, choline, and B Vitamins, supporting bone and brain health.
- Mushrooms: a great source of antioxidants and selenium, helping to boost immunity and reduce inflammation.
- Spinach: rich in magnesium and iron, supporting energy and muscle health.
- Onion: provides antioxidants and support gut health.

## Avocado toast with eggs and spinach

*A delicious and nutrient-packed breakfast or lunch option*

**Ingredients**

*Serves 1*

- ½ avocado, mashed

- 2 eggs: poached or fried
- Spinach: 1 handful, sautéed or fresh
- Sourdough or bread of choice: 1 slice, toasted
- Olive oil or butter :1 teaspoon for sautéing spinach
- Salt and pepper: to taste
- Chilli flakes or seeds (optional): for topping

**Instructions**

1. Toast the sourdough or bread of your choice until golden.
2. While the bread is toasting, mash the avocado with a pinch of salt and pepper.
3. In a pan, heat olive oil or butter over medium heat and lightly sauté the spinach until wilted (optional).
4. Poach or fry the eggs to your desired doneness.
5. Spread the mashed avocado onto the toast.
6. Layer the sautéed spinach over the avocado.
7. Top with the eggs and sprinkle with salt, pepper, and chilli flakes or seeds if desired.
8. Serve immediately and enjoy!

**Nutritional Benefits**

- Avocado: rich in heart-healthy monounsaturated fats, potassium, and fibre, supporting hormonal balance and heart health.
- Eggs: provide high-quality protein, vitamin D, and choline, essential for brain health and muscle maintenance.
- Spinach: high in magnesium, calcium, and iron, promoting energy, strong bones, and muscle function.
- Sourdough or Whole-Grain Bread: a source of complex carbohydrates and fibre to maintain stable energy levels.
- Olive Oil or Butter (optional): adds healthy fats for better absorption of fat-soluble vitamins.

## Cherry almond smoothie

**Ingredients**

- 1 cup unsweetened almond milk
- 1 cup frozen cherries
- ½ banana
- 1-2 cups spinach
- 1 teaspoon chai or hemp hearts

**Instructions:**

Blend all ingredients together in blender and enjoy!

**Nutritional Benefits**

- Cherries: antioxidants (Anthocyanins): Help combat oxidative stress and inflammation, which can worsen menopausal symptoms. Melatonin: Naturally present in cherries, it aids in regulating sleep, often disrupted during menopause.
- Banana: potassium: Helps manage blood pressure, reducing the risk of heart-related issues post-menopause. Magnesium: Supports relaxation and helps combat mood swings or anxiety.
- Spinach: iron and folate help combat fatigue, a common symptom during menopause. Magnesium: Supports bone health, muscle function, and mood regulation. Fibre aids digestion and can help manage weight gain associated with menopause.
- Chia or Hemp Hearts: Omega-3 fatty acids support heart health, reduce inflammation, and may improve brain function and mood stability. Fibre promotes digestive health and helps stabilise blood sugar levels. Protein supports muscle maintenance, particularly important as muscle mass naturally declines with age.

- This smoothie combines nutrient-dense ingredients that can help support energy, mood, and overall health during menopause.

## Berry bliss smoothie

**Ingredients:**

- 1 cup of mixed berries (strawberries, blueberries, raspberries)
- 1 cup of Greek yogurt or plant-based yogurt
- 1 tablespoon of chia seeds
- 1 cup of almond milk (or milk of choice)

**Instructions:**

1. Combine all ingredients in a blender.
2. Blend until smooth.
3. Pour into a glass and enjoy.

**Nutritional Benefits:**

- Berries: packed with antioxidants, which combat oxidative stress linked to ageing and hormonal changes. Berries also provide fibre, Vitamin C, and other essential nutrients.
- Greek Yogurt: high in protein and probiotics, supporting gut health and digestion. Probiotics can help maintain a healthy balance of gut bacteria, which is important for overall health.
- Chia Seeds: provide Omega-3 fatty acids, fibre, and protein. Omega-3s support heart health and reduce inflammation, while fibre aids in digestion.

## LUNCH

### Wholemeal wrap with chicken salad

*A light, protein-packed meal*

**Ingredients**

*Serves 1*

- 1 Wholemeal wrap
- Cooked chicken breast: 100g, sliced or shredded
- Mixed salad leaves: 1 cup (e.g. spinach, lettuce, rocket)
- Cucumber: ¼, sliced
- Tomato: 1 small, sliced
- Avocado: ¼, sliced
- 2 tablespoons Greek yoghurt or hummus: (as a spread or dressing)
- Salt and pepper: To taste
- Lemon juice (optional): A squeeze

**Instructions**

1. Lay the wholemeal wrap flat on a clean surface.
2. Spread the Greek yoghurt or hummus evenly over the wrap.
3. Layer the mixed salad leaves, cucumber, tomato, avocado, and chicken slices on top.
4. Season with salt, pepper, and a squeeze of lemon juice if desired.
5. Fold the sides of the wrap inward, then roll it tightly from the bottom to secure the filling.
6. Slice in half and serve immediately or wrap in foil for on-the-go meals.

**Nutritional Benefits:**

- Wholemeal Wrap: a source of fibre and complex

carbohydrates to keep energy levels steady.

- Chicken Breast: provides lean protein for muscle maintenance and repair.
- Mixed Salad Leaves: rich in antioxidants, Vitamins A and K, and fibre for overall health.
- Cucumber and Tomato: hydrating and full of antioxidants and Vitamin C.
- Avocado: packed with healthy fats and potassium, supporting heart health and hormone balance.
- Greek Yoghurt or hummus: adds probiotics and protein (yoghurt) or plant-based fibre and healthy fats (hummus).

## Lentil and roasted veg warm salad

**Ingredients**

*Serves 2*

- Vegetables for roasting: carrots, courgettes, peppers, sweet potato, beetroot, squash, onion, leek
- 2 tablespoons Extra Virgin Olive Oil
- Kale: A large handful per person
- 220g cooked lentils
- Seeds for topping: 1 tablespoon of pumpkin, sesame, or sunflower seeds

**Dressing**

- Extra virgin olive oil: 50g
- Apple cider vinegar: 3 tablespoons

**Instructions**

1. Preheat the oven to 200°C (400°F).
2. Cut the vegetables into bite-sized pieces and spread them onto a baking tray.
3. Toss the vegetables with olive oil.

4. Roast in the oven for 30-40 minutes, stirring halfway through, until the vegetables are soft and caramelised.
5. Prepare the kale by stripping it into small pieces and placing it on plates or bowls.
6. Warm the lentils (if preferred) and layer them on top of the kale.
7. Add the roasted vegetables over the lentils.
8. Prepare the dressing by mixing all the ingredients in a small jar and shaking well.
9. Drizzle the dressing over the salad.
10. Sprinkle with seeds.

**Nutritional Benefits:**

- Vegetables: packed with fibre, vitamins, and antioxidants to support hormonal balance and overall health.
- Kale: high in calcium, vitamin K, and magnesium, all essential for bone health during menopause.
- Lentils: provide plant-based protein, iron, and fibre to stabilise energy levels and support heart health.
- Seeds: rich in healthy fats and magnesium, which can help alleviate mood swings and improve sleep.

## Mackerel salad with mixed greens

*A heart-healthy and Omega-3-rich dish*

**Ingredients**

*Serves 2*

- 2 Smoked mackerel fillets
- Mixed salad greens: 2 cups (e.g. spinach, rocket, lettuce)
- 1 cup Cherry tomatoes halved
- Cucumber: ½, sliced
- Red onion: ¼, thinly sliced

- Avocado: ½, sliced
- 2 tablespoons olive oil
- Squeeze of lemon
- Salt and pepper: to taste
- Pumpkin or sunflower seeds: 1 tablespoon (optional)

**Instructions**

1. Prepare the salad base by combining mixed greens, cherry tomatoes, cucumber, and red onion in a large bowl.
2. Remove the skin from the smoked mackerel fillets and flake the fish into bite-sized pieces.
3. Add the flaked mackerel and avocado slices to the salad.
4. Drizzle with olive oil and lemon juice, then season with salt and pepper.
5. Sprinkle with seeds for added crunch and nutrients if desired.
6. Serve immediately and enjoy!

**Nutritional Benefits:**

- Mackerel: high in Omega-3 fatty acids, which support heart health, brain function, and reduce inflammation.
- Mixed Greens: packed with fibre, vitamins, and minerals like calcium and magnesium for bone health.
- Tomatoes and Cucumber: provide hydration, antioxidants, and Vitamin C for skin and immune support.
- Avocado: adds heart-healthy fats and potassium to support hormonal balance.
- Olive Oil: a source of monounsaturated fats that promote cardiovascular health.
- Seeds (optional): provide magnesium and zinc, which can help manage stress and support sleep.

## Quinoa salad with roasted veg and chickpeas

*A nutrient-dense and satisfying option for menopause readers.*

**Ingredients**

*Serves 2*

- 1 cup cooked quinoa
- Roasted vegetables: 2 cups (e.g. courgettes, peppers, sweet potato, carrots)
- 1 cup drained and rinsed chickpeas (cooked)
- 1/4 cup feta cheese: crumbled (optional)
- 2 tablespoons olive oil
- Lemon juice: 1 tablespoon
- Dried herbs: 1 teaspoon (e.g. oregano or thyme)
- Salt and pepper: to taste

**Instructions**

1. Preheat the oven to 200°C (400°F).
2. Chop vegetables into bite-sized pieces and toss with 1 tablespoon of olive oil, salt, pepper, and dried herbs. Spread on a baking tray and roast for 25–30 minutes until tender.
3. Cook quinoa according to package instructions and let it cool slightly.
4. In a large bowl, combine the cooked quinoa, roasted vegetables, and chickpeas.
5. Drizzle with the remaining olive oil and lemon juice, mixing gently to combine.
6. Top with crumbled feta cheese if desired.
7. Serve warm or chilled.

**Nutritional Benefits:**

- Quinoa: a complete protein with all nine essential amino acids, plus fibre and magnesium.

- Roasted Vegetables: packed with antioxidants and vitamins to support immune and skin health.
- Chickpeas: high in protein, fibre, and iron for sustained energy and hormonal balance.
- Olive Oil: heart-healthy fats that reduce inflammation.

## Roasted veg and hummus wrap

*A hearty and nutrient-packed lunch option.*

**Ingredients**

*Serves 1*

- 1 Wholemeal wrap
- 1 cup roasted vegetables (e.g., courgettes, peppers, sweet potato)
- 2 tablespoons hummus
- Rocket or spinach leaves: 1 handful
- 1 teaspoon olive oil: (for roasting)
- Salt and pepper: to taste

**Instructions**

1. Preheat the oven to 200°C (400°F).
2. Chop the vegetables into bite-sized pieces, toss with olive oil, salt, and pepper, and roast for 25-30 minutes.
3. Spread hummus evenly over the wrap.
4. Layer the roasted vegetables and fresh rocket or spinach leaves on top.
5. Roll the wrap tightly and slice in half.
6. Serve immediately or pack for on-the-go.

**Nutritional benefits:**

- Roasted Vegetables: high in fibre, antioxidants, and vitamins to support immune health and hormonal balance.

- Hummus: provides plant-based protein, fibre, and healthy fats.
- Wholemeal Wrap: a source of complex carbohydrates to maintain steady energy levels.

## Simple tuna and avocado wrap

*A quick and protein-packed lunch option.*

**Ingredients**

*Serves 1*

- 1 Wholemeal wrap
- Canned tuna (in water): 1 small can (approx. 100g), drained
- ½ Avocado: mashed
- 1 tablespoon Greek yoghurt or mayonnaise
- Mixed salad leaves: 1 handful
- Salt and pepper: to taste

**Instructions**

1. In a bowl, mash the avocado and mix with Greek yoghurt or mayonnaise.
2. Add the drained tuna and stir until combined. Season with salt and pepper.
3. Spread the mixture evenly over the wrap.
4. Top with mixed salad leaves.
5. Roll the wrap tightly, slice in half, and serve.

**Nutritional Benefits:**

- Tuna: high in lean protein and Omega-3 fatty acids for brain **and heart health.**
- Avocado: provides healthy fats to support hormonal balance.
- Greek Yoghurt: adds protein and probiotics for gut health.

## Quinoa and beetroot salad with feta

*A vibrant and energising meal.*

### Ingredients

*Serves 2*

- 1 cup cooked quinoa
- 1 cup cooked beetroot, diced
- ¼ cup feta cheese, crumbled
- 2 cups spinach or mixed greens
- 2 tablespoons olive oil
- 1 tablespoon lemon juice
- Salt and pepper, to taste

### Instructions

1. In a large bowl, combine cooked quinoa, beetroot, and mixed greens.
2. Drizzle with olive oil and lemon juice, then season with salt and pepper.
3. Toss gently to combine.
4. Top with crumbled feta and serve chilled or at room temperature.

### Nutritional Benefits

- Quinoa: a complete protein containing all nine essential amino acids, along with magnesium and fibre to support muscle health and digestion.
- Beetroot: high in antioxidants and nitrates, which enhance blood flow and reduce oxidative stress, improving stamina and energy levels.
- Feta Cheese: provides calcium and protein for strong bones and muscle maintenance.
- Spinach or Mixed Greens: packed with Vitamins A, C, and K, as well as magnesium, supporting hormonal

balance and overall vitality.
- Olive Oil: rich in heart-healthy monounsaturated fats that reduce inflammation.

## DINNER

### Roasted salmon with quinoa and broccoli

**Ingredients**

- 2 salmon fillets
- 1 cup of quinoa
- 2 cups of broccoli florets
- 1 lemon (zested and juiced)
- 2 cloves of garlic, minced
- 1 tablespoon of olive oil
- Salt and pepper to taste

**Instructions**

1. Preheat the oven to 400°F (200°C).
2. Season salmon with lemon zest, garlic, salt, and pepper.
3. Place salmon and broccoli on a baking sheet, drizzle with olive oil.
4. Roast for 15-20 minutes.
5. Cook quinoa according to package instructions.
6. Serve salmon and broccoli over quinoa, drizzle with lemon juice.

**Nutritional Benefits:**

- Salmon: rich in Omega-3 fatty acids, which are beneficial for cardiovascular health and can help reduce inflammation. Omega-3s also support brain health and may help alleviate mood swings and depression.

- Quinoa: a complete protein source, meaning it contains all nine essential amino acids. It's also high in fibre, magnesium, B Vitamins, iron, potassium, calcium, phosphorus, and vitamin E.
- Broccoli: contains Vitamins C and K, fibre, and folate. It's also a good source of calcium, which supports bone health and liver detoxification.

## Avocado & chickpea power bowl

**Ingredients**

- 2 cups of romaine lettuce, chopped
- 1 avocado, sliced
- 1 cup of chickpeas (roasted or cooked)
- 1/2 cup of cherry tomatoes, halved
- 1 cup of cooked quinoa
- 1/4 cup of feta cheese (optional)
- 2 tablespoons of olive oil
- 1 tablespoon of lemon juice

**Instructions**

1. Combine lettuce, avocado, chickpeas, cherry tomatoes, and quinoa in a bowl.
2. Sprinkle with feta cheese, if using.
3. Drizzle with olive oil and lemon juice.
4. Toss gently and serve.

**Nutritional Benefits:**

- Avocado: provides healthy fats that support hormonal health and are beneficial for skin and hair. Avocados are also rich in potassium, which helps control blood pressure.
- Chickpeas: a great source of plant-based protein and fibre, which aid in satiety and digestive health. They also provide important vitamins and minerals such as iron, phosphorus, and B Vitamins.
- Quinoa: high in protein and fibre, and contains iron, magnesium, B Vitamins, calcium, vitamin E, and potassium, making it a nutritious grain alternative.

## Quinoa-stuffed bell peppers

**Ingredients**

- 4 bell peppers, halved and seeded
- 1 cup of cooked quinoa
- 1 cup of black beans, drained and rinsed
- 1 cup of corn kernels
- 1 cup of salsa
- 1/2 cup of shredded cheese
- 2 tablespoons of chopped cilantro

**Instructions**

1. Preheat oven to 375°F (190°C).
2. Mix quinoa, black beans, corn, and salsa in a bowl.
3. Stuff bell pepper halves with the mixture.
4. Place on a baking sheet and top with shredded cheese.
5. Bake for 20-25 minutes.
6. Garnish with cilantro before serving.

**Nutritional Benefits:**

- Quinoa and Black Beans: provide a complete protein source when combined. They are also high in fibre, which helps maintain a healthy digestive system.
- Bell Peppers: rich in Vitamins A and C, which support immune function and skin health. They also contain antioxidants and fibre.
- Salsa: adds flavour with minimal calories and can provide additional vitamins and antioxidants from tomatoes and other ingredients.

## Walnut and spinach stuffed chicken breast

**Ingredients**

- 2 chicken breasts
- 1 cup of spinach leaves
- 1/4 cup of walnuts, chopped
- 2 cloves of garlic, minced
- 1 tablespoon of Dijon mustard
- 1 tablespoon of lemon juice
- Salt and pepper to taste

**Instructions**

1. Preheat oven to 375°F (190°C).
2. Butterfly chicken breasts and season with salt and pepper.
3. In a bowl, mix spinach, walnuts, garlic, mustard, and lemon juice.
4. Stuff the mixture into the chicken breasts.
5. Secure with toothpicks if needed.
6. Bake for 25-30 minutes.
7. Serve immediately.

**Nutritional Benefits:**

- Walnuts: provide Omega-3 fatty acids, supporting heart health and reducing inflammation. They also contain antioxidants and healthy fats.
- Spinach: high in iron, calcium, and Vitamins A, C, and K, supporting bone health and providing antioxidants.
- Provides lean protein necessary for muscle maintenance, which is crucial as muscle mass declines during menopause.

## Pistachio-crusted salmon

**Ingredients:**

- 2 salmon fillets
- 1/2 cup of pistachios, crushed
- 1 tablespoon of Dijon mustard
- 1 lemon (zested)
- Fresh dill for garnish
- Salt and pepper to taste

**Instructions:**

1. Preheat oven to 375°F (190°C).
2. Spread Dijon mustard over the salmon fillets.
3. Press crushed pistachios onto the mustard-coated salmon.
4. Place on a baking sheet and bake for 15-20 minutes.
5. Garnish with lemon zest and fresh dill.
6. Serve immediately.

**Nutritional Benefits:**

- Salmon: Omega-3 fatty acids are essential fats that play a crucial role in brain function, heart health, and reducing inflammation. High-quality protein supports muscle repair and maintenance, which is especially important during ageing. Vitamin D helps with calcium absorption, promoting bone health, and supporting immune function. Vitamins, including B12, B6, and niacin are important for energy metabolism and maintaining healthy skin and nerves.

- Pistachios: healthy fats, mainly monounsaturated and polyunsaturated, which can help reduce bad cholesterol levels and decrease the risk of heart disease.
- Lemon Zest: Vitamin C is a potent antioxidant that supports immune function, skin health, and collagen production. Lemon zest is an antioxidant that contains compounds like limonene, which have anti-inflammatory and antimicrobial properties.

## Vegetable stir fry with tofu and ginger

*A light yet satisfying dinner option.*

### Ingredients

*Serves 2*

- 200g Tofu cubed
- 2 cups mixed vegetables (e.g. broccoli, bell peppers, carrots)
- 1 teaspoon fresh ginger, grated
- 1 clove garlic, minced
- 2 tablespoons soy sauce (low sodium)
- Olive oil or sesame oil: 1 tablespoon

### Instructions

1. Heat oil in a large pan or wok over medium heat.
2. Add tofu cubes and cook until lightly browned. Remove and set aside.
3. Add garlic and ginger to the pan and sauté until fragrant.
4. Add vegetables and stir-fry for 5-7 minutes until tender

but crisp.

5. Return tofu to the pan and drizzle with soy sauce. Toss to coat.
6. Serve warm.

**Nutritional Benefits:**

- Tofu: plant-based protein rich in calcium and iron, supporting bone health.
- Mixed Vegetables: provide fibre, antioxidants, and vitamins for hormonal support.
- Ginger: contains anti-inflammatory properties and aids digestion.

## Mediterranean baked cod

*A light yet flavourful dinner option.*

**Ingredients**

*Serves 2*

- 2 cod fillets (about 150g each)
- 1 cup cherry tomatoes, halved
- ¼ cup Kalamata olives, sliced
- 2 cloves garlic, minced
- 2 tablespoons olive oil
- 1 tablespoon lemon juice
- 2 tablespoons fresh parsley, chopped
- Salt and pepper, to taste

**Instructions**

1. Preheat oven to 190°C (375°F).
2. Place cod fillets on a baking sheet lined with parchment paper.
3. Arrange cherry tomatoes, olives, and garlic around the cod.
4. Drizzle with olive oil and lemon juice, then season with

salt and pepper.

5. Bake for 12-15 minutes, or until the fish flakes easily with a fork.
6. Garnish with fresh parsley and serve warm.

**Nutritional Benefits**

- Cod: a lean source of high-quality protein and Omega-3 fatty acids, which support brain function, reduce inflammation, and improve heart health.
- Cherry Tomatoes: contain lycopene, a powerful antioxidant that protects against oxidative stress and promotes skin health.
- Kalamata Olives: rich in healthy monounsaturated fats and antioxidants that support cardiovascular health.
- Garlic: known for its anti-inflammatory and immune-boosting properties.
- Parsley: provides Vitamin C, vitamin K, and antioxidants, which help reduce inflammation and support detoxification.
- Olive Oil: adds healthy fats to enhance flavour and nutrient absorption.

# SNACKS

## Dark chocolate and nut delight

**Ingredients**

- 1 cup of dark chocolate squares
- 1/2 cup of mixed nuts (almonds, walnuts, pistachios)
- 1/4 cup of dried cherries or cranberries

**Instructions**

1. Melt dark chocolate squares in a microwave-safe bowl, heating in 30-second intervals and stirring until smooth.
2. Mix in the nuts and dried fruit until evenly coated.
3. Spoon the mixture onto a baking sheet lined with parchment paper.
4. Refrigerate until set (about 30 minutes).
5. Break into pieces and enjoy.

**Nutritional Benefits:**

- Dark Chocolate: contains flavonoids and magnesium
- Nuts: provide healthy fats, supporting hormonal balance and offering protein, fibre, vitamins, and minerals.
- Dried Cherries or Cranberries: add natural sweetness and antioxidants, which can help reduce inflammation and support urinary tract health.

## Hummus with carrot and celery sticks

*A light and nutrient-dense snack,*

**Ingredients**

*Serves 1-2*

- ½ cup hummus (store-bought or homemade)
- 1 large carrot, cut into sticks
- 2 stalks celery, cut into sticks
- Olive oil (optional): 1 teaspoon for drizzling

**Instructions**

1. Wash and peel the carrot, then slice into sticks.
2. Wash the celery and slice into sticks.
3. Place the hummus in a small serving bowl.
4. Drizzle olive oil over the hummus if desired

5. Arrange the carrot and celery sticks on a plate around the hummus.
6. Serve fresh as a snack or light meal.

**Nutritional Benefits:**

- Hummus: made from chickpeas, it's high in plant-based protein, fibre, and healthy fats to support energy and digestion. Also provides magnesium and iron.
- Carrots: rich in beta-carotene (vitamin A) for skin and eye health, along with fibre to aid digestion.
- Celery: low in calories but high in antioxidants and water content, helping with hydration and reducing inflammation.
- Olive Oil (optional): adds heart-healthy fats and enhances the absorption of fat-soluble vitamins

## Seed and nut power balls

*A nutritious and energising snack*

**Ingredients**

*Makes 10-12 balls*

- ½ cup peanut butter (unsweetened)
- 2 tablespoons mixed seeds (chia, flax, sunflower)
- 2 tablespoons nuts (chopped almonds, walnuts, or cashews)
- 1 tablespoon cacao powder
- 2 tablespoons honey or maple syrup
- 2 tablespoons coconut (desiccated, optional) (for rolling)

**Instructions**

1. In a large mixing bowl, combine the peanut butter, honey or maple syrup, and cacao powder. Mix until smooth.
2. Add the rolled oats, mixed seeds, and chopped nuts. Stir well to combine.

3. If the mixture is too dry, add a small splash of water or more peanut butter to achieve a sticky consistency.
4. Scoop out small portions of the mixture (about 1 tablespoon) and roll into balls using your hands.
5. Optional: Roll the balls in desiccated coconut for extra flavour and texture.
6. Place the balls on a tray and refrigerate for at least 30 minutes to firm up.
7. Store in an airtight container in the fridge for up to a week.

**Nutritional Benefits:**

- Peanut Butter: source of healthy fats and protein to keep energy levels stable.
- Mixed Seeds: provide Omega-3 fatty acids, magnesium, and zinc, supporting hormonal health and reducing inflammation.
- Nuts: offer healthy fats, protein, and vitamins like vitamin E for skin health.
- Cacao Powder: packed with antioxidants and magnesium to improve mood and support heart health.

## Soothing tumeric infusion

**Ingredients**

- 1 teaspoon of ground turmeric
- 1/2 teaspoon of ginger (freshly grated or powdered)
- 1 tablespoon of honey
- 1 teaspoon of lemon juice
- 2 cups of hot water

**Instructions**

1. Boil 2 cups of water.
2. Add turmeric and ginger to the boiling water.

3. Let it steep for 5-10 minutes.
4. Strain the mixture into a cup.
5. Stir in honey and lemon juice.
6. Enjoy warm.

**Nutritional Benefits:**

- Turmeric: contains curcumin, a potent anti-inflammatory compound that may help alleviate menopausal symptoms such as joint pain and hot flushes. Curcumin also has antioxidant properties that support overall cellular health.
- Ginger: aids in digestive health and has anti-inflammatory effects. Ginger can help reduce nausea and improve digestion, which is beneficial during menopause.
- Honey: provides natural sweetness without refined sugars and has antibacterial and anti-inflammatory properties.
- Lemon Juice: offers a good dose of Vitamin C, which supports immune function and skin health. The acidity of lemon juice also enhances the absorption of iron from other foods.

## Apple slices with almond butter

*A simple and satisfying snack.*

**Ingredients**

*Serves 1*

- 1 apple, sliced
- 2 tablespoons almond butter (unsweetened)

**Instructions**

1. Slice the apple into wedges.
2. Spread almond butter onto each slice or use it as a dip.
3. Serve fresh and enjoy.

**Nutritional Benefits:**

- Apple: high in fibre and antioxidants, supporting digestion and immune health.
- Almond Butter: provides healthy fats to support hormones and sustain energy levels.

## Yoghurt-dipped frozen bluberries

*A refreshing and antioxidant-rich snack.*

**Ingredients**

*Serves 1-2*

- ½ cup Greek yoghurt (unsweetened)
- 1 cup blueberries

**Instructions**

1. Dip each blueberry into the Greek yoghurt, ensuring it is fully coated.
2. Place the coated blueberries on a baking sheet lined with parchment paper.
3. Freeze for at least 1-2 hours until firm.
4. Serve straight from the freezer.

**Nutritional Benefits**

- Blueberries: packed with antioxidants and Vitamin C to combat oxidative stress.
- Greek Yoghurt: high in protein and probiotics for gut health.

## Chia and coconut energy bites

*A quick and energising snack.*

**Ingredients**

*Makes 10-12 bites*

- 2 tablespoons chia seeds

- ¼ cup desiccated coconut
- ½ cup rolled oats
- 2 tablespoons almond butter
- 2 tablespoons honey
- 2 tablespoons dark chocolate chips (optional)

**Instructions**

1. In a bowl, mix chia seeds, coconut, oats, almond butter, and honey until combined.
2. Fold in the chocolate chips if desired.
3. Roll the mixture into small balls (about 1 tablespoon each).
4. Refrigerate for 30 minutes to firm up.
5. Store in an airtight container in the fridge for up to a week.

**Nutritional Benefits:**

- Chia Seeds: Omega-3 fatty acids help reduce inflammation and support heart and brain health. Fibre promotes digestion, helps maintain stable blood sugar levels, and supports weight management.
- Rolled Oats: complex carbohydrates provide sustained energy and support blood sugar regulation. Beta-Glucan is a type of soluble fibre that supports heart health and reduces cholesterol.
- Almond Butter: Vitamin E acts as a powerful antioxidant, supporting skin health and reducing oxidative stress. Protein and healthy fats aid in keeping energy levels stable.
- Dark Chocolate Chips (optional): flavonoids support heart health and improve mood by enhancing brain function. Magnesium helps reduce stress and improve relaxation.

| Breakfast | Lunch | Dinner | Snacks |
|---|---|---|---|
| Berry-Licious Chia Pudding | Wholemeal Wrap with Chicken Salad | Roasted Salmon with Quinoa and Broccoli | Dark Chocolate and Nut Delight |
| Greek Yoghurt with Mixed Berries & Seeds | Lentil and Roasted Veg Warm Salad | Avocado & Chickpea Power Bowl | Hummus with Carrot and Celery Sticks |
| Egg Omelette with Mushrooms | Mackerel Salad with Mixed Greens | Quinoa-Stuffed Bell Peppers | Seed and Nut Power Balls |
| Avocado Toast with Eggs and Spinach | Quinoa Salad with Roasted Veg and Chickpeas | Walnut and Spinach Stuffed Chicken Breast | Soothing Turmeric Infusion |
| Cherry Almond Smoothie | Roasted Veg and Hummus Wrap | Pistachio-Crusted Salmon | Yoghurt-Dipped Frozen Blueberries |
| Berry Bliss Smoothie | Simple Tuna and Avocado Wrap | Vegetable Stir-Fry with Tofu and Ginger | Apple Slices with Almond Butter |
| Sweet Potato Toast With Avocado and Egg | Quinoa and Beetroot Salad | Mediterranean Baked Cod | Chia And Coconut Energy Bites |

## Nutrition for emotional well-being during menopause – a recap:

Nutrition is not just important for our physical health. A balanced diet rich in essential nutrients like Omega-3 fatty acids, B Vitamins, magnesium, vitamin D, and protein plays a vital role in supporting hormonal health, mood stability, and emotional resilience during menopause.

**Protein and amino acids:** Protein-rich foods like lean meats, fish, legumes, tofu, and dairy provide essential amino acids needed for neurotransmitter production, supporting cognitive function and mood stability.

- **B vitamins and omega-3s:** B6, B9 (folate), and B12 are critical for mood regulation and cognitive health. Omega-3 fatty acids, found in fatty fish and flaxseeds, support brain health and neurotransmitter function, aiding emotional resilience.
- **Magnesium:** Magnesium is essential for reducing stress and promoting relaxation by supporting neurotransmitter activity. Found in leafy greens, nuts, seeds, and whole grains, it also helps with energy production and muscle relaxation.
- **Vitamin D:** Often called the "sunshine vitamin", vitamin D supports serotonin production. Vitamin D has become increasingly recognised for its antioxidant, anti-inflammatory, neuroprotective, and neuromodulatory roles, which are thought to underpin its ability to reduce anxiety. Additionally, it has been shown to improve sleep disorders and enhance overall sleep quality. Foods like fatty fish, egg yolks, and fortified dairy, along with safe sun exposure, are great sources of vitamin D.

These recipes are more than just meals; they are tools for self-care, crafted to support you during this time of transition. From the anti-inflammatory properties of turmeric to the healthy fats in avocado and the protein in eggs, every ingredient has been chosen with care to work in harmony with your body's needs.

Remember, this journey is yours, and each bite is an act of self-love and empowerment. Whether you're preparing a quick snack, or a hearty dinner, celebrate the healing and energising qualities of food and allow this to become a cornerstone of your menopausal wellness. Enjoy this culinary exploration and the joy it brings to your plate, your body, and your life.

# *Epilogue*

## The End – And The Beginning

*"Joy is your anchor. It's about finding the things – big or small – that light you up inside and give you purpose."*

If you've made it this far, thank you from the bottom of my heart. Writing this book has been a deeply personal journey and knowing that you've stayed with me through these pages means the world to me. Menopause isn't just a phase; it's a transformation—a time to rediscover the parts of yourself that may have been quieted by life's demands or buried under the weight of expectations. As I've shared my story, my hope is that you've seen glimpses of your own reflected here—moments of struggle, triumph, and the quiet courage to pause and breathe deeply.

When my own menopause journey began, it quickly became clear that the changes weren't just physical; they touched every corner of my life, from energy levels and sleep to emotions and identity; I often felt as though my world had been turned upside down. Yet amidst these challenges, I discovered an opportunity—a chance to reconnect with myself, to focus on what truly mattered, and, most importantly, to rediscover my joy.

It wasn't an easy road. There were moments when it felt overwhelming, but by seeking knowledge, leaning on support, and anchoring myself in key pillars—nutrition, self-care, and stress management—I began to feel stronger, more balanced, and more like myself. What helped most was the strength I found in community, in the stories of other women navigating their own menopause journeys. Knowing I wasn't alone gave me the courage to keep moving forward.

I'll never forget Amanda, a woman I worked with, who once told me, "I feel like I'm completely losing control of my body." Together, we unpacked her story. As she began to understand her hormones and make small, intentional changes, her perspective shifted. Menopause became less of a challenge and more of an opportunity—a phase where she could reclaim her health and well-being. A few months later, Amanda told me, "I feel like I'm getting to know myself all over again—only this time, I'm stronger and wiser."

Just like Amanda, you have the power to turn uncertainty into empowerment. Menopause is not something that happens to you—it's a journey that you can shape on your own terms. Finding joy in menopause doesn't mean trying to recapture who you were; it means embracing who you are now—a woman carrying wisdom, resilience, and untapped strength. Joy begins with the smallest, most intentional steps: reconnecting with the things that bring you lightness, laughter, and peace. Whether it's a walk in the fresh air, dancing to your favourite song, or saying "yes" to something that reignites your vitality, these moments matter.

As we come to the end of this journey together, I want to leave you with a heartfelt reminder: your joy is still within you. Even if it feels buried under exhaustion, self-doubt, or the weight of change, it hasn't disappeared. It's waiting for you—ready to be rediscovered, nurtured, and celebrated in a way that honours the woman you are today. By caring for your health, listening to your body, and prioritising your well-being, you open the door for joy to flourish. These small but meaningful actions will grow into brighter, more frequent moments of happiness, lighting your path and helping you move forward with self-assurance.

Joy and vitality in menopause are not just possibilities—they are within your reach. Thank you for allowing me to walk this path with you. You are not alone, and you never will be. Step forward with self-compassion and confidence, knowing that your joy—your beautiful, radiant joy—is ready to shine once again.

*"You are strong. You are capable. And your joy is still there, waiting for you."*

*Julie Robertson*

*"Menopause is the gateway to the best years of a woman's life."*

*Dr Christine Northrup*

# *Acknowledgements*

This book has been a true labour of love, and it wouldn't have been possible without the extraordinary people who have supported and guided me throughout this journey.

To Sarah Clayton, my incredible writing coach from Write Wild Books —thank you for your endless encouragement, wisdom, and patience. Your insights and belief in me have been pivotal, and I feel so fortunate to have had your expertise and guidance at every step.

To Anne Hamilton, my brilliant editor—your expertise and dedication have shaped this book into something I am truly proud of. Thank you for believing in me and this project, and for always understanding my vision.

To Jane Kerridge from The Balanced Health Clinic and Louise Anderson from Maiya's Light, your contributions to this book have been invaluable. Your knowledge and generosity in sharing your expertise have elevated these pages, and I am endlessly inspired by your passion and commitment to your fields.

To my family and friends—your unwavering encouragement and belief in me have kept me going through the most challenging moments. Thank you for grounding me and reminding me of the bigger picture when I needed it most. Your love and support mean everything to me.

To Gayle and Kate Hamilton, your unwavering courage, remarkable strength, and heartfelt resilience in the face of such a profound loss inspire me every single day.

To all those who have reached out to me for advice on menopause and nutrition—thank you from the bottom of my heart. Your trust, openness, and courage have been the driving force behind this book. You are the reason this project exists, and your stories and resilience continue to inspire me every day. This book is for you—for your strength, your journeys, and the shared determination to navigate this transformative time with confidence and empowerment. You have helped me find my joy, and for that, I am forever grateful.

Lastly, to my husband, Craig—your unwavering love and support have been my foundation through every high and low of this process. You are my cheerleader, my rock, and the calm voice that quiets my inner critic. Thank you for being my constant, for always lifting me up, and for believing in me even when I struggled to believe in myself. You are my soulmate, and my love and gratitude for you are beyond words.

To all of you—thank you for being a part of this journey. It means more to me than you will ever know.

# References

Abdulnour, J., Doucet, É., Brochu, M., Lavoie, J.-M., Strychar, I., Rabasa-Lhoret, R. and Prud'homme, D. (2012). The effect of the menopausal transition on body composition and cardiometabolic risk factors. *Menopause*, 19(7), pp.760–767. doi:https://doi.org/10.1097/gme.0b013e318240f6f3.

AbuMweis, S., Jew, S., Tayyem, R. and Agraib, L. (2018). Eicosapentaenoic acid and docosahexaenoic acid containing supplements modulate risk factors for cardiovascular disease: a meta-analysis of randomised placebo-control human clinical trials. *Journal of Human Nutrition and Dietetics: The Official Journal of the British Dietetic Association*, [online] 31(1), pp.67–84. doi:https://doi.org/10.1111/jhn.12493.

Ağagündüz, D., Şahin, T.Ö., Yılmaz, B., Ekenci, K.D., Duyar Özer, Ş. and Capasso, R. (2022). Cruciferous Vegetables and Their Bioactive Metabolites: from Prevention to Novel Therapies of Colorectal Cancer. *Evidence-Based Complementary and Alternative Medicine*, 2022, pp.1–20. doi:https://doi.org/10.1155/2022/1534083.

Agarwal, A. and Doshi, S. (2013). The role of oxidative stress in menopause. *Journal of Mid-life Health*, 4(3), p.140. doi:https://doi.org/10.4103/0976-

7800.118990.

Aiyer, H.S. and Gupta, R.C. (2010). Berries and Ellagic Acid Prevent Estrogen-Induced Mammary Tumorigenesis by Modulating Enzymes of Estrogen Metabolism. *Cancer Prevention Research*, 3(6), pp.727–737. doi:https://doi.org/10.1158/1940-6207.capr-09-0260.

Akilen, R., Tsiami, A., Devendra, D. and Robinson, N. (2012). Cinnamon in glycaemic control: Systematic review and meta analysis. *Clinical Nutrition*, 31(5), pp.609–615. doi:https://doi.org/10.1016/j.clnu.2012.04.003.

Al-Safi, Z.A. and Santoro, N. (2014). Menopausal hormone therapy and menopausal symptoms. *Fertility and Sterility*, 101(4), pp.905–915. doi:https://doi.org/10.1016/j.fertnstert.2014.02.032.

Alehagen, U., Aaseth, J. and Johansson, P. (2015). Reduced Cardiovascular Mortality 10 Years after Supplementation with Selenium and Coenzyme Q10 for Four Years: Follow-Up Results of a Prospective Randomized Double-Blind Placebo-Controlled Trial in Elderly Citizens. *PLOS ONE*, 10(12), p.e0141641. doi:https://doi.org/10.1371/journal.pone.0141641.

Almey, A., Milner, T.A. and Brake, W.G. (2015). Estrogen receptors in the central nervous system and their implication for dopamine-dependent cognition in females. *Hormones and Behavior*, 74, pp.125–138. doi:https://doi.org/10.1016/j.yhbeh.2015.06.010.

Almohanna, H.M., Ahmed, A.A., Tsatalis, J.P. and Tosti, A. (2019). The Role of Vitamins and Minerals in Hair Loss: A Review. *Dermatology and therapy*, [online] 9(1), pp.51–70. doi:https://doi.org/10.1007/s13555-018-0278-6.

Alqudah, M., Al-Shboul, O., Al-Dwairi, A., Al-U´Dat, D.G. and Alqudah, A. (2022). Progesterone Inhibitory Role on Gastrointestinal Motility. *Physiological*

*Research*, 71(2), pp.193–198. doi:https://doi.org/10.33549/physiolres.934824.

Ambikairajah, A., Walsh, E. and Cherbuin, N. (2019). Lipid profile differences during menopause. *Menopause*, 26(11), pp.1327–1333. doi:https://doi.org/10.1097/gme.0000000000001403.

Ameratunga, D., Goldin, J. and Hickey, M. (2012). Sleep disturbance in menopause. *Internal Medicine Journal*, 42(7), pp.742–747. doi:https://doi.org/10.1111/j.1445-5994.2012.02723.x.

American Heart Association (2017). *The Skinny on Fats.* [online] www.heart.org. Available at: https://www.heart.org/en/health-topics/cholesterol/prevention-and-treatment-of-high-cholesterol-hyperlipidemia/the-skinny-on-fats. [Accessed 13th Jan. 2025]

Anderson, L. Maiya's Light., A, Reiki Master Teacher, (2023). *Silent Counselling.*

Anglin, R.E.S., Samaan, Z., Walter, S.D. and McDonald, S.D. (2013). Vitamin D deficiency and depression in adults: systematic review and meta-analysis. *British Journal of Psychiatry*, [online] 202(2), pp.100–107. doi:https://doi.org/10.1192/bjp.bp.111.106666.

Aranow, C. (2011). Vitamin D and the immune system. *Journal of investigative medicine : the official publication of the American Federation for Clinical Research*, [online] 59(6), pp.881–886. doi:https://doi.org/10.2310/JIM.0b013e31821b8755.

Arevalo, M.-A., Azcoitia, I. and Garcia-Segura, L.M. (2014). The neuroprotective actions of oestradiol and oestrogen receptors. *Nature Reviews Neuroscience*, 16(1), pp.17–29. doi:https://doi.org/10.1038/nrn3856.

Armstrong, M., Asuka, E. and Fingeret, A. (2019). *Physiology, Thyroid*

*Function*. [online] Nih.gov. Available at: https://www.ncbi.nlm.nih.gov/books/NBK537039/.

Ashor, A.W., Lara, J., Siervo, M., Celis-Morales, C., Oggioni, C., Jakovljevic, D.G. and Mathers, J.C. (2014). Exercise Modalities and Endothelial Function: A Systematic Review and Dose–Response Meta-Analysis of Randomized Controlled Trials. *Sports Medicine*, 45(2), pp.279–296. doi:https://doi.org/10.1007/s40279-014-0272-9.

Asltoghiri, M. and Ghodsi, Z. (2012). The effects of Reflexology on sleep disorder in menopausal women. *Procedia - Social and Behavioral Sciences*, 31, pp.242–246. doi:https://doi.org/10.1016/j.sbspro.2011.12.049.

Atabaki, Mahdi., Shariati-Sarabi, Zhaleh., Tavakkol-Afshari, Jalil. and Mohammadi, Mojgan. (2020). Significant immunomodulatory properties of curcumin in patients with osteoarthritis; a successful clinical trial in Iran. *International Immunopharmacology*, 85, p.106607. doi:https://doi.org/10.1016/j.intimp.2020.106607.

Aune, D., Giovannucci, E., Boffetta, P., Fadnes, L.T., Keum, N., Norat, T., Greenwood, D.C., Riboli, E., Vatten, L.J. and Tonstad, S. (2017). Fruit and vegetable intake and the risk of cardiovascular disease, total cancer and all-cause mortality-a systematic review and dose-response meta-analysis of prospective studies. *International journal of epidemiology*, [online] 46(3), pp.1029–1056. doi:https://doi.org/10.1093/ije/dyw319.

Aune, D., Keum, N., Giovannucci, E., Fadnes, L.T., Boffetta, P., Greenwood, D.C., Tonstad, S., Vatten, L.J., Riboli, E. and Norat, T. (2016). Whole grain consumption and risk of cardiovascular disease, cancer, and all cause and cause specific mortality: systematic review and dose-response meta-analysis of prospective studies. *BMJ*, [online] 353(2716), p.i2716. doi:https://doi.org/10.1136/bmj.i2716.

Autoimmune Association. (2025). *About Autoimmunity.* [online] Available at: https://autoimmune.org/resource-center/about-autoimmunity/ [Accessed 17 Jan. 2025].

Avis, N.E., Colvin, A., Bromberger, J.T., Hess, R., Matthews, K.A., Ory, M. and Schocken, M. (2009). Change in health-related quality of life over the menopausal transition in a multiethnic cohort of middle-aged women. *Menopause*, [online] 16(5), pp.860–869. doi:https://doi.org/10.1097/gme.0b013e3181a3cdaf.

Avis, N.E., Crawford, S.L., Greendale, G., Bromberger, J.T., Everson-Rose, S.A., Gold, E.B., Hess, R., Joffe, H., Kravitz, H.M., Tepper, P.G. and Thurston, R.C. (2015). Duration of Menopausal Vasomotor Symptoms Over the Menopause Transition. *JAMA Internal Medicine*, [online] 175(4), p.531. doi:https://doi.org/10.1001/jamainternmed.2014.8063.

Bachman, G. and Pinkerton, J. (n.d.). *Patient education: Vaginal dryness (Beyond the Basics).* [online] www.uptodate.com. Available at: https://www.uptodate.com/contents/vaginal-dryness-beyond-the-basics/print [Accessed 12 Dec. 2024].

Badaeva Anastasiia, Danilov, A., Anastasiia Kosareva, Mariia Lepshina, Novikov, V., Yulia Vorobyeva and Danilov, A. (2024). Neuronutritional Approach to Fibromyalgia Management: A Narrative Review. *Pain and Therapy*, 13(5), pp.1047–1061. doi:https://doi.org/10.1007/s40122-024-00641-2.

Bajalan, Z., Moafi, F., MoradiBaglooei, M. and Alimoradi, Z. (2018a). Mental health and primary dysmenorrhea: a systematic review. *Journal of Psychosomatic Obstetrics & Gynecology*, 40(3), pp.185–194. doi:https://doi.org/10.1080/0167482x.2018.1470619.

Baker, F.C., de Zambotti, M., Colrain, I.M. and Bei, B. (2018). Sleep problems during the menopausal transition: prevalence, impact, and management challenges. *Nature and Science of Sleep*, Volume 10, pp.73–95. doi:https://doi.

org/10.2147/nss.s125807.

Baltacioglu, E., Akalin, F.A., Alver, A., Balaban, F., Unsal, M. and Karabulut, E. (2006). Total antioxidant capacity and superoxide dismutase activity levels in serum and gingival crevicular fluid in post-menopausal women with chronic periodontitis. *Journal of Clinical Periodontology*, 33(6), pp.385–392. doi:https://doi.org/10.1111/j.1600-051x.2006.00923.x.

Barber, T.M., Kabisch, S., Pfeiffer, A.F.H. and Weickert, M.O. (2020). The health benefits of dietary fibre. *Nutrients*, 12(10), p.3209. doi:https://doi.org/10.3390/nu12103209.

Barnea, A., Asghar Hajibeigi, Trant, J.M. and J. Ian Mason (1990). Barnea, A., Hajibeigi, A., Trant, J.M., & Mason, J.I. (1990). Expression of steroid metabolizing enzymes by aggregating fetal brain cells in culture: a model for developmental regulation of the progesterone 5 alpha-reductase pathway. *Endocrinology*, 127(1), pp.500–502. doi:https://doi.org/10.1210/endo-127-1-500.

Barth, C., Villringer, A. and Sacher, J. (2015). Sex Hormones Affect Neurotransmitters and Shape the Adult Female Brain during Hormonal Transition Periods. *Frontiers in Neuroscience*, [online] 9(37). doi:https://doi.org/10.3389/fnins.2015.00037.

Bathina, S. and Das, U.N. (2015). Brain-derived neurotrophic factor and its clinical implications. *Archives of Medical Science*, [online] 11(6), pp.1164–1178. doi:https://doi.org/10.5114/aoms.2015.56342.

Baumgartner RN, Koehler KM, Gallagher D, Romero L, Heymsfield SB, Ross RR, Garry PJ, Lindeman RD. Epidemiology of sarcopenia among the elderly in New Mexico. Am J Epidemiol. 1998;147:755–763. doi: 10.1093/oxfordjournals.aje.a009520.

Baxter, R. (2022). *Migraine and perimenopause.* [online] The Migraine Trust. Available at: https://migrainetrust.org/news/migraine-and-perimenopause/.

Beaudry, K.M. and Devries, M.C. (2019). Nutritional Strategies to Combat Type 2 Diabetes in Aging Adults: The Importance of Protein. *Frontiers in Nutrition*, [online] 6. doi:https://doi.org/10.3389/fnut.2019.00138.

Belujon, P. and Grace, A.A. (2017). Dopamine System Dysregulation in Major Depressive Disorders. *International Journal of Neuropsychopharmacology*, [online] 20(12), pp.1036–1046. doi:https://doi.org/10.1093/ijnp/pyx056.

Bendis, P.C., Zimmerman, S., Onisiforou, A., Zanos, P. and Georgiou, P. (2024). The impact of estradiol on serotonin, glutamate, and dopamine systems. *Frontiers in neuroscience*, 18. doi:https://doi.org/10.3389/fnins.2024.1348551.

Benjamin, E.J., Muntner, P., Alonso, A., Bittencourt, M.S., Callaway, C.W., Carson, A.P., Chamberlain, A.M., Chang, A.R., Cheng, S., Das, S.R., Delling, F.N., Djousse, L., Elkind, M.S.V., Ferguson, J.F., Fornage, M., Jordan, L.C., Khan, S.S., Kissela, B.M., Knutson, K.L. and Kwan, T.W. (2019). Heart Disease and Stroke Statistics—2019 Update: A Report from the American Heart Association. *Circulation*, [online] 139(10). doi:https://doi.org/10.1161/cir.0000000000000659.

Benjamin, J., Levine, J., Fux, M., Aviv, A., Levy, D. and Belmaker, R. (1995). Double-blind, placebo-controlled, crossover trial of inositol treatment for panic disorder. *American Journal of Psychiatry*, 152(7), pp.1084–1086. doi:https://doi.org/10.1176/ajp.152.7.1084.

Bergman, E.A., Massey, L.K., Wise, K.J. and Sherrard, D.J. (1990). Effects of dietary caffeine on renal handling of minerals in adult women. *Life Sciences*, 47(6), pp.557–564. doi:https://doi.org/10.1016/0024-3205(90)90616-y.

Berk, M., Sanders, K.M., Pasco, J.A., Jacka, F.N., Williams, L.J., Hayles, A.L. and Dodd, S. (2007). Vitamin D deficiency may play a role in depression. *Medical Hypotheses*, [online] 69(6), pp.1316–1319. doi:https://doi.org/10.1016/j.mehy.2007.04.001.

Berná, G. and Romero-Gomez, M. (2020). The role of nutrition in non-alcoholic fatty liver disease: Pathophysiology and management. *Liver International*, 40(S1), pp.102–108. doi:https://doi.org/10.1111/liv.14360.

Berto, R. (2014). The Role of Nature in Coping with Psycho-Physiological Stress: A Literature Review on Restorativeness. *Behavioral Sciences*, [online] 4(4), pp.394–409. doi:https://doi.org/10.3390/bs4040394.

Bethea, C.L., Lu, N.Z., Gundlah, C. and Streicher, J.M. (2002). Diverse Actions of Ovarian Steroids in the Serotonin Neural System. *Frontiers in Neuroendocrinology*, 23(1), pp.41–100. doi:https://doi.org/10.1006/frne.2001.0225.

Biason-Lauber, A. and Lang-Muritano, M. (2022). Estrogens: Two nuclear receptors, multiple possibilities. *Molecular and Cellular Endocrinology*, 554, p.111710. doi:https://doi.org/10.1016/j.mce.2022.111710.

Binic, I., Lazarevic, V., Ljubenovic, M., Mojsa, J. and Sokolovic, D. (2013). Skin Ageing: Natural Weapons and Strategies. *Evidence-based Complementary and Alternative Medicine : eCAM*, [online] 2013. doi:https://doi.org/10.1155/2013/827248.

Bischoff, S.C., Barbara, G., Buurman, W., Ockhuizen, T., Schulzke, J.-D., Serino, M., Tilg, H., Watson, A. and Wells, J.M. (2014). Intestinal permeability – a new target for disease prevention and therapy. *BMC Gastroenterology*, [online] 14(1). doi:https://doi.org/10.1186/s12876-014-0189-7.

Bitran, D., Shiekh, M. and McLeod, M. (1995). Anxiolytic Effect of Progesterone is Mediated by the Neurosteroid Allopregnanolone at Brain GABAAReceptors. *Journal of Neuroendocrinology*, 7(3), pp.171–177. doi:https://doi.org/10.1111/j.1365-2826.1995.tb00744.x.

Bittner, V. (2009). Menopause, Age, and Cardiovascular Risk. *Journal of the American College of Cardiology*, 54(25), pp.2374–2375. doi:https://doi.org/10.1016/j.jacc.2009.10.008.

Blair, R.M. (2000). The Estrogen Receptor Relative Binding Affinities of 188 Natural and Xenochemicals: Structural Diversity of Ligands. *Toxicological Sciences*, 54(1), pp.138–153. doi:https://doi.org/10.1093/toxsci/54.1.138.

BoehmG. and Moro, G. (2008). Structural and Functional Aspects of Prebiotics Used in Infant Nutrition. *The Journal of Nutrition*, 138(9), pp.1818S1828S. doi:https://doi.org/10.1093/jn/138.9.1818s.

Bommer, S., Klein, P. and Suter, A. (2011). First time proof of sage's tolerability and efficacy in menopausal women with hot flushes. *Advances in Therapy*, [online] 28(6), pp.490–500. doi:https://doi.org/10.1007/s12325-011-0027-z.

Bonds, R.S. and Midoro-Horiuti, T. (2013). Estrogen effects in allergy and asthma. *Current Opinion in Allergy & Clinical Immunology*, 13(1), pp.92–99. doi:https://doi.org/10.1097/aci.0b013e32835a6dd6.

Bopp, M.J., Houston, D.K., Lenchik, L., Easter, L., Kritchevsky, S.B. and Nicklas, B.J. (2008). Lean Mass Loss Is Associated with Low Protein Intake during Dietary-Induced Weight Loss in Postmenopausal Women. *Journal of the American Dietetic Association*, 108(7), pp.1216–1220. doi:https://doi.org/10.1016/j.jada.2008.04.017.

Bouhnik, Y., Raskine, L., Simoneau, G., Vicaut, E., Neut, C., Flourié, B., Brouns,

F. and Bornet, F.R. (2004). The capacity of nondigestible carbohydrates to stimulate fecal bifidobacteria in healthy humans: a double-blind, randomized, placebo-controlled, parallel-group, dose-response relation study. *The American Journal of Clinical Nutrition*, 80(6), pp.1658–1664. doi:https://doi.org/10.1093/ajcn/80.6.1658.

Bourre, J.-M. (2007). Dietary omega-3 fatty acids for women. *Biomedicine & Pharmacotherapy*, 61(2-3), pp.105–112. doi:https://doi.org/10.1016/j.biopha.2006.09.015.

Boyle, N., Lawton, C. and Dye, L. (2017). The Effects of Magnesium Supplementation on Subjective Anxiety and Stress—A Systematic Review. *Nutrients*, 9(5), p.429. doi:https://doi.org/10.3390/nu9050429.

Božina, N., Bradamante, V. and Lovrić, M. (2009). Genetic Polymorphism of Metabolic Enzymes P450 (CYP) as a Susceptibility Factor for Drug Response, Toxicity, and Cancer Risk. *Archives of Industrial Hygiene and Toxicology*, 60(2), pp.217–242. doi:https://doi.org/10.2478/10004-1254-60-2009-1885.

Bozzetto, L., Costabile, G., Della Pepa, G., Ciciola, P., Vetrani, C., Vitale, M., Rivellese, A.A. and Annuzzi, G. (2018). Dietary Fibre as a Unifying Remedy for the Whole Spectrum of Obesity-Associated Cardiovascular Risk. *Nutrients*, [online] 10(7). doi:https://doi.org/10.3390/nu10070943.

Braith, R.W. and Stewart, K.J. (2006). Resistance Exercise Training. *Circulation*, 113(22), pp.2642–2650. doi:https://doi.org/10.1161/circulationaha.105.584060.

Brian A. Ference, Henry N. Ginsberg, Ian Graham, Kausik K. Ray, Chris J. Packard, Eric Bruckert, Robert A. Hegele, Ronald M. Krauss, Frederick J. Raal, Heribert Schunkert, Gerald F. Watts, Jan Borén, Sergio Fazio, Jay D. Horton, Luis Masana, Stephen J. Nicholls, Børge G. Nordestgaard, Bart van de Sluis, Marja-Riitta Taskinen, Lale Tokgözoğlu, Ulf Landmesser, Ulrich Laufs, Olov

Wiklund, Jane K. Stock, M. John Chapman, Alberico L. Catapano, Low-density lipoproteins cause atherosclerotic cardiovascular disease. 1. Evidence from genetic, epidemiologic, and clinical studies. A consensus statement from the European Atherosclerosis Society Consensus Panel, *European Heart Journal*, Volume 38, Issue 32, 21 August 2017, Pages 2459–2472, https://doi.org/10.1093/eurheartj/ehx144

Briden, L. (2020). *The Curious Link Between Estrogen, Mast Cells, and Histamine.* [online] Lara Briden - The Period Revolutionary. Available at: https://www.larabriden.com/the-curious-link-between-estrogen-and-histamine-intolerance/ [Accessed Dec. 2024].

Briden, L. (2021). *Hormone repair manual : every woman's guide to healthy hormones after 40.* Greenpeak Publishing.

Brighten, D.J. (2016). *How to Increase Progesterone Levels Naturally.* [online] Dr. Jolene Brighten. Available at: https://drbrighten.com/boost-low-progesterone/. [Accessed Dec. 2024].

Brinton, R.D. (2008). The healthy cell bias of estrogen action: mitochondrial bioenergetics and neurological implications. *Trends in Neurosciences*, 31(10), pp.529–537. doi:https://doi.org/10.1016/j.tins.2008.07.003.

Brinton, R.D., Thompson, R.F., Foy, M.R., Baudry, M., Wang, J., Finch, C.E., Morgan, T.E., Pike, C.J., Mack, W.J., Stanczyk, F.Z. and Nilsen, J. (2008). Progesterone receptors: Form and function in brain. *Frontiers in Neuroendocrinology*, 29(2), pp.313–339. doi:https://doi.org/10.1016/j.yfrne.2008.02.001.

British Association of Dermotoligists (2020). *British Association of Dermatologists.* [online] www.bad.org.uk. Available at: https://www.bad.org.uk/pils/telogen-effluvium/ [Accessed 11 Jan. 2025].

British Heart Foundation (2024). *Understanding your cholesterol levels.* [online] British Heart Foundation. Available at: https://www.bhf.org.uk/informationsupport/risk-factors/high-cholesterol/understanding-your-cholesterol-levels. [Accessed 03 Jan. 2025].

British Menopause Society (2020). *BRITISH MENOPAUSE SOCIETY FACT SHEET Information for GPs and other healthcare professionals, for women and for media.* [online] Available at: https://www.womens-health-concern.org/wp-content/uploads/2020/09/BMS-Infographic-A-womans-relationship-with-the-menopause-SEPT2020-B.pdf.

British Menopause Society (n.d.). *https://www.womens-health-concern.org/wp-content/uploads/2020/09/BMS-Infographic-A-womans-relationship-with-the-menopause-SEPT2020-B.pdf.* [Accessed 10 Dec. 2024].

British Menopause Society Tool for clinicians Information for GPs and other health professionals Surgical menopause: a toolkit for healthcare professionals. (n.d.). Available at: https://thebms.org.uk/wp-content/uploads/2024/10/13-BMS-TfC-Surgical-Menopause-SEPT2024-D.pdf [Accessed 10 Dec. 2024].

British Thyroid Foundation (2019). *Thyroid function tests.* [online] British Thyroid Foundation. Available at: https://www.btf-thyroid.org/thyroid-function-tests [Accessed 5 May 2024].

British Thyroid Foundation (2024). *Hair loss and thyroid disorders.* [online] British Thyroid Foundation. Available at: https://www.btf-thyroid.org/hair-loss-and-thyroid-disorders. [Accessed 5 May 2024].

Brodowska Katarzyna, Brodowska Agnieszka Joanna, Śmigielski Krzysztof and Łodyga-Chruścińska Elżbieta (2016). Antioxidant profile of essential oils and extracts of cinnamon bark (Cinnamomum cassia). *European Journal of Biological Research.*, 6. doi:https://doi.org/10.5281/zenodo.197200.

Bromberger, J.T. and Epperson, C.N. (2018). Depression During and After the Perimenopause. *Obstetrics and Gynecology Clinics of North America*, [online] 45(4), pp.663–678. doi:https://doi.org/10.1016/j.ogc.2018.07.007.

Bromberger, J.T., Kravitz, H.M., Chang, Y., Randolph, J.F., Avis, N.E., Gold, E.B. and Matthews, K.A. (2013). Does risk for anxiety increase during the menopausal transition? Study of Women's Health Across the Nation. *Menopause: The Journal of The North American Menopause Society*, 20(5), p.1. doi:https://doi.org/10.1097/gme.0b013e3182730599.

Brossaud, J., Pallet, V. and Corcuff, J-B. (2017). Vitamin A, endocrine tissues and hormones: interplay and interactions. *Endocrine Connections*, 6(7), pp.R121–R130. doi:https://doi.org/10.1530/ec-17-0101.

Bull, J.R., Rowland, S.P., Scherwitzl, E.B., Scherwitzl, R., Danielsson, K.G. and Harper, J. (2019). Real-world menstrual cycle characteristics of more than 600,000 menstrual cycles. *npj Digital Medicine*, 2(1). doi:https://doi.org/10.1038/s41746-019-0152-7.

Burger, H.G. (1999). The endocrinology of the menopause. *The Journal of Steroid Biochemistry and Molecular Biology*, [online] 69(1-6), pp.31–35. doi:https://doi.org/10.1016/s0960-0760(98)00145-9.

Cagnacci, A., Cannoletta, M., Caretto, S., Zanin, R., Xholli, A. and Volpe, A. (2011). Increased cortisol level. *Menopause*, 18(3), pp.273–278. doi:https://doi.org/10.1097/gme.0b013e3181f31947.

Callan, N.G.L., Mitchell, E.S., Heitkemper, M.M. and Woods, N.F. (2018). Constipation and diarrhea during the menopause transition and early postmenopause. *Menopause*, 25(6), pp.615–624. doi:https://doi.org/10.1097/gme.0000000000001057.

Canty, D.J. and Zeisel, S.H. (2009). Lecithin and Choline in Human Health and Disease. *Nutrition Reviews*, 52(10), pp.327–339. doi:https://doi.org/10.1111/j.1753-4887.1994.tb01357.x.

Carbone, E.A., Menculini, G., de Filippis, R., D'Angelo, M., De Fazio, P., Tortorella, A. and Steardo, L. (2023). Sleep Disturbances in Generalized Anxiety Disorder: The Role of Calcium Homeostasis Imbalance. *International Journal of Environmental Research and Public Health*, 20(5), p.4431. doi:https://doi.org/10.3390/ijerph20054431.

Carr, A.C. and Frei, B. (1999). Toward a new recommended dietary allowance for vitamin C based on antioxidant and health effects in humans. *The American Journal of Clinical Nutrition*, [online] 69(6), pp.1086–1107. doi:https://doi.org/10.1093/ajcn/69.6.1086.

Carr, A.C. and Maggini, S. (2017). Vitamin C and immune function. *Nutrients*, [online] 9(11), p.1211. doi:https://doi.org/10.3390/nu9111211.

Castillo-Bustamante, M., Neşe Çelebisoy, Echavarria, L.G., Franco, I., Valencia, S., Gonzalez, S. and García, A. (2024). Balance in Transition: Unraveling the Link Between Menopause and Vertigo. *Cureus*. [online] doi:https://doi.org/10.7759/cureus.59277.

Castro-Marrero, J., Segundo, M.J., Lacasa, M., Martinez-Martinez, A., Sentañes, R.S. and Alegre-Martin, J. (2021). Effect of Dietary Coenzyme Q10 Plus NADH Supplementation on Fatigue Perception and Health-Related Quality of Life in Individuals with Myalgic Encephalomyelitis/Chronic Fatigue Syndrome: A Prospective, Randomized, Double-Blind, Placebo-Controlled Trial. *Nutrients*, 13(8), p.2658. doi:https://doi.org/10.3390/nu13082658.

Cattell, J. and Marsden , K. (2024). *To HRT or Not to HRT (Webinar). Biocare*. [online] Available at: https://www.biocare.co.uk/news/to-hrt-or-not-hrt-webinar.

html [Accessed 22 Oct. 2024].

Cazzaniga, A., Fedele, G., Castiglioni, S. and Maier, J.A. (2022). The Presence of Blood–Brain Barrier Modulates the Response to Magnesium Salts in Human Brain Organoids. *International Journal of Molecular Sciences*, 23(9), p.5133. doi:https://doi.org/10.3390/ijms23095133.

Chaker, L., Bianco, A.C., Jonklaas, J. and Peeters, R.P. (2020). Hypothyroidism. *The Lancet*, 390(10101), pp.1550–1562. doi:https://doi.org/10.1016/s0140-6736(17)30703-1.

Chalasani, N., Younossi, Z., Lavine, J., Diehl, A., Brunt, E., Cusi, K., Charlton, M. and Sanyal, A. (2012). AASLD PRACTICE GUIDELINE The Diagnosis and Management of Non-Alcoholic Fatty. *American Gastroenterological Association*. [online] doi:https://doi.org/10.1002/hep.25762.

Chavda, V.P., Chaudhari, A.Z., Balar, P.C., Amol Gholap and Vora, L.K. (2024). Phytoestrogens: Chemistry, potential health benefits, and their medicinal importance. *PTR. Phytotherapy research/Phytotherapy research*. doi:https://doi.org/10.1002/ptr.8196.

Chen, C., Zhang, J.-Q., Li, L., Guo, M., He, Y., Dong, Y., Meng, H. and Yi, F. (2022). Advanced Glycation End Products in the Skin: Molecular Mechanisms, Methods of Measurement, and Inhibitory Pathways. *Frontiers in Medicine*, 9. doi:https://doi.org/10.3389/fmed.2022.837222.

Chen, Y. and Lyga, J. (2014). Brain-Skin Connection: Stress, Inflammation and Skin Aging. *Inflammation & Allergy-Drug Targets*, [online] 13(3), pp.177–190. doi:https://doi.org/10.2174/1871528113666140522104422.

Chidi-Ogbolu, N. and Baar, K. (2019). Effect of Estrogen on Musculoskeletal Performance and Injury Risk. *Frontiers in Physiology*, [online] 9(1). doi:https://

doi.org/10.3389/fphys.2018.01834.

Cho, H.-C., Kim, J., Kim, S., Son, Y.H., Lee, N. and Jung, S.H. (2012). The concentrations of serum, plasma and platelet BDNF are all increased by treadmill $VO_2$max performance in healthy college men. *Neuroscience Letters*, [online] 519(1), pp.78–83. doi:https://doi.org/10.1016/j.neulet.2012.05.025.

Chung, S.M., Moriyama, T., Eiko Uezu, Kayoko Uezu, Hirata, R., Yohena, N., Masuda, Y., Yoyohiko Kokubu and Yamamoto, S. (1995). Administration of phosphatidylcholine increases brain acetylcholine concentration and improves memory in mice with dementia. *J Nutr*, 125(6), pp.1484–9. doi:https://doi.org/10.1093/jn/125.6.1484.

Ciesielska, A., Kusiak, A., Ossowska, A. and Grzybowska, M.E. (2021). Changes in the Oral Cavity in Menopausal Women—A Narrative Review. *International Journal of Environmental Research and Public Health*, 19(1), p.253. doi:https://doi.org/10.3390/ijerph19010253.

Clayton, A.H., Goldstein, I., Kim, N.N., Althof, S.E., Faubion, S.S., Faught, B.M., Parish, S.J., Simon, J.A., Vignozzi, L., Christiansen, K., Davis, S.R., Freedman, M.A., Kingsberg, S.A., Kirana, P.-S., Larkin, L., McCabe, M. and Sadovsky, R. (2018). The International Society for the Study of Women's Sexual Health Process of Care for Management of Hypoactive Sexual Desire Disorder in Women. *Mayo Clinic Proceedings*, [online] 93(4), pp.467–487. doi:https://doi.org/10.1016/j.mayocp.2017.11.002.

Clayton, S., MA(HONS), MLitt (2025). *Nature, Writing and Menopause*. Write Wild Books. Available at: https://www.writewildbooks.com [Accessed 17 Jan. 2025].

Cleveland Clinic (2022). *Estrogen: Hormone, Function, Levels & Imbalances*. [online] Cleveland Clinic. Available at: https://my.clevelandclinic.org/health/

body/22353-estrogen [Accessed May 30 2024].

Colorado Womens Health (n.d.). *Hypoactive Sexual Desire Disorder (HSDD) | CU OB-GYN | Denver, CO.* [online] University of Colorado OB-GYN. Available at: https://obgyn.coloradowomenshealth.com/health-info/conditions/hypoactive-sexual-desire-disorder [Accessed Dec. 2024].

Contreras, C.M. and Gutierrez-Garcia, A.G. (2018). Cortisol Awakening Response: An Ancient Adaptive Feature. *Journal of Psychiatry and Psychiatric Disorders*, 02(01), pp.29–40. doi:https://doi.org/10.26502/jppd.2572-519x0038.

Cook, N.R. (2007). A Randomized Factorial Trial of Vitamins C and E and Beta Carotene in the Secondary Prevention of Cardiovascular Events in Women. *Archives of Internal Medicine*, [online] 167(15), p.1610. doi:https://doi.org/10.1001/archinte.167.15.1610.

Cordts, E.B., Christofolini, D.M., dos Santos, A.A., Bianco, B. and Barbosa, C.P. (2010). Genetic aspects of premature ovarian failure: a literature review. *Archives of Gynecology and Obstetrics*, 283(3), pp.635–643. doi:https://doi.org/10.1007/s00404-010-1815-4.

Cornelissen, V.A., Fagard, R.H., Coeckelberghs, E. and Vanhees, L. (2011). Impact of Resistance Training on Blood Pressure and Other Cardiovascular Risk Factors. *Hypertension*, 58(5), pp.950–958. doi:https://doi.org/10.1161/hypertensionaha.111.177071.

Corso, S.D. (2024). *Frozen Shoulder during Menopause - Your Shoulder*. [online] Your Shoulder. Available at: https://your-shoulder.com/frozen-shoulder-during-menopause/ [Accessed 14 Jan. 2025]

Craig, W.Y., Palomaki, G.E. and Haddow, J.E. (1989). Cigarette smoking and serum lipid and lipoprotein concentrations: an analysis of published data. *BMJ*, [online] 298(6676), pp.784–788. doi:https://doi.org/10.1136/bmj.298.6676.784.

Cryan, J.F. and Dinan, T.G. (2012). Mind-altering microorganisms: the Impact of the Gut Microbiota on Brain and Behaviour. *Nature Reviews Neuroscience*, 13(10), pp.701–712. doi:https://doi.org/10.1038/nrn3346.

Cui, J., Shen, Y. and Li, R. (2013). Estrogen synthesis and signaling pathways during aging: from periphery to brain. *Trends in Molecular Medicine*, [online] 19(3), pp.197–209. doi:https://doi.org/10.1016/j.molmed.2012.12.007.

Cunningham, A.C., Pal, L., Wickham, A.P., Prentice, C., Frederick, Klepchukova, A. and Liudmila Zhaunova (2024). Chronicling menstrual cycle patterns across the reproductive lifespan with real-world data. *Scientific reports*, 14(1). doi:https://doi.org/10.1038/s41598-024-60373-3.

Currie, H. and Williams, C. (2008). Menopause, Cholesterol and Cardiovascular Disease. *US Cardiology Review*, 5(1), pp.12–14. doi:https://doi.org/10.15420/usc.2008.5.1.12.

D'Alessio, L., Korman, G.P., Sarudiansky, M., Guelman, L.R., Scévola, L., Pastore, A., Obregón, A. and Roldán, E.J.A. (2020). Reducing Allostatic Load in Depression and Anxiety Disorders: Physical Activity and Yoga Practice as Add-On Therapies. *Frontiers in Psychiatry*, 11. doi:https://doi.org/10.3389/fpsyt.2020.00501.

Dabek, M., McCrae, S.I., Stevens, V.J., Duncan, S.H. and Louis, P. (2008). Distribution of beta-glucosidase and beta-glucuronidase activity and of beta-glucuronidase gene gus in human colonic bacteria. *FEMS microbiology ecology*, [online] 66(3), pp.487–95. doi:https://doi.org/10.1111/j.1574-6941.2008.00520.x.

Dai, J., Jones, D.P., Goldberg, J., Ziegler, T.R., Bostick, R.M., Wilson, P.W.,

Manatunga, A.K., Shallenberger, L., Jones, L. and Vaccarino, V. (2008). Association between adherence to the Mediterranean diet and oxidative stress. *The American Journal of Clinical Nutrition*, [online] 88(5), pp.1364–1370. doi:https://doi.org/10.3945/ajcn.2008.26528.

Dalal, P. and Agarwal, M. (2015). Postmenopausal Syndrome. *Indian Journal of Psychiatry*, 57(6), p.222. doi:https://doi.org/10.4103/0019-5545.161483.

Daubenmier, J., Kristeller, J., Hecht, F.M., Maninger, N., Kuwata, M., Jhaveri, K., Lustig, R.H., Kemeny, M., Karan, L. and Epel, E. (2011). Mindfulness Intervention for Stress Eating to Reduce Cortisol and Abdominal Fat among Overweight and Obese Women: An Exploratory Randomized Controlled Study. *Journal of Obesity*, [online] 2011, pp.1–13. doi:https://doi.org/10.1155/2011/651936.

Davenport, D.M. and Wargovich, M.J. (2005). Modulation of cytochrome P450 enzymes by organosulfur compounds from garlic. *Food and Chemical Toxicology*, 43(12), pp.1753–1762. doi:https://doi.org/10.1016/j.fct.2005.05.018.

Davis, S.R., Castelo-Branco, C., Chedraui, P., Lumsden, M.A., Nappi, R.E., Shah, D., Villaseca, P. and Writing Group of the International Menopause Society for World Menopause Day 2012 (2012). Understanding weight gain at menopause. *Climacteric: The Journal of the International Menopause Society*, [online] 15(5), pp.419–429. doi:https://doi.org/10.3109/13697137.2012.707385.

Davis, S.R., Lambrinoudaki, I., Lumsden, M., Mishra, G.D., Pal, L., Rees, M., Santoro, N. and Simoncini, T. (2015). Menopause. *Nature Reviews Disease Primers*, [online] 1(1). doi:https://doi.org/10.1038/nrdp.2015.4.

Davis, S.R., Worsley, R., Miller, K.K., Parish, S.J. and Santoro, N. (2016). Androgens and Female Sexual Function and Dysfunction—Findings from the Fourth International Consultation of Sexual Medicine. *The Journal of Sexual Medicine*, 13(2), pp.168–178. doi:https://doi.org/10.1016/j.jsxm.2015.12.033.

de Bruin, J.P., Bovenhuis, H., van Noord, P. a. H., Pearson, P.L., van Arendonk, J. a. M., te Velde, E.R., Kuurman, W.W. and Dorland, M. (2001). The role of genetic factors in age at natural menopause. *Human Reproduction*, [online] 16(9), pp.2014–2018. doi:https://doi.org/10.1093/humrep/16.9.2014.

de Novaes Soares, C., Almeida, O.P., Joffe, H. and Cohen, L.S. (2001). Efficacy of Estradiol for the Treatment of Depressive Disorders in Perimenopausal Women. *Archives of General Psychiatry*, 58(6), p.529. doi:https://doi.org/10.1001/archpsyc.58.6.529.

Defries, D., Shariati, S., Blewett, H. and Aliani, M. (2021). Expression of Cytochrome P450 Enzymes Is Induced by Flaxseed Enterolignans. *Current Developments in Nutrition*, 5(Supplement_2), pp.312–312. doi:https://doi.org/10.1093/cdn/nzab037_022.

Del Río, J.P., Alliende, M.I., Molina, N., Serrano, F.G., Molina, S. and Vigil, P. (2018). Steroid Hormones and Their Action in Women's Brains: The Importance of Hormonal Balance. *Frontiers in Public Health*, [online] 6. doi:https://doi.org/10.3389/fpubh.2018.00141.

Delgado, B.J. and Lopez-Ojeda, W. (2019). *Estrogen*. [online] National Library of Medicine. Available at: https://www.ncbi.nlm.nih.gov/books/NBK538260/. [Accessed 5 July 2024].

Dennerstein, L., Koochaki, P., Barton, I. and Graziottin, A. (2006). Hypoactive Sexual Desire Disorder in Menopausal Women: A Survey of Western European Women. *The Journal of Sexual Medicine*, 3(2), pp.212–222. doi:https://doi.org/10.1111/j.1743-6109.2006.00215.x.

Department of Health and Social Care (2022). *Results of the 'Women's Health – Let's talk about it' survey*. [online] GOV.UK. Available at: https://www.gov.uk/government/calls-for-evidence/womens-health-strategy-call-for-evidence/

outcome/3fa4a313-f7a5-429a-b68d-0eb0be15e696.

Devirian, T.A. and Volpe, S.L. (2003). The Physiological Effects of Dietary Boron. *Critical Reviews in Food Science and Nutrition*, 43(2), pp.219–231. doi:https://doi.org/10.1080/10408690390826491.

Dinan, T.G. and Cryan, J.F. (2016). Gut instincts: microbiota as a key regulator of brain development, ageing and neurodegeneration. *The Journal of Physiology*, 595(2), pp.489–503. doi:https://doi.org/10.1113/jp273106.

DiNicolantonio, J.J. and O'Keefe, J.H. (2018). Effects of dietary fats on blood lipids: a review of direct comparison trials. *Open Heart*, [online] 5(2), p.e000871. doi:https://doi.org/10.1136/openhrt-2018-000871.

DiNicolantonio, J.J. and O'Keefe, J.H. (2018). Importance of maintaining a low omega–6/omega–3 ratio for reducing inflammation. *Open Heart*, [online] 5(2), p.e000946. doi:https://doi.org/10.1136/openhrt-2018-000946.

DiStefano, J.K. (2020). NAFLD and NASH in Postmenopausal Women: Implications for Diagnosis and Treatment. *Endocrinology*, 161(10). doi:https://doi.org/10.1210/endocr/bqaa134.

Djebaili, M., Hoffman, S.W. and Stein, D.G. (2004). Allopregnanolone and progesterone decrease cell death and cognitive deficits after a contusion of the rat pre-frontal cortex. *Neuroscience*, 123(2), pp.349–359. doi:https://doi.org/10.1016/j.neuroscience.2003.09.023.

Dolinko, A.V. and Ginsburg, E.S. (2015). Hyperandrogenism in menopause: a case report and literature review. *Fertility Research and Practice*, 1(1). doi:https://doi.org/10.1186/2054-7099-1-7.

Doostdar, H., Burke, M.Danny. and Mayer, R.T. (2000). Bioflavonoids: selective substrates and inhibitors for cytochrome P450 CYP1A and CYP1B1. *Toxicology*, 144(1-3), pp.31–38. doi:https://doi.org/10.1016/s0300-483x(99)00215-2.

Duralde, E.R., Sobel, T.H. and Manson, J.E. (2023). Management of perimenopausal and menopausal symptoms. *BMJ*, 382, pp.e072612–e072612. doi:https://doi.org/10.1136/bmj-2022-072612.

Dutt, P., Chaudhary, S. and Kumar, P. (2013). Oral Health and menopause: A comprehensive review on current knowledge and associated dental management. *Annals of Medical and Health Sciences Research*, 3(3), p.320. doi:https://doi.org/10.4103/2141-9248.117926.

Eaker, E.D., Chesebro, J.H., Sacks, F.M., Wenger, N.K., Whisnant, J.P. and Winston, M. (1993). Cardiovascular disease in women. *Circulation*, 88(4), pp.1999–2009. doi:https://doi.org/10.1161/01.cir.88.4.1999.

Ebeling, P.R., Atley, L.M., Guthrie, J.R., Burger, H.G., Dennerstein, L., Hopper, J.L. and Wark, J.D. (1996). Bone turnover markers and bone density across the menopausal transition. *The Journal of Clinical Endocrinology & Metabolism*, 81(9), pp.3366–3371. doi:https://doi.org/10.1210/jcem.81.9.8784098.

Ede, G. (n.d.). *Histamine Intolerance: Understanding the Science*. [online] Diagnosis Diet. Available at: https://www.diagnosisdiet.com/full-article/histamine-intolerance-science [Accessed 20 Dec. 2024].

El Khoudary, S.R. (2017). Gaps, limitations and new insights on endogenous estrogen and follicle stimulating hormone as related to risk of cardiovascular disease in women traversing the menopause: A narrative review. *Maturitas*, 104, pp.44–53. doi:https://doi.org/10.1016/j.maturitas.2017.08.003.

El Khoudary, S.R., Aggarwal, B., Beckie, T.M., Hodis, H.N., Johnson, A.E., Langer, R.D., Limacher, M.C., Manson, J.E., Stefanick, M.L. and Allison, M.A.

(2020). Menopause Transition and Cardiovascular Disease Risk: Implications for Timing of Early Prevention: A Scientific Statement from the American Heart Association. *Circulation*, [online] 142(25). doi:https://doi.org/10.1161/cir.0000000000000912.

El Khoudary, S.R., Greendale, G., Crawford, S.L., Avis, N.E., Brooks, M.M., Thurston, R.C., Karvonen-Gutierrez, C., Waetjen, L.E. and Matthews, K. (2019). The menopause transition and women's health at midlife. *Menopause*, [online] 26(10), pp.1213–1227. doi:https://doi.org/10.1097/gme.0000000000001424.

El, R., Brahim Tighilet, Stéphane Besnard and Chabbert, C. (2023). Vestibular Disorders and Hormonal Dysregulations: State of the Art and Clinical Perspectives. *Cells*, 12(4), pp.656–656. doi:https://doi.org/10.3390/cells12040656.

ELDerawi, W., Naser, I., Taleb, M. and Abutair, A. (2018). The Effects of Oral Magnesium Supplementation on Glycemic Response among Type 2 Diabetes Patients. *Nutrients*, 11(1), p.44.

Elgar , K. (2022). Curcumin: A Review of Clinical Use and Efficacy. Nutr Med J., 1 (1): 10-31.

Endocrine Society (2022). *Menopause and Bone Loss*. [online] www.endocrine.org. Available at: https://www.endocrine.org/patient-engagement/endocrine-library/menopause-and-bone-loss. [Accessed 13 October 2024].

Ervin, S.M., Li, H., Lim, L., Roberts, L.R., Liang, X., Mani, S. and Redinbo, M.R. (2019). Gut microbial β-glucuronidases reactivate estrogens as components of the estrobolome that reactivate estrogens. *The Journal of Biological Chemistry*, [online] 294(49), pp.18586–18599. doi:https://doi.org/10.1074/jbc.RA119.010950.

Espinosa-Salas, S. and Gonzalez-Arias, M. (2023). *Nutrition: Micronutrient*

*Intake, Imbalances, and Interventions*. [online] PubMed. Available at: https://www.ncbi.nlm.nih.gov/books/NBK597352/ [Accessed 23 Dec. 2024].

Esposito, K., Kastorini, C.-M., Panagiotakos, D.B. and Giugliano, D. (2013). Mediterranean diet and metabolic syndrome: An updated systematic review. *Reviews in Endocrine and Metabolic Disorders*, 14(3), pp.255–263. doi:https://doi.org/10.1007/s11154-013-9253-9.

Evcili, G. (2018). Early and Long Period Follow-up Results of Low-Glycemic Index Diet for Migraine Prophylaxis. *Ağrı - The Journal of The Turkish Society of Algology*. doi:https://doi.org/10.5505/agri.2017.62443.

Evernow (2022). *How Your Period Flow Changes in Perimenopause*. [online] Evernow.com. Available at: https://www.evernow.com/learn/how-your-period-flow-changes-in-perimenopause?srsltid=AfmBOoqgksIKO_GKFln6uxGQBaawGsJre-BlaC_nF37tpmpxpvkiDIZR [Accessed 20 Dec. 2024].

Faddy, M.J., Gosden, R.G., Gougeon, A., Richardson, S.J. and Nelson, J.F. (1992). Accelerated disappearance of ovarian follicles in mid-life: implications for forecasting menopause. *Human Reproduction*, [online] 7(10), pp.1342–1346. doi:https://doi.org/10.1093/oxfordjournals.humrep.a137570.

Fahed, G., Aoun, L., Bou Zerdan, M., Allam, S., Bou Zerdan, M., Bouferraa, Y. and Assi, H.I. (2022). Metabolic Syndrome: Updates on Pathophysiology and Management in 2021. *International Journal of Molecular Sciences*, 23(2), p.786. doi:https://doi.org/10.3390/ijms23020786.

Falahati-Nini, A., Riggs, B.L., Atkinson, E.J., O'Fallon, W.M., Eastell, R. and Khosla, S. (2000). Relative contributions of testosterone and estrogen in regulating bone resorption and formation in normal elderly men. *Journal of Clinical Investigation*, 106(12), pp.1553–1560. doi:https://doi.org/10.1172/jci10942.

Farage, M.A., Miller, K.W. and Maibach, H.I. (2012). Effects of menopause on autoimmune diseases. *Expert Review of Obstetrics & Gynecology*, 7(6), pp.557–571. doi:https://doi.org/10.1586/eog.12.63.

Farrar, M.D. (2016). Advanced glycation end products in skin ageing and photoageing: what are the implications for epidermal function? *Experimental Dermatology*, 25(12), pp.947–948. doi:https://doi.org/10.1111/exd.13076.

Farzaneh, S. and Zarghi, A. (2016). Estrogen Receptor Ligands: A Review (2013–2015). *Scientia Pharmaceutica*, [online] 84(3), pp.409–427. doi:https://doi.org/10.3390/scipharm84030409.

Farzi, A., Fröhlich, E.E. and Holzer, P. (2018). Gut Microbiota and the Neuroendocrine System. *Neurotherapeutics*, [online] 15(1), pp.5–22. doi:https://doi.org/10.1007/s13311-017-0600-5.

Faubion, S.S., Batur, P. and Calhoun, A.H. (2018). Migraine Throughout the Female Reproductive Life Cycle. *Mayo Clinic Proceedings*, [online] 93(5), pp.639–645. doi:https://doi.org/10.1016/j.mayocp.2017.11.027.

Faubion, S.S., Sood, R., Thielen, J.M. and Shuster, L.T. (2015). Caffeine and menopausal symptoms: what is the association? *Menopause (New York, N.Y.)*, [online] 22(2), pp.155–8. doi:https://doi.org/10.1097/GME.0000000000000301.

Fawcett (2022). *Menopause and the Workplace*. [online] The Fawcett Society. Available at: https://www.fawcettsociety.org.uk/menopauseandtheworkplace [Accessed 5 Jun. 2024].

Feingold KR. Introduction to Lipids and Lipoproteins. [Updated 2024 Jan 14]. In: Feingold KR, Anawalt B, Blackman MR, et al., editors. Endotext [Internet]. South Dartmouth (MA): MDText.com, Inc.; 2000-. Available from: https://www.ncbi.nlm.nih.gov/books/NBK305896/ [Accessed 16th Jan.2025]

Félix-Soriano, E., Martínez-Gayo, A., María José Cobo, Pérez-Chávez, A., Ibáñez-Santos, J., Natalia Palacios Samper, Iñaki Goikoetxea Galarza, Cuervo, M., García-Unciti, M., González-Muniesa, P., Lorente-Cebrián, S. and Moreno-Aliaga, M.J. (2021). Effects of DHA-Rich n-3 Fatty Acid Supplementation and/or Resistance Training on Body Composition and Cardiometabolic Biomarkers in Overweight and Obese Post-Menopausal Women. *Nutrients*, [online] 13(7), pp.2465–2465. doi:https://doi.org/10.3390/nu13072465.

Ferreira, N.R., Vitorino, C. and Fortuna, A. (2022). From antioxidant to neuromodulator: The role of ascorbate in the management of major depression disorder. *Biochemical Pharmacology*, [online] 206, p.115300. doi:https://doi.org/10.1016/j.bcp.2022.115300.

Figueiro MG, Wood B, Plitnick B, Rea MS. The impact of light from computer monitors on melatonin levels in college students. Neuro Endocrinol Lett. 2011;32(2):158-63. PMID: 21552190. (n.d.).

Fink, G., Sumner, B.E.H., Rosie, R., Grace, O. and Quinn, J.P. (1996). Estrogen control of central neurotransmission: Effect on mood, mental state, and memory. *Cellular and Molecular Neurobiology*, 16(3), pp.325–344. doi:https://doi.org/10.1007/bf02088099.

Finkelstein, J.S., Brockwell, S.E., Mehta, V., Greendale, G.A., Sowers, M.R., Ettinger, B., Lo, J.C., Johnston, J.M., Cauley, J.A., Danielson, M.E. and Neer, R.M. (2008). Bone Mineral Density Changes during the Menopause Transition in a Multiethnic Cohort of Women. *The Journal of Clinical Endocrinology & Metabolism*, [online] 93(3), pp.861–868. doi:https://doi.org/10.1210/jc.2007-1876.

Finner, A.M. (2013). Nutrition and Hair. *Dermatologic Clinics*, 31(1), pp.167–172. doi:https://doi.org/10.1016/j.det.2012.08.015.

Fischer, L.M., da Costa, K.-A., Kwock, L., Galanko, J. and Zeisel, S.H. (2010). Dietary choline requirements of women: effects of estrogen and genetic variation. *The American Journal of Clinical Nutrition*, 92(5), pp.1113–1119. doi:https://doi.org/10.3945/ajcn.2010.30064.

Flack, K.D., Davy, K.P., Hulver, M.W., Winett, R.A., Frisard, M.I. and Davy, B.M. (2011). Aging, Resistance Training, and Diabetes Prevention. *Journal of Aging Research*, 2011, pp.1–12. doi:https://doi.org/10.4061/2011/127315.

Ford, E.S. (2005). Risks for All-Cause Mortality, Cardiovascular Disease, and Diabetes Associated with the Metabolic Syndrome: A summary of the evidence. *Diabetes Care*, [online] 28(7), pp.1769–1778. doi:https://doi.org/10.2337/diacare.28.7.1769.

Foster, K., Roche, M., Delgado, C., Cuzzillo, C., Giandinoto, J.-A. and Furness, T. (2019). Resilience and mental health nursing: An integrative review of international literature. *International Journal of Mental Health Nursing*, [online] 28(1), pp.71–85. doi:https://doi.org/10.1111/inm.12548.

Fowke, J., Longcope, C. and Hebert, J. (n.d.). Fowke JH, Longcope C, Hebert JR. Brassica vegetable consumption shifts estrogen metabolism in healthy postmenopausal women. Cancer Epidemiol Biomarkers Prev. 2000 Aug;9(8):773-9. PMID: 10952093.

Francois, M.E., Myette-Cote, E., Bammert, T.D., Durrer, C., Neudorf, H., DeSouza, C.A. and Little, J.P. (2018). Carbohydrate restriction with postmeal walking effectively mitigates postprandial hyperglycemia and improves endothelial function in type 2 diabetes. *American Journal of Physiology-Heart and Circulatory Physiology*, 314(1), pp.H105–H113. doi:https://doi.org/10.1152/ajpheart.00524.2017.

Freedman, R.R. (2005). Hot flashes: behavioral treatments, mechanisms, and relation to sleep Freedman. *The American Journal of Medicine*, Volume 118 (Suppl.12B) Issue 12, 124 - 130.

Freeman, E.W., Sammel, M.D., Lin, H., Gracia, C.R., Pien, G.W., Nelson, D.B. and Sheng, L. (2007). Symptoms Associated with Menopausal Transition and Reproductive Hormones in Midlife Women. *Obstetrics & Gynecology*, [online] 110(2, Part 1), pp.230–240. doi:https://doi.org/10.1097/01.AOG.0000270153.59102.40.

Frei, B., England, L. and Ames, B.N. (1989). Ascorbate is an outstanding antioxidant in human blood plasma. *Proceedings of the National Academy of Sciences*, [online] 86(16), pp.6377–6381. doi:https://doi.org/10.1073/pnas.86.16.6377.

Fritzen, R., Davies, A., Veenhuizen, M., Campbell, M., Pitt, S.J., Ajjan, R.A. and Stewart, A.J. (2023). Magnesium Deficiency and Cardiometabolic Disease. *Nutrients*, [online] 15(10), pp.2355–2355. doi:https://doi.org/10.3390/nu15102355.

Fuh, J.-L., Wang, S.-J., Lee, S.-J., Lu, S.-R. and Juang, K.-D. (2006). A longitudinal study of cognition change during early menopausal transition in a rural community. *Maturitas*, [online] 53(4), pp.447–453. doi:https://doi.org/10.1016/j.maturitas.2005.07.009.

Gambacciani, M. and Levancini, M. (2014). Management of postmenopausal osteoporosis and the prevention of fractures. *Panminerva Med. 2014 Jun*, pp.56(2):115-31.

Ganguly, R. and Pierce, G.N. (2015). The toxicity of dietary trans fats. *Food and Chemical Toxicology*, 78, pp.170–176. doi:https://doi.org/10.1016/j.fct.2015.02.004.

Gannon, M.C., Nuttall, J.A., Damberg, G., Gupta, V. and Nuttall, F.Q. (2001). Effect of Protein Ingestion on the Glucose Appearance Rate in People with Type 2 Diabetes[1]. *The Journal of Clinical Endocrinology & Metabolism*, 86(3), pp.1040–1047. doi:https://doi.org/10.1210/jcem.86.3.7263.

Gans, I.M. and Coffman, J.A. (2021). Glucocorticoid-Mediated Developmental Programming of Vertebrate Stress Responsivity. *Frontiers in Physiology*, 12. doi:https://doi.org/10.3389/fphys.2021.812195.

Gao, T., Wang, X., Li, Y. and Ren, F. (2023). The Role of Probiotics in Skin Health and Related Gut–Skin Axis: A Review. *Nutrients*, [online] 15(14), pp.3123–3123. doi:https://doi.org/10.3390/nu15143123.

Garrett, D.A. (2024). *Estrogen Dominance: The Good, Bad & Ugly of Estrogen Metabolites*. [online] Anna Garrett. Available at: https://drannagarrett.com/estrogen-dominance-the-good-bad-ugly-of-estrogen-metabolites/ [Accessed 22 Dec. 2024].

Gautam, M., Agrawal, M., Gautam, M., Sharma, P., Gautam, A. and Gautam, S. (2012). Role of antioxidants in generalised anxiety disorder and depression. *Indian Journal of Psychiatry*, 54(3), p.244. doi:https://doi.org/10.4103/0019-5545.102424.

Geleijnse, J.M., Vermeer, C., Grobbee, D.E., Schurgers, L.J., Knapen, M.H.J., van der Meer, I.M., Hofman, A. and Witteman, J.C.M. (2004). Dietary Intake of Menaquinone Is Associated with a Reduced Risk of Coronary Heart Disease: The Rotterdam Study. *The Journal of Nutrition*, 134(11), pp.3100–3105. doi:https://doi.org/10.1093/jn/134.11.3100.

Genova Diagnostics (n.d.). *Estrogens Order Number: Estrogen Metabolism Plus 24hr Urine*. [online] Available at: https://www.gdx.net/uk/core-uk/sample-reports-uk/Oestrogen-Metabolism-Plus-Sample-Report-END20.pdf [Accessed

22 Dec. 2024].

Ghavami, A., Ziaei, R., Talebi, S., Barghchi, H., Nattagh-Eshtivani, E., Moradi, S., Rahbarinejad, P., Mohammadi, H., Ghasemi-Tehrani, H., Marx, W. and Askari, G. (2023). Soluble Fiber Supplementation and Serum Lipid Profile: A Systematic Review and Dose-Response Meta-Analysis of Randomized Controlled Trials. *Advances in Nutrition (Bethesda, Md.)*, [online] 14(3), pp.465–474. doi:https://doi.org/10.1016/j.advnut.2023.01.005.

Gil-Cardoso, K., Ginés, I., Pinent, M., Ardévol, A., Blay, M. and Terra, X. (2016). Effects of flavonoids on intestinal inflammation, barrier integrity and changes in gut microbiota during diet-induced obesity. *Nutrition Research Reviews*, 29(2), pp.234–248. doi:https://doi.org/10.1017/s0954422416000159.

Gilbrech, K. (2020). *The Impact of Stress on the Menstrual Cycle.* [online] Available at: https://scholarworks.uark.edu/cgi/viewcontent.cgi?article=1102&context=nursuht [Accessed Dec. 2024].

Gillett, J.E. and Crisp, D.A. (2017). Examining coping style and the relationship between stress and subjective well-being in Australia's 'sandwich generation'. *Australasian Journal on Ageing*, 36(3), pp.222–227. doi:https://doi.org/10.1111/ajag.12439.

Giugliano, D. and Esposito, K. (2008). Mediterranean diet and metabolic diseases. *Current Opinion in Internal Medicine*, 7(2), pp.149–154. doi:https://doi.org/10.1097/mol.0b013e3282f2fa4d.

Gold, E.B., Colvin, A., Avis, N., Bromberger, J., Greendale, G.A., Powell, L., Sternfeld, B. and Matthews, K. (2006). Longitudinal Analysis of the Association Between Vasomotor Symptoms and Race/Ethnicity Across the Menopausal Transition: Study of Women's Health Across the Nation. *American Journal of Public Health*, 96(7), pp.1226–1235. doi:https://doi.org/10.2105/

ajph.2005.066936.

Goldberg, T., Cai, W., Peppa, M., Dardaine, V., Baliga, B.S., Uribarri, J. and Vlassara, H. (2004). Advanced glycoxidation end products in commonly consumed foods. *Journal of the American Dietetic Association*, 104(8), pp.1287–1291. doi:https://doi.org/10.1016/j.jada.2004.05.214.

González-Orozco, J.C. and Camacho-Arroyo, I. (2019). Progesterone Actions During Central Nervous System Development. *Frontiers in Neuroscience*, 13. doi:https://doi.org/10.3389/fnins.2019.00503.

Gou, Y., Cheng, S., Kang, M., Zhou, R., Liu, C., Hui, J., Liu, Y., Wang, B., Shi, P. and Zhang, F. (2024). Association of allostatic load with depression, anxiety, and suicide: a prospective cohort study. *Biological Psychiatry*. doi:https://doi.org/10.1016/j.biopsych.2024.09.026.

Goyal, M., Singh, S., Sibinga, E.M.S., Gould, N.F., Rowland-Seymour, A., Sharma, R., Berger, Z., Sleicher, D., Maron, D.D., Shihab, H.M., Ranasinghe, P.D., Linn, S., Saha, S., Bass, E.B. and Haythornthwaite, J.A. (2014). Meditation Programs for Psychological Stress and Well-being. *JAMA Internal Medicine*, [online] 174(3), p.357. doi:https://doi.org/10.1001/jamainternmed.2013.13018.

Gozuyesil, E. and Baser, M. (2016). The effect of foot reflexology applied to women aged between 40 and 60 on vasomotor complaints and quality of life. *Complementary Therapies in Clinical Practice*, [online] 24, pp.78–85. doi:https://doi.org/10.1016/j.ctcp.2016.05.011.

Green, D.J., Hopman, M.T.E., Padilla, J., Laughlin, M.H. and Thijssen, D.H.J. (2017). Vascular Adaptation to Exercise in Humans: Role of Hemodynamic Stimuli. *Physiological Reviews*, [online] 97(2), pp.495–528. doi:https://doi.org/10.1152/physrev.00014.2016.

Greendale, G.A., Huang, M.-H. ., Wight, R.G., Seeman, T., Luetters, C., Avis, N.E., Johnston, J. and Karlamangla, A.S. (2009). Effects of the menopause transition and hormone use on cognitive performance in midlife women. *Neurology*, [online] 72(21), pp.1850–1857. doi:https://doi.org/10.1212/WNL.0b013e3181a71193.

Greendale, G.A., Sternfeld, B., Huang, M., Han, W., Karvonen-Gutierrez, C., Ruppert, K., Cauley, J.A., Finkelstein, J.S., Jiang, S.-F. and Karlamangla, A.S. (2019). Changes in body composition and weight during the menopause transition. *JCI Insight*, 4(5). doi:https://doi.org/10.1172/jci.insight.124865.

Greenspan, S.L., Maitland, L.A., Myers, E.R., Krasnow, M.B. and Kido, T.H. (2009). Femoral bone loss progresses with age: A longitudinal study in women over age 65. *Journal of Bone and Mineral Research*, 9(12), pp.1959–1965. doi:https://doi.org/10.1002/jbmr.5650091216.

Gregersen, I., Høibraaten, E., Holven, K.B., Løvdahl, L., Ueland, T., Mowinckel, M.-C., Dahl, T.B., Aukrust, P., Halvorsen, B. and Sandset, P.M. (2019). Effect of hormone replacement therapy on atherogenic lipid profile in postmenopausal women. *Thrombosis Research*, 184, pp.1–7. doi:https://doi.org/10.1016/j.thromres.2019.10.005.

Gregorio, L., Brindisi, J., Kleppinger, A., Sullivan, R., Mangano, K.M., Bihuniak, J.D., Kenny, A.M., Kerstetter, J.E. and Insogn, K.L. (2013). Adequate dietary protein is associated with better physical performance among post-menopausal women 60–90 years. *The journal of nutrition, health & aging*, 18(2), pp.155–160. doi:https://doi.org/10.1007/s12603-013-0391-2.

Gregson, C.L., Armstrong, D.J., Bowden, J., Cooper, C., Edwards, J., Gittoes, N.J.L., Harvey, N., Kanis, J., Leyland, S., Low, R., McCloskey, E., Moss, K., Parker, J., Paskins, Z., Poole, K., Reid, D.M., Stone, M., Thomson, J., Vine, N. and Compston, J. (2022). UK clinical guideline for the prevention and treatment of osteoporosis. *Archives of Osteoporosis*, 17(1). doi:https://doi.org/10.1007/s11657-022-01061-5.

Grewal, K., MacIntyre, David A. and Bennett, Phillip R. (2021). The reproductive tract microbiota in pregnancy. *Bioscience Reports*, 41(9). doi:https://doi.org/10.1042/bsr20203908.

Grishina, I. (2014). Gender Differences, Aging and Hormonal Status in Mucosal Injury and Repair. *Aging and Disease*, pp.160–169. doi:https://doi.org/10.14336/ad.2014.0500160.

Gröber, U., Schmidt, J. and Kisters, K. (2015). Magnesium in Prevention and Therapy. *Nutrients*, 7(9), pp.8199–8226. doi:https://doi.org/10.3390/nu7095388.

Grundy, S.M., Hansen, B., Smith, S.C., Cleeman, J.I. and Kahn, R.A. (2004). Clinical Management of Metabolic Syndrome. *Arteriosclerosis, Thrombosis, and Vascular Biology*, 24(2). doi:https://doi.org/10.1161/01.atv.0000112379.88385.67.

Grymowicz, M., Rudnicka, E., Podfigurna, A., Napierala, P., Smolarczyk, R., Smolarczyk, K. and Meczekalski, B. (2020). Hormonal Effects on Hair Follicles. *International Journal of Molecular Sciences*, 21(15), p.5342. doi:https://doi.org/10.3390/ijms21155342.

Guerrera, M., Volpe, S. and Mao, J. (n.d.). Therapeutic uses of magnesium. Am Fam Physician. 2009 Jul 15;80(2):157-62. PMID: 19621856.

Guidi, J., Lucente, M., Sonino, N. and Fava, Giovanni A. (2020). Allostatic Load and Its Impact on Health: A Systematic Review. *Psychotherapy and Psychosomatics*, [online] 90(1), pp.1–17. doi:https://doi.org/10.1159/000510696.

Gunnerud, U.J., Östman, E.M. and Björck, I.M.E. (2013). Effects of whey proteins on glycaemia and insulinaemia to an oral glucose load in healthy adults; a dose–response study. *European Journal of Clinical Nutrition*, 67(7), pp.749–753. doi:https://doi.org/10.1038/ejcn.2013.88.

Guo, C., Huo, Y.-J., Li, Y., Han, Y. and Zhou, D. (2022). Gut-brain axis: Focus on gut metabolites short-chain fatty acids. *World Journal of Clinical Cases*, 10(6), pp.1754–1763. doi:https://doi.org/10.12998/wjcc.v10.i6.1754.

Guo, E.L. and Katta, R. (2017). Diet and hair loss: effects of nutrient deficiency and supplement use. *Dermatology practical & conceptual*, 7(1), pp.1–10. doi:https://doi.org/10.5826/dpc.0701a01.

Guo, S., Woo Jean Kim, Lok, J., Sun Ryung Lee, Besancon, E., Bing Hao Luo, Stins, M.F., Wang, X., Shoukat Dedhar and Lo, E.H. (2008). Neuroprotection via matrix-trophic coupling between cerebral endothelial cells and neurons. *Proceedings of the National Academy of Sciences of the United States of America*, 105(21), pp.7582–7587. doi:https://doi.org/10.1073/pnas.0801105105.

Guo, Y., Zhu, X., Zeng, M., Qi, L., Tang, X., Wang, D., Zhang, M., Xie, Y., Li, H., Yang, X. and Chen, D. (2021). A diet high in sugar and fat influences neurotransmitter metabolism and then affects brain function by altering the gut microbiota. *Translational Psychiatry*, 11(1). doi:https://doi.org/10.1038/s41398-021-01443-2.

Gutierrez-Mariscal, F.M., Yubero-Serrano, E.M., Villalba, J.M. and Lopez-Miranda, J. (2018). Coenzyme Q10: From bench to clinic in aging diseases, a translational review. *Critical Reviews in Food Science and Nutrition*, 59(14), pp.2240–2257. doi:https://doi.org/10.1080/10408398.2018.1442316.

Gyorkos, A., Baker, M.H., Miutz, L.N., Lown, D.A., Jones, M.A. and Houghton-Rahrig, L.D. (2019). Carbohydrate-restricted Diet and Exercise Increase Brain-derived Neurotrophic Factor and Cognitive Function: A Randomized Crossover Trial. *Cureus*, 11(9). doi:https://doi.org/10.7759/cureus.5604.

Hagel, A.F., Layritz, C.M., Hagel, W.H., Hagel, H.-J., Hagel, E., Dauth, W., Kressel, J., Regnet, T., Rosenberg, A., Neurath, M.F., Molderings, G.J. and Raithel, M. (2013). Intravenous infusion of ascorbic acid decreases serum histamine concentrations in patients with allergic and non-allergic diseases. *Naunyn-Schmiedeberg's Archives of Pharmacology*, 386(9), pp.789–793. doi:https://doi.org/10.1007/s00210-013-0880-1.

Hand GC, Athanasou NA, Matthews T, Carr AJ. The pathology of frozen shoulder. J Bone Joint Surg Br. 2007 Jul;89(7):928-32. doi: 10.1302/0301-620X.89B7.19097. PMID: 17673588.

Hannafin J. A., Chiaia T. A. (2000). Adhesive capsulitis. A treatment approach. *Clin. Orthop. Relat. Res.* 372, 95–109. doi:10.1097/00003086-200003000-00012

Hara, Y., Waters, E.M., McEwen, B.S. and Morrison, J.H. (2015). Estrogen Effects on Cognitive and Synaptic Health Over the Lifecourse. *Physiological Reviews*, [online] 95(3), pp.785–807. doi:https://doi.org/10.1152/physrev.00036.2014.

Harding, A.T. and Heaton, N.S. (2022). The Impact of Estrogens and Their Receptors on Immunity and Inflammation during Infection. *Cancers*, [online] 14(4), p.909. doi:https://doi.org/10.3390/cancers14040909.

Harlow, S.D., Gass, M., Hall, J.E., Lobo, R., Maki, P., Rebar, R.W., Sherman, S., Sluss, P.M. and de Villiers, T.J. (2012). Executive Summary of the Stages of Reproductive Aging Workshop + 10: Addressing the Unfinished Agenda of Staging Reproductive Aging. *The Journal of Clinical Endocrinology & Metabolism*, 97(4), pp.1159–1168. doi:https://doi.org/10.1210/jc.2011-3362.

Harper-Harrison, G. and Shanahan, M.M. (2023). *Hormone replacement therapy*. [online] National Library of Medicine. Available at: https://www.ncbi.nlm.nih.gov/books/NBK493191/ [Accessed Dec. 2024].

Harris, R.B., Fonseca, F.L.A., Sharp, M.H. and Ottinger, C.R. (2021). Functional Characterization of Undenatured Type II Collagen Supplements: Are They Interchangeable? *Journal of Dietary Supplements*, pp.1–16. doi:https://doi.org/10.1080/19390211.2021.1931621.

Haufe, A. and Leeners, B. (2023). Sleep disturbances across a woman's lifespan: What is the role of reproductive hormones? *Journal of the Endocrine Society*, 7(5). doi:https://doi.org/10.1210/jendso/bvad036.

Hayes, R.D., Bennett, C.M., Fairley, C.K. and Dennerstein, L. (2006). ORIGINAL RESEARCH—EPIDEMIOLOGY: What can Prevalence Studies Tell Us about Female Sexual Difficulty and Dysfunction? *The Journal of Sexual Medicine*, 3(4), pp.589–595. doi:https://doi.org/10.1111/j.1743-6109.2006.00241.x.

HealthDay (2024). *Female Whales Undergo Menopause, and Scientists Now Know Why*. [online] US News & World Report. Available at: https://www.usnews.com/news/health-news/articles/2024-03-13/female-whales-undergo-menopause-and-scientists-now-know-why [Accessed 3 Dec. 2024].

Heldring, N., Pike, A., Andersson, S., Matthews, J., Cheng, G., Hartman, J., Tujague, M., Ström, A., Treuter, E., Warner, M. and Gustafsson, J.-Å. (2007). Estrogen Receptors: How Do They Signal and What Are Their Targets. *Physiological Reviews*, 87(3), pp.905–931. doi:https://doi.org/10.1152/physrev.00026.2006.

Henmi, H., Endo, T., Kitajima, Y., Manase, K., Hata, H. and Kudo, R. (2003). Effects of ascorbic acid supplementation on serum progesterone levels in patients with a luteal phase defect. *Fertility and Sterility*, 80(2), pp.459–461. doi:https://

doi.org/10.1016/s0015-0282(03)00657-5.

Henri Déchaud, Ravard, C., Claustrat, F., Aude and Pugeat, M. (1999). Xenoestrogen interaction with human sex hormone-binding globulin (hSHBG)1. *Steroids*, 64(5), pp.328–334. doi:https://doi.org/10.1016/s0039-128x(98)00114-7.

Herber-Gast, G.-C.M. and Mishra, G.D. (2013). Fruit, Mediterranean-style, and high-fat and -sugar diets are associated with the risk of night sweats and hot flushes in midlife: results from a prospective cohort study. *The American Journal of Clinical Nutrition*, [online] 97(5), pp.1092–1099. doi:https://doi.org/10.3945/ajcn.112.049965.

Hernández-Hernández, O.T., Martínez-Mota, L., Herrera-Pérez, J.J. and Jiménez-Rubio, G. (2019). Role of Estradiol in the Expression of Genes Involved in Serotonin Neurotransmission: Implications for Female Depression. *Current Neuropharmacology*, 17(5), pp.459–471. doi:https://doi.org/10.2174/1570159x16666180628165107.

Hewison, M. (2011). Vitamin D and immune function: an overview. *Proceedings of the Nutrition Society*, [online] 71(1), pp.50–61. doi:https://doi.org/10.1017/s0029665111001650.

Higashi, Y., Maruhashi, T., Noma, K. and Kihara, Y. (2014). Oxidative stress and endothelial dysfunction: Clinical evidence and therapeutic implications. *Trends in Cardiovascular Medicine*, 24(4), pp.165–169. doi:https://doi.org/10.1016/j.tcm.2013.12.001.

Hindiyeh, N.A., Zhang, N., Farrar, M., Banerjee, P., Lombard, L. and Aurora, S.K. (2020). The Role of Diet and Nutrition in Migraine Triggers and Treatment: A Systematic Literature Review. *Headache: The Journal of Head and Face Pain*, [online] 60(7), pp.1300–1316. doi:https://doi.org/10.1111/head.13836.

Hirahatake, K.M., Jiang, L., Wong, N.D., Shikany, J.M., Eaton, C.B., Allison, M.A., Martin, L., Garcia, L., Zaslavsky, O. and Odegaard, A.O. (2019). Diet Quality and Cardiovascular Disease Risk in Postmenopausal Women with Type 2 Diabetes Mellitus: The Women's Health Initiative. *Journal of the American Heart Association*, 8(19). doi:https://doi.org/10.1161/jaha.119.013249.

Hirotsu, C., Tufik, S. and Andersen, M.L. (2015). Interactions between sleep, stress, and metabolism: From physiological to pathological conditions. *Sleep Science*, [online] 8(3), pp.143–152. doi:https://doi.org/10.1016/j.slsci.2015.09.002.

Ho, S.-M. (2003). Estrogen, Progesterone and Epithelial Ovarian Cancer. *Reproductive biology and endocrinology : RB&E*, [online] 1, p.73. doi:https://doi.org/10.1186/1477-7827-1-73.

Hodges, R.E. and Minich, D.M. (2015). Modulation of Metabolic Detoxification Pathways Using Foods and Food-Derived Components: A Scientific Review with Clinical Application. *Journal of Nutrition and Metabolism*, 2015(760689), pp.1–23.

Hoffmann, J. and Recober, A. (2013). Migraine and Triggers: Post Hoc Ergo Propter Hoc? *Current Pain and Headache Reports*, 17(10). doi:https://doi.org/10.1007/s11916-013-0370-7.

Hoga, L., Rodolpho, J., Gonçalves, B. and Quirino, B. (2015). Women's experience of menopause: a systematic review of qualitative evidence. *JBI Database of Systematic Reviews and Implementation Reports*, 13(8), pp.250–337. doi:https://doi.org/10.11124/jbisrir-2015-1948.

Holick, M.F. (2007). Vitamin D deficiency. *The New England journal of medicine*, [online] 357(3), pp.266–81. doi:https://doi.org/10.1056/NEJMra070553.

Hormones Australia (2023). *Pituitary Gland.* [online] Hormones Australia.

Available at: https://www.hormones-australia.org.au/the-endocrine-system/pituitary/.

Hsieh, Y.-W., Huang, C.-Y., Yang, S.-Y., Peng, Y.-H., Yu, C.-P., Chao, P.-D.L. and Hou, Y.-C. (2014). Oral intake of curcumin markedly activated CYP 3A4: in vivo and ex-vivo studies. *Scientific Reports*, [online] 4(1), p.6587. doi:https://doi.org/10.1038/srep06587.

Hughes, G.C. (2012). Progesterone and autoimmune disease. *Autoimmunity Reviews*, 11(6-7), pp.A502–A514. doi:https://doi.org/10.1016/j.autrev.2011.12.003.

Huh, A.J.H., Chen, J.-W., Bakland, L. and Goodacre, C. (2021). Comparison of Different Clinical Decision Support Tools in Aiding Dental and Medical Professionals in Managing Primary Dentition Traumatic Injuries. *Pediatric Emergency Care*, 38(2), pp.e534–e539. doi:https://doi.org/10.1097/pec.0000000000002409.

Huskisson, E., Maggini, S. and Ruf, M. (2007). The Role of Vitamins and Minerals in Energy Metabolism and Well-Being. *Journal of International Medical Research*, [online] 35(3), pp.277–289. doi:https://doi.org/10.1177/147323000703500301.

Hwang, W.J., Lee, T.Y., Kim, N.S. and Kwon, J.S. (2020). The Role of Estrogen Receptors and Their Signaling across Psychiatric Disorders. *International Journal of Molecular Sciences*, [online] 22(1), p.373. doi:https://doi.org/10.3390/ijms22010373.

Institute of Medicine (US) Standing Committee on the Scientific Evaluation of Dietary Reference Intakes. (1997). *Dietary Reference Intakes for Calcium, Phosphorus, Magnesium, Vitamin D, and Fluoride.* [online] Washington, D.C.: National Academies Press. doi:https://doi.org/10.17226/5776.

Ipsen, D.H., Lykkesfeldt, J. and Tveden-Nyborg, P. (2018). Molecular mechanisms of hepatic lipid accumulation in non-alcoholic fatty liver disease. *Cellular and Molecular Life Sciences*, [online] 75(18), pp.3313–3327. doi:https://doi.org/10.1007/s00018-018-2860-6.

Ishihara, Y., Fujitani, N., Sakurai, H., Takemoto, T., Ikeda-Ishihara, N., Mori-Yasumoto, K., Nehira, T., Ishida, A. and Yamazaki, T. (2016). Effects of sex steroid hormones and their metabolites on neuronal injury caused by oxygen-glucose deprivation/reoxygenation in organotypic hippocampal slice cultures. *Steroids*, 113, pp.71–77. doi:https://doi.org/10.1016/j.steroids.2016.06.004.

Ivanny Carolina Marchant, Chabert, S., Martínez-Pinto, J., Ramón Sotomayor-Zárate, Ramírez-Barrantes, R., Acevedo, L., Córdova, C. and Olivero, P. (2022). Estrogen, Cognitive Performance, and Functional Imaging Studies: What Are We Missing About Neuroprotection? *Frontiers in cellular neuroscience*, 16. doi:https://doi.org/10.3389/fncel.2022.866122.

Jacob, R.A. and Sotoudeh, G. (2002). Vitamin C Function and Status in Chronic Disease. *Nutrition in Clinical Care*, [online] 5(2), pp.66–74. doi:https://doi.org/10.1046/j.1523-5408.2002.00005.x.

Jacqueline, Grobbee, D.E., Kok, F.J., Hofman, A. and Valkenburg, H.A. (1989). Increased risk of atherosclerosis in women after the menopause. *BMJ*, 298(6674), pp.642–644. doi:https://doi.org/10.1136/bmj.298.6674.642.

Jafferany, M. and Patel, A. (2019). Understanding psychocutaneous disease: psychosocial & psychoneuroimmunologic perspectives. *International Journal of Dermatology*, 59(1), pp.8–15. doi:https://doi.org/10.1111/ijd.14629.

James, D., Devaraj, S., Bellur, P., Lakkanna, S., Vicini, J. and Boddupalli, S. (2012). Novel concepts of broccoli sulforaphanes and disease: induction of phase II antioxidant and detoxification enzymes by enhanced-glucoraphanin broccoli. *Nutrition Reviews*, [online] 70(11), pp.654–665. doi:https://doi.org/10.1111/

j.1753-4887.2012.00532.x.

James, K.A., Stromin, J.I., Steenkamp, N. and Combrinck, M.I. (2023). Understanding the relationships between physiological and psychosocial stress, cortisol and cognition. *Frontiers in Endocrinology*, 14(1085950), p.1085950. doi:https://doi.org/10.3389/fendo.2023.1085950.

Jenkins, D.J.A., Kendall, C.W.C., Axelsen, M., Augustin, L.S.A. and Vuksan, V. (2000). Viscous and nonviscous fibres, nonabsorbable and low glycaemic index carbohydrates, blood lipids and coronary heart disease. *Current Opinion in Lipidology*, 11(1), pp.49–56. doi:https://doi.org/10.1097/00041433-200002000-00008.

Jensen, M.D. (2008). Role of Body Fat Distribution and the Metabolic Complications of Obesity. *The Journal of Clinical Endocrinology & Metabolism*, 93(11_supplement_1), pp.s57–s63. doi:https://doi.org/10.1210/jc.2008-1585.

Jeong, H.G. and Park, H. (2022). Metabolic Disorders in Menopause. *Metabolites*, 12(10), p.954. doi:https://doi.org/10.3390/metabo12100954.

Ji, M.-X. and Yu, Q. (2015). Primary osteoporosis in postmenopausal women. *Chronic Diseases and Translational Medicine*, [online] 1(1), pp.9–13. doi:https://doi.org/10.1016/j.cdtm.2015.02.006.

Jiang, Y., Greenwood-Van Meerveld, B., Johnson, A.C. and Travagli, R.A. (2019). Role of estrogen and stress on the brain-gut axis. *American Journal of Physiology-Gastrointestinal and Liver Physiology*, 317(2), pp.G203–G209. doi:https://doi.org/10.1152/ajpgi.00144.2019.

Jochems, C., Islander, U., Erlandsson, M., Verdrengh, M., Ohlsson, C. and Carlsten, H. (2005). Osteoporosis in experimental postmenopausal polyarthritis: the relative contributions of estrogen deficiency and inflammation. *Arthritis*

*Research & Therapy*, 7(4), p.R837. doi:https://doi.org/10.1186/ar1753.

Joffe, H., Massler, A. and Sharkey, K.M. (2010). Evaluation and Management of Sleep Disturbance During the Menopause Transition. *Seminars in reproductive medicine*, [online] 28(5), pp.404–421. doi:https://doi.org/10.1055/s-0030-1262900.

Johnson, C., Martin, L. and Cai, x (n.d.). Antihistamine effect of supplemental ascorbic acid and neutrophil chemotaxis. J. Am. Coll. Nutr. 1992;11:172–176.

Ju, W., Li, X., Li, Z., Wu, G.R., Fu, X.F., Yang, X.M., Zhang, X.Q. and Gao, X.B. (2017). The effect of selenium supplementation on coronary heart disease: A systematic review and meta-analysis of randomized controlled trials. *Journal of Trace Elements in Medicine and Biology*, 44, pp.8–16. doi:https://doi.org/10.1016/j.jtemb.2017.04.009.

Kacharava, T., Giorgadze, E., Janjgava, S., Lomtadze, N. and Iamze, T. (2022). Correlation between Vitamin B12 Deficiency and Autoimmune Thyroid Diseases. *Endocrine, Metabolic & Immune Disorders - Drug Targets,* 22. doi:https://doi.org/10.2174/1871530322666220627145635.

Kadir, A., Rabbi, A. and Rahman, M. (2021). CoEnzyme Q10: A new horizon in the treatment of periodontal diseases. *International Dental Journal of Student's Research*, 5(1), pp.1–6. doi:https://doi.org/10.18231/2278-3784.2017.0001

Kalantaridou, S.N., & Nelson, L. M. (2006). *Premature Ovarian Failure Is Not Premature Menopause. Annals of the New York Academy of Sciences, 900(1), 393–402.*doi:10.1111/j.1749-6632.2000.tb06251.x

Kalmbach, D.A., Anderson, J.R. and Drake, C.L. (2018). The impact of stress on sleep: Pathogenic sleep reactivity as a vulnerability to insomnia and circadian disorders. *Journal of sleep research*, [online] 27(6), p.e12710. doi:https://doi.

org/10.1111/jsr.12710.

Kamp, E., Musbahi, E., Ashraf, M. and DeGiovanni, C. (2022). Menopause, skin and common dermatosis: part 1. *Clinical and Experimental Dermatology*. doi:https://doi.org/10.1111/ced.15327.

Kandola, A., Vancampfort, D., Herring, M., Rebar, A., Hallgren, M., Firth, J. and Stubbs, B. (2018). Moving to Beat Anxiety: Epidemiology and Therapeutic Issues with Physical Activity for Anxiety. *Current Psychiatry Reports*, [online] 20(8). doi:https://doi.org/10.1007/s11920-018-0923-x.

Kanis, J.A., McCloskey, E.V., Johansson, H., Oden, A., Melton, L.J. and Khaltaev, N. (2008). A reference standard for the description of osteoporosis. *Bone*, 42(3), pp.467–475. doi:https://doi.org/10.1016/j.bone.2007.11.001.

Kanis, J.A., Melton, L.J., Christiansen, C., Johnston, C.C. and Khaltaev, N. (2009). The diagnosis of osteoporosis. *Journal of Bone and Mineral Research*, 9(8), pp.1137–1141. doi:https://doi.org/10.1002/jbmr.5650090802.

Kantor, J., Kessler, L.J., Brooks, D.G. and Cotsarelis, G. (2003). Decreased serum ferritin is associated with alopecia in women. *The Journal of Investigative Dermatology*, [online] 121(5), pp.985–988. doi:https://doi.org/10.1046/j.1523-1747.2003.12540.x.

Kapoor, E., Collazo-Clavell, M.L. and Faubion, S.S. (2017). Weight Gain in Women at Midlife: A Concise Review of the Pathophysiology and Strategies for Management. *Mayo Clinic Proceedings*, [online] 92(10), pp.1552–1558. doi:https://doi.org/10.1016/j.mayocp.2017.08.004.

Karaçam, Z. and Şeker, S.E. (2007). Factors associated with menopausal symptoms and their relationship with the quality of life among Turkish women. *Maturitas*, 58(1), pp.75–82. doi:https://doi.org/10.1016/j.maturitas.2007.06.004.

Karvonen-Gutierrez, C. and Kim, C. (2016). Association of Mid-Life Changes in Body Size, Body Composition and Obesity Status with the Menopausal Transition. *Healthcare*, 4(3), p.42. doi:https://doi.org/10.3390/healthcare4030042.

Kassam, A., Overstreet, J.W., Snow-Harter, C., De Souza, M.J., Gold, E.B. and Lasley, B.L. (1996). Identification of anovulation and transient luteal function using a urinary pregnanediol-3-glucuronide ratio algorithm. *Environmental Health Perspectives*, 104(4), pp.408–413. doi:https://doi.org/10.1289/ehp.96104408.

Kastorini, C.-M., Milionis, H.J., Esposito, K., Giugliano, D., Goudevenos, J.A. and Panagiotakos, D.B. (2011). The Effect of Mediterranean Diet on Metabolic Syndrome and its Components. *Journal of the American College of Cardiology*, [online] 57(11), pp.1299–1313. doi:https://doi.org/10.1016/j.jacc.2010.09.073.

Kennedy, D. (2016). B Vitamins and the Brain: Mechanisms, Dose and Efficacy—A Review. *Nutrients*, [online] 8(2), p.68. doi:https://doi.org/10.3390/nu8020068.

Kennedy, D.O., Pace, S., Haskell, C., Okello, E.J., Milne, A. and Scholey, A.B. (2006). Effects of Cholinesterase Inhibiting Sage ( Salvia officinalis ) on Mood, Anxiety and Performance on a Psychological Stressor Battery. *Neuropsychopharmacology*, [online] 31(4), pp.845–852. doi:https://doi.org/10.1038/sj.npp.1300907.

Kenny, A.M. and Prestwood, K.M. (2000). OSTEOPOROSIS. *Rheumatic Disease Clinics of North America*, 26(3), pp.569–591. doi:https://doi.org/10.1016/s0889-857x(05)70157-5.

Kerridge, J. (Bsc(Hons), DipCNM, mBANT, rCNHC, ITEC, mFHT. BalancedHEALTH. Nutritional Therapy | Holistic Massage | Reflexology (2024). *Reflexology and Menopause*. [Accessed 5 Nov. 2024].

Kim, B.K., Kim, B.S., An, S.-Y., Lee, M.S., Choi, Y.J., Han, S.J., Chung, Y., Lee, K.-W. and Kim, D.J. (2013). Sleep Duration and Glycemic Control in Patients with Diabetes Mellitus: Korea National Health and Nutrition Examination Survey 2007-2010. *Journal of Korean Medical Science*, 28(9), p.1334. doi:https://doi.org/10.3346/jkms.2013.28.9.1334.

Kim, T.W. Jeong, J.H. Hong, S.C. (2015). 'The Impact of Sleep and Circadian Disturbance on Hormones and Metabolism', International Journal of Endocrinology, 2015(), 1–9. doi:10.1155/2015. (n.d.).

King, E.M., Kaida, A., Prior, J., Albert, A., Frank, P., Abdul-Noor, R., Kwaramba, G., Gormley, R., de Pokomandy, A., Loutfy, M. and Murray, M.C.M. (2022). Resilience and psychosocial factors linked to symptom experience during the menopause transition for women living with HIV*. *Menopause*, Publish Ahead of Print. doi:https://doi.org/10.1097/gme.0000000000001926.

Knezevic, J., Starchl, C., Tmava Berisha, A. and Amrein, K. (2020). Thyroid-Gut-Axis: How Does the Microbiota Influence Thyroid Function? *Nutrients*, [online] 12(6), p.1769. doi:https://doi.org/10.3390/nu12061769.

Knox, S. and O'Boyle, N.M. (2021). Skin lipids in health and disease: A review. *Chemistry and Physics of Lipids*, 236, p.105055. doi:https://doi.org/10.1016/j.chemphyslip.2021.105055.

Knudsen, J.K., Bundgaard-Nielsen, C., Hjerrild, S., Nielsen, R.E., Leutscher, P. and Sørensen, S. (2021). Gut microbiota variations in patients diagnosed with major depressive disorder—A systematic review. Brain and Behavior. doi:https://doi.org/10.1002/brb3.2177.

Kocaadam, B. and Şanlier, N. (2017). Curcumin, an active component of turmeric (Curcuma longa), and its effects on health. *Critical reviews in food science and nutrition*, [online] 57(13), pp.2889–2895. doi:https://doi.org/10.1080/1040839

8.2015.1077195.

Köhrle, J. (2023). Selenium, Iodine and Iron–Essential Trace Elements for Thyroid Hormone Synthesis and Metabolism. *International Journal of Molecular Sciences*, 24(4), p.3393. doi:https://doi.org/10.3390/ijms24043393.

Koothirezhi, R. and Ranganathan, S. (2021). *Postmenopausal Syndrome.* [online] PubMed. Available at: https://www.ncbi.nlm.nih.gov/books/NBK560840/ [Accessed 4 Jan. 2025].

Koran.MD, A. (2014). *VA.gov | Veterans Affairs.* [online] Va.gov. Available at: https://www.va.gov/WHOLEHEALTHLIBRARY/tools/estrogen-dominance.asp#ref-1 [Accessed 23 Dec. 2024].

Kostoglou-Athanassiou, I., Athanassiou, L. and Athanassiou, P. (2020). The Effect of Omega-3 Fatty Acids on Rheumatoid Arthritis. *Mediterranean Journal of Rheumatology*, 31(2), pp.190–194. doi:https://doi.org/10.31138/mjr.31.2.190.

Kouba, B.R., Camargo, A., Gil-Mohapel, J. and Rodrigues, A.L.S. (2022). Molecular Basis Underlying the Therapeutic Potential of Vitamin D for the Treatment of Depression and Anxiety. *International Journal of Molecular Sciences*, 23(13), p.7077. doi:https://doi.org/10.3390/ijms23137077.

Kraal T, Lübbers J, van den Bekerom MPJ, Alessie J, van Kooyk Y, Eygendaal D, Koorevaar RCT. The puzzling pathophysiology of frozen shoulders - a scoping review. J Exp Orthop. 2020 Nov 18;7(1):91. doi: 10.1186/s40634-020-00307-w. PMID: 33205235; PMCID: PMC7672132.

Kraus, W.E., Houmard, J.A., Duscha, B.D., Knetzger, K.J., Wharton, M.B., McCartney, J.S., Bales, C.W., Henes, S., Samsa, G.P., Otvos, J.D., Kulkarni, K.R. and Slentz, C.A. (2002). Effects of the amount and intensity of exercise on plasma lipoproteins. *The New England journal of medicine*, [online] 347(19), pp.1483–92. doi:https://doi.org/10.1056/NEJMoa020194.

Kravitz HM, Zhao X, Bromberger JT, Gold EB, Hall MH, Matthews KA, Sowers MR. Sleep disturbance during the menopausal transition in a multi-ethnic community sample of women. Sleep. 2008 Jul;31(7):979-90. Erratum in: (n.d.).

Kravitz, H.M., Ganz, P.A., Bromberger, J., Powell, L.H., Sutton-Tyrrell, K. and Meyer, P.M. (2003). Sleep difficulty in women at midlife: a community survey of sleep and the menopausal transition *. *Menopause*, 10(1), pp.19–28. doi:https://doi.org/10.1097/00042192-200310010-00005.

Kravitz, H.M., Schott, L.L., Joffe, H., Cyranowski, J.M. and Bromberger, J.T. (2014). Do anxiety symptoms predict major depressive disorder in midlife women? The Study of Women's Health Across the Nation (SWAN) Mental Health Study (MHS). *Psychological Medicine*, 44(12), pp.2593–2602. doi:https://doi.org/10.1017/s0033291714000075.

Kronenberg, F. (2010). Menopausal Hot Flashes: A Review of Physiology and Biosociocultural Perspective on Methods of Assessment. *The Journal of Nutrition*, [online] 140(7), pp.1380S1385S. doi:https://doi.org/10.3945/jn.109.120840.

Kruger, M.C., Coetzer, H., de Winter, R., Gericke, G. and van Papendorp, D.H. (1998). Calcium, gamma-linolenic acid and eicosapentaenoic acid supplementation in senile osteoporosis. *Aging Clinical and Experimental Research*, [online] 10(5), pp.385–394. doi:https://doi.org/10.1007/bf03339885.

Kuiper, G.G.J.M., Lemmen, J.G., Carlsson, B., Corton, J.C., Safe, S.H., van der Saag, P.T., van der Burg, B. and GustafssonJ.-A. (1998). Interaction of Estrogenic Chemicals and Phytoestrogens with Estrogen Receptor β. *Endocrinology*, [online] 139(10), pp.4252–4263. doi:https://doi.org/10.1210/endo.139.10.6216.

Kumar, R., Rathi, H., Haq, A., Wimalawansa, S.J. and Sharma, A. (2021). Putative roles of vitamin D in modulating immune response and immunopathology associated with COVID-19. *Virus Research*, 292, p.198235. doi:https://doi.org/10.1016/j.virusres.2020.198235.

Kuptniratsaikul, V., Dajpratham, P., Taechaarpornkul, W., Buntragulpoontawee, M., Lukkanapichonchut, P., Chootip, C., Saengsuwan, J., Tantayakom, K. and Laongpech, S. (2014). Efficacy and safety of Curcuma domestica extracts compared with ibuprofen in patients with knee osteoarthritis: a multicenter study. *Clinical Interventions in Aging*, [online] 9, p.451. doi:https://doi.org/10.2147/cia.s58535.

Kuryłowicz, A. (2023). Estrogens in Adipose Tissue Physiology and Obesity-Related Dysfunction. *Biomedicines*, 11(3), p.690. doi:https://doi.org/10.3390/biomedicines11030690.

Kuszewski, J. C. Wong, R. Howe, P. (2017). (2017). Effects of Long-Chain Omega-3 Polyunsaturated Fatty Acids on Endothelial Vasodilator Function and Cognition—Are They Interrelated? *Nutrients*, 9(5), p.487. doi:https://doi.org/10.3390/nu9050487.

Kwa, M., Plottel, C., Blaser, M. and Adams, S. (2016). The Intestinal Microbiome and Estrogen Receptor–Positive Female Breast Cancer. *JNCI: Journal of the National Cancer Institute*, 108(8). doi:https://doi.org/10.1093/jnci/djw029.

Laima Ķimse, Reinis, A., Lāsma Miķelsone-Jansone, Gintere, S. and Krūmiņa, A. (2024). A Narrative Review of Psychobiotics: Probiotics That Influence the Gut–Brain Axis. *Medicina*, 60(4), pp.601–601. doi:https://doi.org/10.3390/medicina60040601.

Laitinen, K. and Välimäki, M. (1991). Alcohol and bone. *Calcified Tissue International*, 49(S1), pp.S70–S73. doi:https://doi.org/10.1007/bf02555094.

Lara, L.A.S., Ramos, F.K.P., Kogure, G.S., Costa, R.S., Silva de Sá, M.F., Ferriani, R.A. and dos Reis, R.M. (2015). Impact of Physical Resistance Training on the Sexual Function of Women with Polycystic Ovary Syndrome. *The Journal of Sexual Medicine*, 12(7), pp.1584–1590. doi:https://doi.org/10.1111/jsm.12909.

Larmo PS, Yang B, Hyssälä J, Kallio HP, Erkkola R. Effects of sea buckthorn oil intake on vaginal atrophy in postmenopausal women: a randomized, double-blind, placebo-controlled study. Maturitas. 2014 Nov;79(3):316-21. doi: 10.1016/j.maturitas.2014.07.010. Epub 2014 Jul 21. PMID: 25104582.

Larrieu, T. and Layé, S. (2018). Food for Mood: Relevance of Nutritional Omega-3 Fatty Acids for Depression and Anxiety. *Frontiers in Physiology*, [online] 9(1047). doi:https://doi.org/10.3389/fphys.2018.01047.

Le Floc'h, C., Cheniti, A., Connétable, S., Piccardi, N., Vincenzi, C. and Tosti, A. (2015). Effect of a nutritional supplement on hair loss in women. *Journal of Cosmetic Dermatology*, 14(1), pp.76–82. doi:https://doi.org/10.1111/jocd.12127.

Leimola-Virtanen, R., Salo, T., Toikkanen, S., Pulkkinen, J. and Syrjänen, S. (2000). Expression of estrogen receptor (ER) in oral mucosa and salivary glands. *Maturitas*, [online] 36(2), pp.131–137. doi:https://doi.org/10.1016/S0378-5122(00)00138-9.

Lejri, I., Grimm, A. and Eckert, A. (2018). Mitochondria, Estrogen and Female Brain Aging. *Frontiers in Aging Neuroscience*, 10. doi:https://doi.org/10.3389/fnagi.2018.00124.

LEJSKOVÁ, M., ALUŠÍK, Š., VALENTA, Z., ADÁMKOVÁ, S. and PIŤHA, J. (2012). Natural Postmenopause Is Associated With an Increase in Combined Cardiovascular Risk Factors. *Physiological Research*, pp.587–596. doi:https://doi.org/10.33549/physiolres.932313.

Lemlem Gebremariam Aregawi, Teferi Gebru Gebremeskel and Zoltan, C. (2024). Preventive and Therapeutic Effects of Ginger on Bowel Disease: A Review of Clinical Trials. *Pharmacological research. Modern Chinese medicine*, pp.100457–100457. doi:https://doi.org/10.1016/j.prmcm.2024.100457.

Lenhart, A., Naliboff, B., Shih, W., Gupta, A., Tillisch, K., Liu, C., Mayer, E.A. and Chang, L. (2020). Postmenopausal women with irritable bowel syndrome (IBS) have more severe symptoms than premenopausal women with IBS. *Neurogastroenterology & Motility*, 32(10). doi:https://doi.org/10.1111/nmo.13913.

Lephart, E.D. (2021). Phytoestrogens (Resveratrol and Equol) for Estrogen-Deficient Skin—Controversies/Misinformation versus Anti-Aging In Vitro and Clinical Evidence via Nutraceutical-Cosmetics. *International Journal of Molecular Sciences*, 22(20), p.11218. doi:https://doi.org/10.3390/ijms222011218.

Lephart, E.D. and Naftolin, F. (2020). Menopause and the Skin: Old Favorites and New Innovations in Cosmeceuticals for Estrogen-Deficient Skin. *Dermatology and Therapy*, [online] 11(1), pp.53–69. doi:https://doi.org/10.1007/s13555-020-00468-7.

Lerner, U.H. (2006). Bone remodeling in post-menopausal osteoporosis. *Journal of Dental Research*, [online] 85(7), pp.584–595. doi:https://doi.org/10.1177/154405910608500703.

Leventhal, J. (n.d.). Management of Libido Problems in Menopause. Perm J. 2000 Summer;4(3):29–34. PMCID: PMC6220606.

LeWine, H.E. (2024). *Understanding the stress response.* [online] Harvard Health. Available at: https://www.health.harvard.edu/staying-healthy/understanding-the-stress-response [Accessed 15 Dec. 2024].

Lewis, A.L. and Gilbert, N.M. (2020). Roles of the vagina and the vaginal microbiota in urinary tract infection: evidence from clinical correlations and experimental models. *GMS infectious diseases*, [online] 8, p.Doc02. doi:https://doi.org/10.3205/id000046.

Ley, R.E., Hamady, M., Lozupone, C., Turnbaugh, P.J., Ramey, R.R., Bircher, J.S., Schlegel, M.L., Tucker, T.A., Schrenzel, M.D., Knight, R. and Gordon, J.I. (2008). Evolution of Mammals and Their Gut Microbes. *Science*, [online] 320(5883), pp.1647–1651. doi:https://doi.org/10.1126/science.1155725.

Li, B., Lv, J., Wang, W. and Zhang, D. (2016). Dietary magnesium and calcium intake and risk of depression in the general population: A meta-analysis. *Australian & New Zealand Journal of Psychiatry*, 51(3), pp.219–229. doi:https://doi.org/10.1177/0004867416676895.

Li, Y. and Schellhorn, H.E. (2007). New developments and novel therapeutic perspectives for vitamin C. *The Journal of nutrition*, [online] 137(10), pp.2171–84. doi:https://doi.org/10.1093/jn/137.10.2171.

Lindsay, J. and May, D.R. (2022). *NHS England» NHS England signs Menopause Workplace Pledge*. [online] www.england.nhs.uk. Available at: https://www.england.nhs.uk/blog/nhs-england-signs-menopause-workplace-pledge/ [Accessed 5 Jun. 2024].

Livesey, G., Taylor, R., Livesey, H.F., Buyken, A.E., Jenkins, D.J.A., Augustin, L.S.A., Sievenpiper, J.L., Barclay, A.W., Liu, S., Wolever, T.M.S., Willett, W.C., Brighenti, F., Salas-Salvadó, J., Björck, I., Rizkalla, S.W., Riccardi, G., Vecchia, C.L., Ceriello, A., Trichopoulou, A. and Poli, A. (2019). Dietary Glycemic Index and Load and the Risk of Type 2 Diabetes: A Systematic Review and Updated Meta-Analyses of Prospective Cohort Studies. *Nutrients*, [online] 11(6), p.1280. doi:https://doi.org/10.3390/nu11061280.

Lobo, R.A. (2016). Hormone-replacement therapy: current thinking. *Nature Reviews Endocrinology*, 13(4), pp.220–231. doi:https://doi.org/10.1038/nrendo.2016.164.

Lobo, R.A., Pickar, J.H., Stevenson, J.C., Mack, W.J. and Hodis, H.N. (2016). Back to the future: Hormone replacement therapy as part of a prevention strategy for women at the onset of menopause. *Atherosclerosis*, 254, pp.282–290. doi:https://doi.org/10.1016/j.atherosclerosis.2016.10.005.

Locatelli, C., Nardi, G., anuário, A. de F., Freire, C., Megiolaro, F., Schneider, K., Perazzoli, M.A., Do Nascimento, S., Gon, A., Mariano, L.B., Wagner, G. and Niero, R. (2016). Anti-inflammatory activity of berry fruits in mice model of inflammation is based on oxidative stress modulation. *Pharmacognosy Research*, 8(5), p.42. doi:https://doi.org/10.4103/0974-8490.178642.

Lovejoy, J.C., Champagne, C.M., de Jonge, L., Xie, H. and Smith, S.R. (2008). Increased visceral fat and decreased energy expenditure during the menopausal transition. *International Journal of Obesity*, 32(6), pp.949–958. doi:https://doi.org/10.1038/ijo.2008.25.

Ludwig, D.S., Hu, F.B., Tappy, L. and Brand-Miller, J. (2018). Dietary carbohydrates: role of quality and quantity in chronic disease. *BMJ*, 361, p.k2340. doi:https://doi.org/10.1136/bmj.k2340.

Luksys, G. and Sandi, C. (2011). Neural mechanisms and computations underlying stress effects on learning and memory. *Current Opinion in Neurobiology*, 21(3), pp.502–508. doi:https://doi.org/10.1016/j.conb.2011.03.003.

LUPUS UK. (n.d.). *What is Lupus?* [online] Available at: https://lupusuk.org.uk/what-is-lupus/ [Accessed 17 Jan. 2025].

Lyne, S.A., Goldblatt, F.M. & Shanahan, E.M. Living with a frozen shoulder – a phenomenological inquiry. *BMC Musculoskelet Disord* **23**, 318 (2022). https://doi.org/10.1186/s12891-022-05251-7

Ma, X., Yue, Z.-Q., Gong, Z.-Q., Zhang, H., Duan, N.-Y., Shi, Y.-T., Wei, G.-X. and Li, Y.-F. (2017). The Effect of Diaphragmatic Breathing on Attention, Negative Affect and Stress in Healthy Adults. *Frontiers in Psychology*, 8(874), pp.1–12. doi:https://doi.org/10.3389/fpsyg.2017.00874.

MacDonald, R.S. (2000). The role of zinc in growth and cell proliferation. *The Journal of nutrition*, [online] 130(5S Suppl), pp.1500S8S. doi:https://doi.org/10.1093/jn/130.5.1500S.

MacGregor, E.A., Frith, A., Ellis, J., Aspinall, L. and Hackshaw, A. (2006). Incidence of migraine relative to menstrual cycle phases of rising and falling estrogen. *Neurology*, 67(12), pp.2154–2158. doi:https://doi.org/10.1212/01.wnl.0000233888.18228.19.

Magliano, M. (2010). Menopausal arthralgia: Fact or fiction. *Maturitas*, 67(1), pp.29–33. doi:https://doi.org/10.1016/j.maturitas.2010.04.009.

Mahdavipour, F., Rahemi, Z., Sadat, Z. and Ajorpaz, N.M. (2019). The effects of foot reflexology on depression during menopause: A randomized controlled clinical trial. *Complementary Therapies in Medicine*, [online] 47, p.102195. doi:https://doi.org/10.1016/j.ctim.2019.102195.

Maier, J.A.M., Locatelli, L., Fedele, G., Cazzaniga, A. and Mazur, A. (2023). Magnesium and the Brain: A Focus on Neuroinflammation and Neurodegeneration. *International Journal of Molecular Sciences*, [online] 24(1), p.223. doi:https://doi.org/10.3390/ijms24010223.

Maintz, L. and Novak, N. (2007). Histamine and histamine intolerance. *The American Journal of Clinical Nutrition*, [online] 85(5), pp.1185–1196.

doi:https://doi.org/10.1093/ajcn/85.5.1185.

Mallampalli, M.P. and Carter, C.L. (2014). Exploring Sex and Gender Differences in Sleep Health: A Society for Women's Health Research Report. *Journal of Women's Health*, [online] 23(7), pp.553–562. doi:https://doi.org/10.1089/jwh.2014.4816.

Manthena S, Rao MV, Penubolu LP, Putcha M, Harsha AV. Effectiveness of CoQ10 Oral Supplements as an Adjunct to Scaling and Root Planing in Improving Periodontal Health. J Clin Diagn Res. 2015 Aug;9(8):ZC26-8. doi: 10.7860/JCDR/2015/13486.6291. Epub 2015 Aug 1. PMID: 26436041; PMCID: PMC4576635.

Mariette (n.d.). *Menopause in the Workplace.* [online] Women's Health Concern. Available at: https://www.womens-health-concern.org/help-and-advice/menopause-in-the-workplace/ [Accessed 4 May 2024].

Mariette-JB (2016). *Bioidentical HRT | British Menopause Society.* [online] British Menopause Society. Available at: https://thebms.org.uk/publications/consensus-statements/bioidentical-hrt/ [Accessed Dec. 2024].

Mariette-JB (2024). *Premature ovarian insufficiency.* [online] British Menopause Society. Available at: https://thebms.org.uk/publications/consensus-statements/premature-ovarian-insufficiency/ [Accessed 2 Sep. 2024].

Marike Lancel, Faulhaber, J., Florian Holsboer and Rupprecht, R. (1996). Progesterone induces changes in sleep comparable to those of agonistic GABAA receptor modulators. *Am J Physiol*, 271(4), pp. E763–E772. doi:https://doi.org/10.1152/ajpendo.1996.271.4.e763.

Mariotti, A. (2015). The effects of chronic stress on health: new insights into the molecular mechanisms of brain–body communication. *Future Science OA*, [online] 1(3). doi:https://doi.org/10.4155/fso.15.21.

Martinelli, D., Pocora, M.M., De Icco, R., Putortì, A. and Tassorelli, C. (2022). Triggers of migraine: where do we stand? *Current Opinion in Neurology*, 35(3), pp.360–366. doi:https://doi.org/10.1097/wco.0000000000001065.

Martínez Steele, E., Baraldi, L.G., Louzada, M.L. da C., Moubarac, J.-C., Mozaffarian, D. and Monteiro, C.A. (2016). Ultra-processed foods and added sugars in the US diet: evidence from a nationally representative cross-sectional study. *BMJ Open*, [online] 6(3), p.e009892. doi:https://doi.org/10.1136/bmjopen-2015-009892.

Mashhadi, N.S., Ghiasvand, R., Askari, G., Hariri, M., Darvishi, L. and Mofid, M.R. (2013). Anti-oxidative and anti-inflammatory effects of ginger in health and physical activity: review of current evidence. *International journal of preventive medicine*, [online] 4(Suppl 1), pp.S36-42. Available at: https://www.ncbi.nlm.nih.gov/pmc/articles/PMC3665023 [Accessed Dec. 2024].

Mason, A.E., Epel, E.S., Kristeller, J., Moran, P.J., Dallman, M., Lustig, R.H., Acree, M., Bacchetti, P., Laraia, B.A., Hecht, F.M. and Daubenmier, J. (2016). Effects of a mindfulness-based intervention on mindful eating, sweets consumption, and fasting glucose levels in obese adults: data from the SHINE randomized controlled trial. *Journal of Behavioral Medicine*, [online] 39(2), pp.201–213. doi:https://doi.org/10.1007/s10865-015-9692-8.

Massé, P.G., Dosy, J., Jougleux, J.-L., Caissie, M. and Howell, D.S. (2005). Bone Mineral Density and Metabolism at an Early Stage of Menopause When Estrogen and Calcium Supplement Are Not Used and without the Interference of Major Confounding Variables. *Journal of the American College of Nutrition*, 24(5), pp.354–360. doi:https://doi.org/10.1080/07315724.2005.10719485.

Mathieu, S., Soubrier, M., Peirs, C., Monfoulet, L.-E., Boirie, Y. and Tournadre,

A. (2022). A Meta-Analysis of the Impact of Nutritional Supplementation on Osteoarthritis Symptoms. *Nutrients*, 14(8), p.1607. doi:https://doi.org/10.3390/nu14081607.

Matsuzawa, Y., Funahashi, T. and Nakamura, T. (2011). The Concept of Metabolic Syndrome: Contribution of Visceral Fat Accumulation and Its Molecular Mechanism. *Journal of Atherosclerosis and Thrombosis*, 18(8), pp.629–639. doi:https://doi.org/10.5551/jat.7922.

Matthews, K., Abrams, B., Crawford, S., Miles, T., Neer, R., Powell, L. and Wesley, D. (2001). Body mass index in mid-life women: relative influence of menopause, hormone use, and ethnicity. *International Journal of Obesity*, 25(6), pp.863–873. doi:https://doi.org/10.1038/sj.ijo.0801618.

Mauvais-Jarvis, F., Clegg, D.J. and Hevener, A.L. (2013). The Role of Estrogens in Control of Energy Balance and Glucose Homeostasis. *Endocrine Reviews*, [online] 34(3), pp.309–338. doi:https://doi.org/10.1210/er.2012-1055.

McCabe, D. and Colbeck, M. (2015). The effectiveness of essential fatty acid, B vitamin, Vitamin C, magnesium and zinc supplementation for managing stress in women: a systematic review protocol. *The JBI Database of Systematic Reviews and Implementation Reports*, 13(7), p.104. doi:https://doi.org/10.11124/jbisrir-2015-2298.

McCabe;Karolina, D. (2013). The impact of essential fatty acid, B vitamins, vitamin C, magnesium and zinc supplementation on stress levels in women. *Jbi Database of Systematic Reviews and Implementation Reports*, [online] 15(2), pp.402–453. doi:https://doi.org/10.11124/JBISRIR-2016-002965.

McCarthy, M. and Raval, A.P. (2020). The perimenopause in a woman's life: a systemic inflammatory phase that enables later neurodegenerative disease. *Journal of Neuroinflammation*, 17(1). doi:https://doi.org/10.1186/s12974-020-

01998-9.

MCEwen, B.S. (2004). Protection and Damage from Acute and Chronic Stress: Allostasis and Allostatic Overload and Relevance to the Pathophysiology of Psychiatric Disorders. *Annals of the New York Academy of Sciences*, 1032(1), pp.1–7. doi:https://doi.org/10.1196/annals.1314.001.

Medagama, A.B. (2015). The glycaemic outcomes of Cinnamon, a review of the experimental evidence and clinical trials. *Nutrition Journal*, [online] 14(1). doi:https://doi.org/10.1186/s12937-015-0098-9.

Medline (2022). *Cancer treatment - early menopause: MedlinePlus Medical Encyclopedia*. [online] medlineplus.gov. Available at: https://medlineplus.gov/ency/patientinstructions/000912.htm [Accessed 22 Sep. 2024].

Mehta, J., Kling, J.M. and Manson, J.E. (2021). Risks, Benefits, and Treatment Modalities of Menopausal Hormone Therapy: Current Concepts. *Frontiers in Endocrinology*, 12(564781). doi:https://doi.org/10.3389/fendo.2021.564781.

Melton, L.J., Chrischilles, E.A., Cooper, C., Lane, A.W. and Riggs, B.L. (2009). Perspective how many women have osteoporosis? *Journal of Bone and Mineral Research*, 7(9), pp.1005–1010. doi:https://doi.org/10.1002/jbmr.5650070902.

Mendelsohn, M.E. and Karas, R.H. (1999). The Protective Effects of Estrogen on the Cardiovascular System. *New England Journal of Medicine*, 340(23), pp.1801–1811. doi:https://doi.org/10.1056/nejm199906103402306.

Mendoza-León, M.J. Mangalam, A.K., Regaldiz, A., González-Madrid, E., Ma. Andreina Rangel-Ramírez, Álvarez-Mardonez, O., Vallejos, O.P., Constanza Méndez, Bueno, S.M., Melo-González, F., Duarte, Y., María Cecilia Opazo, Kalergis, A.M. and Riedel, C.A. (2023). Gut microbiota short-chain fatty acids and their impact on the host thyroid function and diseases. *Frontiers in*

*Endocrinology*, 14. doi:https://doi.org/10.3389/fendo.2023.1192216

Mezian, K. and Chang, K.-V. (2020). *Frozen Shoulder*. [online] PubMed. Available at: https://www.ncbi.nlm.nih.gov/books/NBK482162/ [Accessed 13 Jan. 2025].

Michaud, D.S., Fu, Z., Shi, J. and Chung, M. (2017). Periodontal Disease, Tooth Loss, and Cancer Risk. *Epidemiologic Reviews*, 39(1), pp.49–58. doi:https://doi.org/10.1093/epirev/mxx006.

Michnovicz, J.J., Adlercreutz, H. and Bradlow, H.L. (1997a). Changes in Levels of Urinary Estrogen Metabolites After Oral Indole-3-Carbinol Treatment in Humans. *JNCI Journal of the National Cancer Institute*, [online] 89(10), pp.718–723. doi:https://doi.org/10.1093/jnci/89.10.718.

Mid-Nottinghamshire Integrated Care Partnership (2022). *Menopause-Why do I feel fatigued?* [online] Available at: https://www.nhsemployers.org/system/files/2022-03/Fatigue%20%26%20Menopause%20Leaflet.pdf [Accessed Dec. 2024].

Miller, H. (2024). *Estrogen Metabolism 101 A Practical Guide to Understanding and Measuring*. [online] Available at: https://shop.dutchtest.com/wp-content/uploads/2024/04/Estrogen-Metabolism-March-2024-HM.pdf [Accessed 22 Dec. 2024].

Minich, D.M. (2019). A Review of the Science of Colorful, Plant-Based Food and Practical Strategies for 'Eating the Rainbow'. *Journal of Nutrition and Metabolism*, 2019, pp.1–19. doi:https://doi.org/10.1155/2019/2125070.

Miquel, J., Ramírez-Boscá, A., Ramírez-Bosca, J.V. and Alperi, J.D. (2006). Menopause: A review on the role of oxygen stress and favorable effects of dietary antioxidants. *Archives of Gerontology and Geriatrics*, [online] 42(3), pp.289–

306. doi:https://doi.org/10.1016/j.archger.2005.08.005.

Miranda, M., Morici, J.F., Zanoni, M.B. and Bekinschtein, P. (2019). Brain-Derived Neurotrophic Factor: A Key Molecule for Memory in the Healthy and the Pathological Brain. *Frontiers in Cellular Neuroscience*, 13(363). doi:https://doi.org/10.3389/fncel.2019.00363.

Mirończuk-Chodakowska, I., Witkowska, A.M. and Zujko, M.E. (2018). Endogenous non-enzymatic antioxidants in the human body. *Advances in Medical Sciences*, [online] 63(1), pp.68–78. doi:https://doi.org/10.1016/j.advms.2017.05.005.

Misso, M.L., Jang, C., Adams, J., Tran, J., Murata, Y., Bell, R., Boon, W.C., Simpson, E.R. and Davis, S.R. (2005). Differential expression of factors involved in fat metabolism with age and the menopause transition. *Maturitas*, [online] 51(3), pp.299–306. doi:https://doi.org/10.1016/j.maturitas.2004.08.013.

Molska, M., Kinga Mruczyk, Cisek-Woźniak, A., Prokopowicz, W., Patrycja Szydełko, Zuzanna Jakuszewska, Marzec, K. and Martyna Trocholepsza (2024). The Influence of Intestinal Microbiota on BDNF Levels. *Nutrients*, [online] 16(17), pp.2891–2891. doi:https://doi.org/10.3390/nu16172891.

Moretti, R. and Caruso, P. (2019). The Controversial Role of Homocysteine in Neurology: From Labs to Clinical Practice. *International Journal of Molecular Sciences*, [online] 20(1), p.231. doi:https://doi.org/10.3390/ijms20010231.

Mosconi, L., Nerattini, M., Matthews, D.C., Jett, S., Andy, C., Williams, S., Yepez, C.B., Zarate, C., Carlton, C., Fauci, F., Ajila, T., Pahlajani, S., Andrews, R., Pupi, A., Ballon, D., Kelly, J., Osborne, J.R., Nehmeh, S., Fink, M. and Berti, V. (2024). In vivo brain estrogen receptor density by neuroendocrine aging and relationships with cognition and symptomatology. *Scientific Reports*, [online] 14(1), p.12680. doi:https://doi.org/10.1038/s41598-024-62820-7.

Mottillo, S., Filion, K.B., Genest, J., Joseph, L., Pilote, L., Poirier, P., Rinfret, S., Schiffrin, E.L. and Eisenberg, M.J. (2010). The Metabolic Syndrome and Cardiovascular Risk: A Systematic Review and Meta-Analysis. *Journal of the American College of Cardiology*, [online] 56(14), pp.1113–1132. doi:https://doi.org/10.1016/j.jacc.2010.05.034.

MTHFR Support (2016). *HER-stamine? The Link Between Histamine and Estrogen – MTHFR Support Australia.* [online] mthfrsupport.com.au/. Available at: https://mthfrsupport.com.au/2016/09/her-stamine-the-link-between-histamine-and-estrogen/ [Accessed 19 Nov. 2024].

Mukherjee, A. (2023). *Thyroid and menopause article.* [online] British Thyroid Foundation. Available at: https://www.btf-thyroid.org/thyroid-and-menopause-article [Accessed 10 Jan. 2025].

Mumford, S.L., Schisterman, E.F., Siega-Riz, A.M., Browne, R.W., Gaskins, A.J., Trevisan, M., Steiner, A.Z., Daniels, J.L., Zhang, C., Perkins, N.J. and Wactawski-Wende, J. (2010). A Longitudinal Study of Serum Lipoproteins in Relation to Endogenous Reproductive Hormones during the Menstrual Cycle: Findings from the BioCycle Study. *The Journal of Clinical Endocrinology & Metabolism*, 95(9), pp.E80–E85. doi:https://doi.org/10.1210/jc.2010-0109.

Mumford, S.L.Ph.D. and Schisterman, E.F.Ph.D. (2015). *Women's cholesterol levels vary with phase of menstrual cycle.* [online] National Institutes of Health (NIH). Available at: https://www.nih.gov/news-events/news-releases/womens-cholesterol-levels-vary-phase-menstrual-cycle [Accessed 30 Dec. 2024].

Mutlu, M., Argun, M., Kilic, E., Saraymen, R. and Yazar, S. (2007). Magnesium, Zinc and Copper Status in Osteoporotic, Osteopenic and Normal Postmenopausal Women. *Journal of International Medical Research*, 35(5), pp.692–695. doi:https://doi.org/10.1177/147323000703500514.

Myers, M.G., Leibel, R.L., Seeley, R.J. and Schwartz, M.W. (2010). Obesity and leptin resistance: distinguishing cause from effect. *Trends in Endocrinology & Metabolism*, [online] 21(11), pp.643–651. doi:https://doi.org/10.1016/j.tem.2010.08.002.

Nagy, B., Szekeres-Barthó, J., Kovács, G.L., Sulyok, E., Farkas, B., Várnagy, Á., Vértes, V., Kovács, K. and Bódis, J. (2021). Key to Life: Physiological Role and Clinical Implications of Progesterone. *International Journal of Molecular Sciences*, 22(20), p.11039. doi:https://doi.org/10.3390/ijms222011039.

Nair, A.R., Pillai, A.J. and Nair, N. (2020). Cardiovascular Changes in Menopause. *Current Cardiology Reviews*, 16(4). doi:https://doi.org/10.2174/1573403x16666201106141811.

Nakai, K. and Tsuruta, D. (2021). What Are Reactive Oxygen Species, Free Radicals, and Oxidative Stress in Skin Diseases? *International Journal of Molecular Sciences*, 22(19), p.10799. doi:https://doi.org/10.3390/ijms221910799.

NAMS Hormone Therapy Position Statement Advisory Panel (2017). The 2017 hormone therapy position statement of The North American Menopause Society. *Menopause (2017)*, [online] 24(7):728–53. doi:https://doi.org/10.1097/GME.0000000000000921 NAMS 2017 Hormone Therapy Position Statement Advisory Panel.

Nappi, R.E. and Palacios, S. (2014). Impact of vulvovaginal atrophy on sexual health and quality of life at postmenopause. *Climacteric*, 17(1), pp.3–9. doi:https://doi.org/10.3109/13697137.2013.871696.

Nappi, R.E. and Simoncini, T. (2021). Menopause transition: a golden age to prevent cardiovascular disease. *The Lancet Diabetes & Endocrinology*, [online] 9(3), pp.135–137. doi:https://doi.org/10.1016/S2213-8587(21)00018-8.

National Institute of Diabetes and Digestive and Kidney Diseases (2021). *Hypothyroidism (underactive thyroid).* [online] National Institute of Diabetes and Digestive and Kidney Diseases. Available at: https://www.niddk.nih.gov/health-information/endocrine-diseases/hypothyroidism.

National Institute of Health (2024). *National Institutes of Health Office of Dietary Supplements: Iron Fact Sheet for Health Professionals https://ods.od.nih.gov/factsheets/Iron-HealthProfessional/.*

National Institutes of Health (2022). *Office of Dietary Supplements - Iodine.* [online] Nih.gov. Available at: https://ods.od.nih.gov/factsheets/Iodine-HealthProfessional/ [Accessed 28 Dec. 2024].

Nattagh-Eshtivani, E., Sani, M.A., Dahri, M., Ghalichi, F., Ghavami, A., Arjang, P. and Tarighat-Esfanjani, A. (2018). The role of nutrients in the pathogenesis and treatment of migraine headaches: Review. *Biomedicine & Pharmacotherapy*, 102, pp.317–325. doi:https://doi.org/10.1016/j.biopha.2018.03.059.

Navab M, Berliner JA, Watson AD, Hama SY, Territo MC, Lusis AJ, Shih DM, Van Lenten BJ, Frank JS, Demer LL, Edwards PA, Fogelman AM. The Yin and Yang of oxidation in the development of the fatty streak. A review based on the 1994 George Lyman Duff Memorial Lecture. *Arterioscler Thromb Vasc Biol.* 1996; *16*: 831–842

Negar Bafkar, Sheida Zeraattalab-Motlagh, Jayedi, A. and Sakineh Shab-Bidar (2024). Efficacy and safety of omega-3 fatty acids supplementation for anxiety symptoms: a systematic review and dose-response meta-analysis of randomized controlled trials. *BMC Psychiatry*, 24(1). doi:https://doi.org/10.1186/s12888-024-05881-2.

Nettore, I.C., Albano, L., Ungaro, P., Colao, A. and Macchia, P.E. (2017). Sunshine vitamin and thyroid. *Reviews in Endocrine and Metabolic Disorders*,

18(3), pp.347–354. doi:https://doi.org/10.1007/s11154-017-9406-3.

Neumann, A.-M., Schmidt, C.X., Brockmann, R.M. and Oster, H. (2019). Circadian regulation of endocrine systems. *Autonomic Neuroscience*, [online] 216, pp.1–8. doi:https://doi.org/10.1016/j.autneu.2018.10.001.

NeuroLaunch Editorial Team (2024). *DHEA and Cortisol: The Intricate Relationship and Its Role in Stress Management.* [online] NeuroLaunch.com. Available at: https://neurolaunch.com/dhea-and-cortisol-relationship/ [Accessed 8 Jan. 2025].

New, S.A., Robins, S.P., Campbell, M.K., Martin, J.C., Garton, M.J., Bolton-Smith, C., Grubb, D.A., Lee, S.J. and Reid, D.M. (2000). Dietary influences on bone mass and bone metabolism: further evidence of a positive link between fruit and vegetable consumption and bone health? *The American Journal of Clinical Nutrition*, [online] 71(1), pp.142–151. doi:https://doi.org/10.1093/ajcn/71.1.142.

Newnham, R.E. (1994). Essentiality of boron for healthy bones and joints. *Environmental Health Perspectives*, 102(suppl 7), pp.83–85. doi:https://doi.org/10.1289/ehp.94102s783.

Newson, D.L. (n.d.). *Resources.* [online] Newson Health Menopause and Wellbeing Centre. Available at: https://www.newsonhealth.co.uk/resources/ [Accessed Jun. 2024].

Nguyen, H. and Gupta, V. (2021). *Alpha-Lipoic Acid.* [online] PubMed. Available at: https://www.ncbi.nlm.nih.gov/books/NBK564301/ [Accessed 19 Jan. 2025].

Nguyen, N.D., Ahlborg, H.G., Center, J.R., Eisman, J.A. and Nguyen, T.V. (2007). Residual Lifetime Risk of Fractures in Women and Men. *Journal of Bone and Mineral Research*, [online] 22(6), pp.781-788. doi:https://doi.org/10.1359/jbmr.070315.

NHS (2020). *Doing a pregnancy test.* [online] nhs.uk. Available at: https://www.nhs.uk/pregnancy/trying-for-a-baby/doing-a-pregnancy-test/ [Accessed 8 Jan. 2025].

NHS (2023). *Types of hormone replacement therapy (HRT).* [online] nhs.uk. Available at: https://www.nhs.uk/medicines/hormone-replacement-therapy-hrt/types-of-hormone-replacement-therapy-hrt/ [Accessed Dec. 2024].

NICE (2019). *Overview | Menopause: diagnosis and management | Guidance | NICE.* [online] Nice.org.uk. Available at: https://www.nice.org.uk/guidance/ng23 [Accessed Dec. 2024].

NICE. (2022). *CKS is only available in the UK.* [online] Available at: https://cks.nice.org.uk/topics/menopause/prescribing-information/hormone-replacement-therapy-hrt/ [Accessed Dec. 2024].

Nie, X., Xie, R. and Tuo, B. (2018). Effects of Estrogen on the Gastrointestinal Tract. *Digestive Diseases and Sciences*, [online] 63(3), pp.583–596. doi:https://doi.org/10.1007/s10620-018-4939-1.

Nielsen, F.H. (2010). Magnesium, inflammation, and obesity in chronic disease. *Nutrition Reviews*, 68(6), pp.333–340. doi:https://doi.org/10.1111/j.1753-4887.2010.00293.x.

Noah, L., Dye, L., Bois De Fer, B., Mazur, A., Pickering, G. and Pouteau, E. (2021). Effect of magnesium and vitamin B6 supplementation on mental health and quality of life in stressed healthy adults: Post-hoc analysis of a randomised controlled trial. *Stress and Health*, 37(5). doi:https://doi.org/10.1002/smi.3051.

North American Menopause Society (2022). The 2022 hormone therapy position statement of The North American Menopause Society. *Menopause (New York, N.Y.)*, [online] 29(7), pp.767–794. doi:https://doi.org/10.1097/GME.0000000000002028.

Novella, S., Dantas, A.P., Segarra, G., Medina, P. and Hermenegildo, C. (2012). Vascular Aging in Women: is Estrogen the Fountain of Youth? *Frontiers in Physiology*, 3. doi:https://doi.org/10.3389/fphys.2012.00165.

NPR (2024). *Most animals don't go through menopause. So why do these whales? : Short Wave*. [online] NPR. Available at: https://www.npr.org/2024/03/22/1198909539/menopause-humans-whales-evolution [Accessed 8 Mar. 2024].

Nuss, P. (2015). Anxiety disorders and GABA neurotransmission: a disturbance of modulation. *Neuropsychiatric Disease and Treatment*, [online] 11(11), p.165. doi:https://doi.org/10.2147/ndt.s58841.

O'Connor, Á. and Crosswaite, S. (2018). Can healthy motivated British adults achieve the revised UK government fibre recommendations of 30 g per day? Results from a preliminary study. *Nutrition and Health*, 24(4), pp.211–215. doi:https://doi.org/10.1177/0260106018794558.

O'Kane, S.M., Mulhern, M.S., Pourshahidi, L.K., Strain, J.J. and Yeates, A.J. (2018). Micronutrients, iodine status and concentrations of thyroid hormones: a systematic review. *Nutrition Reviews*, [online] 76(6), pp.418–431. doi:https://doi.org/10.1093/nutrit/nuy008.

O'Sullivan, T.A., Bremner, A.P., O'Neill, S. and Lyons-Wall, P. (2010). Glycaemic load is associated with insulin resistance in older Australian women. *European Journal of Clinical Nutrition*, [online] 64(1), pp.80–87. doi:https://doi.org/10.1038/ejcn.2009.115.

Odai, T., Terauchi, M., Hirose, A., Kato, K., Akiyoshi, M. and Miyasaka, N. (2019). Severity of hot flushes is inversely associated with dietary intake of vitamin B6 and oily fish. *Climacteric*, 22(6), pp.617–621. doi:https://doi.org/10.1080/13697137.2019.1609440.

Office of the Surgeon General (US) (2024). *Office of the Surgeon General (US). Bone Health and Osteoporosis: A Report of the Surgeon General. Rockville (MD): Office of the Surgeon General (US); 2004. 2, The Basics of Bone in Health and Disease. Available from: https://www.ncbi.nlm.nih.gov/books/NBK45504/).*

Ogun, O.A., Büki, B., Cohn, E.S., Janky, K.L. and Lundberg, Y.W. (2014). Menopause and benign paroxysmal positional vertigo. *Menopause*, 21(8), pp.886–889. doi:https://doi.org/10.1097/gme.0000000000000190.

Ojo, O., Feng, Q.-Q., Ojo, O.O. and Wang, X.-H. (2020). The Role of Dietary Fibre in Modulating Gut Microbiota Dysbiosis in Patients with Type 2 Diabetes: A Systematic Review and Meta-Analysis of Randomised Controlled Trials. *Nutrients*, 12(11), p.3239. doi:https://doi.org/10.3390/nu12113239.

Oliveira, N.S. de, Lima, A.B.F. de, Brito, J.C.R. de, Sarmento, A.C.A., Gonçalves, A.K.S. and Eleutério, J. (2022). Postmenopausal Vaginal Microbiome and Microbiota. *Frontiers in Reproductive Health*, 3. doi:https://doi.org/10.3389/frph.2021.780931.

Oregon State University (2019). *Glycemic Index and Glycemic Load.* [online] Linus Pauling Institute. Available at: https://lpi.oregonstate.edu/mic/food-beverages/glycemic-index-glycemic-load [Accessed 11 Jan. 2025].

Oren, I., Fleishman, S.J., Kessel, A. and Ben-Tal, N. (2004). Free Diffusion of Steroid Hormones Across Biomembranes: A Simplex Search with Implicit Solvent Model Calculations. *Biophysical Journal*, 87(2), pp.768–779. doi:https://doi.org/10.1529/biophysj.103.035527.

Organization, W.H. (1994). *Assessment of fracture risk and its application to screening for postmenopausal osteoporosis : report of a WHO study group [meeting held in Rome from 22 to 25 June 1992]*. [online] *iris.who.int*. World Health Organization. Available at: https://iris.who.int/handle/10665/39142.

Otberg, N., Finner, A.M. and Shapiro, J. (2007). Androgenetic Alopecia. *Endocrinology and Metabolism Clinics of North America*, 36(2), pp.379–398. doi:https://doi.org/10.1016/j.ecl.2007.03.004.

Ouchi, N., Ohishi, M., Kihara, S., Funahashi, T., Nakamura, T., Nagaretani, H., Kumada, M., Ohashi, K., Okamoto, Y., Nishizawa, H., Kishida, K., Maeda, N., Nagasawa, A., Kobayashi, H., Hiraoka, H., Komai, N., Kaibe, M., Rakugi, H., Ogihara, T. and Matsuzawa, Y. (2003). Association of Hypoadiponectinemia With Impaired Vasoreactivity. *Hypertension*, 42(3), pp.231–234. doi:https://doi.org/10.1161/01.hyp.0000083488.67550.b8.

Oyola, M.G. and Handa, R.J. (2017). Hypothalamic-pituitary-adrenal and hypothalamic-pituitary-gonadal axes: sex differences in regulation of stress responsivity. *Stress (Amsterdam, Netherlands)*, [online] 20(5), pp.476–494. doi:https://doi.org/10.1080/10253890.2017.1369523.

Paddon-Jones D, Rasmussen BB. Dietary protein recommendations and the prevention of sarcopenia. *Curr Opin Clin Nutr Metab Care*. 2009 Jan;12(1):86-90. doi: 10.1097/MCO.0b013e32831cef8b. PMID: 19057193; PMCID: PMC2760315.

Palatnik, A., Frolov, K., Fux, M. and Benjamin, J. (2001). Double-Blind, Controlled, Crossover Trial of Inositol Versus Fluvoxamine for the Treatment of Panic Disorder. *Journal of Clinical Psychopharmacology*, 21(3), pp.335–339. doi:https://doi.org/10.1097/00004714-200106000-00014.

Panay, N., Ang, S.B., Cheshire, R., Goldstein, S.R., Maki, P. and Nappi, R.E. (2024). Menopause and MHT in 2024: addressing the key controversies – an International Menopause Society White Paper. *Climacteric*, 27(5), pp.441–457. doi:https://doi.org/10.1080/13697137.2024.2394950.

Papavagelis, C., Avgeraki, E., Augoulea, A., Stamatelopoulos, K., Lambrinoudaki, I. and Yannakoulia, M. (2018). Dietary patterns, Mediterranean diet and obesity in postmenopausal women. *Maturitas*, [online] 110, pp.79–85. doi:https://doi.org/10.1016/j.maturitas.2018.02.001.

Paramsothy, P., Harlow, S.D., Elliott, M.R., Yosef, M., Lisabeth, L.D., Greendale, G.A., Gold, E.B., Crawford, S.L. and Randolph, J.F. (2015). Influence of race/ethnicity, body mass index, and proximity of menopause on menstrual cycle patterns in the menopausal transition. *Menopause*, 22(2), pp.159–165. doi:https://doi.org/10.1097/gme.0000000000000293.

Park, C., Lee, J., Kong, B., Park, J., Song, H., Choi, K., Guon, T. and Lee, Y. (2019). The effects of bisphenol A, benzyl butyl phthalate, and di(2-ethylhexyl) phthalate on estrogen receptor alpha in estrogen receptor-positive cells under hypoxia. *Environmental Pollution*, 248, pp.774–781. doi:https://doi.org/10.1016/j.envpol.2019.02.069.

Pascoe, M.C., Thompson, D.R., Jenkins, Z.M. and Ski, C.F. (2017). Mindfulness mediates the physiological markers of stress: Systematic review and meta-analysis. *Journal of Psychiatric Research*, 95, pp.156–178. doi:https://doi.org/10.1016/j.jpsychires.2017.08.004.

Patak, P., Willenberg, H.S. and Bornstein, S.R. (2004). Vitamin C Is an Important Cofactor for Both Adrenal Cortex and Adrenal Medulla. *Endocrine Research*, 30(4), pp.871–875. doi:https://doi.org/10.1081/erc-200044126.

Patel, D.P., Swink, S.M. and Castelo-Soccio, L. (2017). A Review of the Use of Biotin for Hair Loss. *Skin Appendage Disorders*, [online] 3(3), pp.166–169. doi:https://doi.org/10.1159/000462981.

Patel, R. and DuPont, H.L. (2015). New Approaches for Bacteriotherapy: Prebiotics, New-Generation Probiotics, and Synbiotics. *Clinical Infectious Diseases*, 60(suppl_2), pp.S108–S121. doi:https://doi.org/10.1093/cid/civ177.

Pavlović, J.M. (2020). The impact of midlife on migraine in women: summary of current views. *Women's Midlife Health*, 6(1). doi:https://doi.org/10.1186/s40695-020-00059-8.

Pazaiti, A. and Fentiman, I.S. (2011). Basal Phenotype Breast Cancer: Implications for Treatment and Prognosis. *Women's Health*, 7(2), pp.181–202. doi:https://doi.org/10.2217/whe.11.5.

PE, K. (2017). Good Mood Foods. *Journal of Nutritional Health & Food Engineering*, 7(4). doi:https://doi.org/10.15406/jnhfe.2017.07.00246.

Pelczyńska, M., Moszak, M. and Bogdański, P. (2022). The Role of Magnesium in the Pathogenesis of Metabolic Disorders. *Nutrients*, 14(9), p.1714. doi:https://doi.org/10.3390/nu14091714.

Pereira, J.C. and Andersen, M.L. (2014). The role of thyroid hormone in sleep deprivation. *Medical Hypotheses*, [online] 82(3), pp.350–355. doi:https://doi.org/10.1016/j.mehy.2014.01.003.

Pertyńska-Marczewska, M. and Pertyński, T. (2021). Postmenopausal women in gynecological care. *Menopausal Review*, 20(2), pp.88–98. doi:https://doi.org/10.5114/pm.2021.107103.

Peter, A., Kantartzis, K., Machann, J., Schick, F., Staiger, H., Machicao, F., Schleicher, E., Fritsche, A., Haring, H.-U. . and Stefan, N. (2010). Relationships of Circulating Sex Hormone-Binding Globulin With Metabolic Traits in Humans. *Diabetes*, 59(12), pp.3167–3173. doi:https://doi.org/10.2337/db10-0179.

Peters, B., Santoro, N., Kaplan, R. and Qi, Q. (2022). Spotlight on the Gut Microbiome in Menopause: Current Insights. *International Journal of Women's Health*, Volume 14(14), pp.1059–1072. doi:https://doi.org/10.2147/ijwh.s340491.

Pettigrew, J.A. and Novick, A.M. (2021). Hypoactive Sexual Desire Disorder in Women: Physiology, Assessment, Diagnosis, and Treatment. *Journal of Midwifery & Women's Health*, 66(6). doi:https://doi.org/10.1111/jmwh.13283.

Phan, M.L., Renshaw, T.L., Caramanico, J., Greeson, J.M., MacKenzie, E., Atkinson-Diaz, Z., Doppelt, N., Tai, H., Mandell, D.S. and Nuske, H.J. (2022). Mindfulness-Based School Interventions: a Systematic Review of Outcome Evidence Quality by Study Design. *Mindfulness*, 13(7). doi:https://doi.org/10.1007/s12671-022-01885-9.

Pi-Sunyer, F.X. (2002). The Obesity Epidemic: Pathophysiology and Consequences of Obesity. *Obesity Research*, 10(S12), pp.97S104S. doi:https://doi.org/10.1038/oby.2002.202.

Pickering, G., Mazur, A., Trousselard, M., Bienkowski, P., Yaltsewa, N., Amessou, M., Noah, L. and Pouteau, E. (2020). Magnesium status and stress: The vicious circle concept revisited. *Nutrients*, [online] 12(12), p.3672. doi:https://doi.org/10.3390/nu12123672.

Pierdominici, M., Maselli, A., Colasanti, T., Giammarioli, A.M., Delunardo, F., Vacirca, D., Sanchez, M., Giovannetti, A., Malorni, W. and Ortona, E. (2010). Estrogen receptor profiles in human peripheral blood lymphocytes. *Immunology Letters*, 132(1-2), pp.79–85. doi:https://doi.org/10.1016/j.imlet.2010.06.003.

Pike, C.J. (2012). Sex hormones aging and Alzheimer s disease. *Frontiers in Bioscience*, E4(3), pp.976–997. doi:https://doi.org/10.2741/e434.

Pinkerton, J.V. and Santoro, N. (2015). Compounded bioidentical hormone therapy. *Menopause*, 22(9), pp.926–936. doi:https://doi.org/10.1097/gme.0000000000000420.

Pizzorno L. (2015)Nothing Boring About Boron. Integr Med (Encinitas). 2015

Aug;14(4):35-48. PMID: 26770156; PMCID: PMC4712861.

Plottel, Claudia S. and Blaser, Martin J. (2011). Microbiome and Malignancy. *Cell Host & Microbe*, 10(4), pp.324–335. doi:https://doi.org/10.1016/j.chom.2011.10.003.

Pludowski, P., Grant, W.B., Karras, S.N., Zittermann, A. and Pilz, S. (2024). Vitamin D Supplementation: A Review of the Evidence Arguing for a Daily Dose of 2000 International Units (50 µg) of Vitamin D for Adults in the General Population. *Nutrients*, [online] 16(3), p.391. doi:https://doi.org/10.3390/nu16030391.

Pochwat, B., Sowa-Kucma, M., Kotarska, K., Misztak, P., Nowak, G. and Szewczyk, B. (2014). Antidepressant-like activity of magnesium in the olfactory bulbectomy model is associated with the AMPA/BDNF pathway. *Psychopharmacology*, 232(2), pp.355–367. doi:https://doi.org/10.1007/s00213-014-3671-6.

Poirier, P., Giles, T.D., Bray, G.A., Hong, Y., Stern, J.S., Pi-Sunyer, F.X. and Eckel, R.H. (2006). Obesity and Cardiovascular Disease: Pathophysiology, Evaluation, and Effect of Weight Loss. *Circulation*, [online] 113(6), pp.898–918. doi:https://doi.org/10.1161/circulationaha.106.171016.

Polo-Kantola, P. (2011). Sleep problems in midlife and beyond. *Maturitas*, 68(3), pp.224–232. doi:https://doi.org/10.1016/j.maturitas.2010.12.009.

Popkin, B.M. D'Anci, K.E. Rosenberg, I.H. (2010). Water, hydration, and health , Nutrition Reviews ,68(8), 439–458. doi:10.1111/j.1753-4887.2010.00304. (n.d.).

Portman, D.J. and Gass, M.L.S. (2014). Genitourinary syndrome of menopause. *Menopause*, 21(10), pp.1063–1068. doi:https://doi.org/10.1097/gme.0000000000000329.

Pouilles, J.M., Tremollieres, F. and Ribot, C. (2009). Effect of menopause on femoral and vertebral bone loss. *Journal of Bone and Mineral Research*, 10(10), pp.1531–1536. doi:https://doi.org/10.1002/jbmr.5650101014.

Practitioners, T.R.A.C. of general and Farrell AM, E. (2017). *Genitourinary syndrome of menopause.* [online] Australian Family Physician. Available at: https://www.racgp.org.au/afp/2017/july/genitourinary-syndrome-of-menopause [Accessed 11 Jan. 2025].

Prakash, R., Fu, L. and Doreswamy, V. (2014). The biochemical pathways of central nervous system neural degeneration in niacin deficiency. *Neural Regeneration Research*, 9(16), p.1509. doi:https://doi.org/10.4103/1673-5374.139475.

Prasad, A.S. and Bao, B. (2019). Molecular Mechanisms of Zinc as a Pro-Antioxidant Mediator: Clinical Therapeutic Implications. *Antioxidants*, 8(6), p.164. doi:https://doi.org/10.3390/antiox8060164.

Price, V.H. (2003). Androgenetic Alopecia in Women. *Journal of Investigative Dermatology Symposium Proceedings*, [online] 8(1), pp.24–27. doi:https://doi.org/10.1046/j.1523-1747.2003.12168.x.

Prior, J.C. (2018). Progesterone for the prevention and treatment of osteoporosis in women. *Climacteric*, 21(4), pp.366–374. doi:https://doi.org/10.1080/13697137.2018.1467400.

Prior, J.C. (2018). Progesterone for treatment of symptomatic menopausal women. *Climacteric*, 21(4), pp.358–365. doi:https://doi.org/10.1080/13697137.2018.1472567.

Prousky, J. and Seely, D. (2005). The treatment of migraines and tension-type headaches with intravenous and oral niacin (nicotinic acid): systematic review of the literature. *Nutrition Journal*, 4(1). doi:https://doi.org/10.1186/1475-2891-4-3.

Rachner, T.D., Khosla, S. and Hofbauer, L.C. (2011). Osteoporosis: now and the future. *The Lancet*, [online] 377(9773), pp.1276–1287. doi:https://doi.org/10.1016/s0140-6736(10)62349-5.

Radahmadi, M., Hosseini, N., Alaei, H. and Sharifi, M.R. (2016). The Effect of Preventive, Therapeutic and Protective Exercises on Hippocampal memory Mediators in Stressed Rats. *Malaysian Journal of Medical Sciences*, 23(5), pp.29–37. doi:https://doi.org/10.21315/mjms2016.23.5.4.

Rajaei, E., Mowla, K., Ghorbani, A., Bahadoram, S., Bahadoram, M. and Dargahi-Malamir, M. (2015). The Effect of Omega-3 Fatty Acids in Patients With Active Rheumatoid Arthritis Receiving DMARDs Therapy: Double-Blind Randomized Controlled Trial. *Global Journal of Health Science*, [online] 8(7), p.18. doi:https://doi.org/10.5539/gjhs.v8n7p18.

Rangel-Huerta, O.D., Aguilera, C.M., Mesa, M.D. and Gil, A. (2012). Omega-3 long-chain polyunsaturated fatty acids supplementation on inflammatory biomakers: a systematic review of randomised clinical trials. *British Journal of Nutrition*, [online] 107(S2), pp.S159–S170. doi:https://doi.org/10.1017/s0007114512001559.

Rao, S.S.C., Yu, S. and Fedewa, A. (2015). Systematic review: dietary fibre and FODMAP-restricted diet in the management of constipation and irritable bowel syndrome. *Alimentary Pharmacology & Therapeutics*, 41(12), pp.1256–1270. doi:https://doi.org/10.1111/apt.13167.

Reiter, R.J. (1991). Pineal melatonin: cell biology of its synthesis and of its physiological interactions. *Endocrine Reviews*, [online] 12(2), pp.151–180. doi:https://doi.org/10.1210/edrv-12-2-151.

Ricker, M.A. and Haas, W.C. (2017). Anti-Inflammatory Diet in Clinical Practice: A Review. *Nutrition in Clinical Practice: Official Publication of the American Society for Parenteral and Enteral Nutrition*, [online] 32(3), pp.318–325. doi:https://doi.org/10.1177/0884533617700353.

Riegel, B., Dunbar, S.B., Fitzsimons, D., Freedland, K.E., Lee, C.S., Middleton, S., Stromberg, A., Vellone, E., Webber, D.E. and Jaarsma, T. (2019). Self-care research: Where are we now? Where are we going? *International Journal of Nursing Studies*, [online] 116(103402), p.103402. doi:https://doi.org/10.1016/j.ijnurstu.2019.103402.

Riggs, B.L. (2000). The mechanisms of estrogen regulation of bone resorption. *Journal of Clinical Investigation*, [online] 106(10), pp.1203–1204. doi:https://doi.org/10.1172/jci11468.

Rinaldi, F., Trink, A., Giorgia Mondadori, Giuliani, G. and Pinto, D. (2023). The Menopausal Transition: Is the Hair Follicle 'Going through Menopause'? *Biomedicines*, [online] 11(11), pp.3041–3041. doi:https://doi.org/10.3390/biomedicines11113041.

Rizzoli, R. (2014). Nutritional aspects of bone health. *Best Practice & Research Clinical Endocrinology & Metabolism*, 28(6), pp.795–808. doi:https://doi.org/10.1016/j.beem.2014.08.003.

Roberfroid, M., Gibson, G.R., Hoyles, L., McCartney, A.L., Rastall, R., Rowland, I., Wolvers, D., Watzl, B., Szajewska, H., Stahl, B., Guarner, F., Respondek, F., Whelan, K., Coxam, V., Davicco, M.-J., Léotoing, L., Wittrant, Y., Delzenne, N.M., Cani, P.D. and Neyrinck, A.M. (2010). Prebiotic effects: metabolic and health benefits. *British Journal of Nutrition*, 104(S2), pp.S1–S63. doi:https://doi.org/10.1017/s0007114510003363.

Roberto Cosimo Melcangi, Garcia-Segura, L.M. and Ayikoe Guy Mensah-

Nyagan (2008). Neuroactive steroids: State of the art and new perspectives. *Cellular and Molecular Life Sciences*, 65(5), pp.777–797. doi:https://doi.org/10.1007/s00018-007-7403-5.

Robinson, L. (2023). *https://www.womens-health-concern.org/wp-content/uploads/2022/12/11-WHC-FACTSHEET-HRT-BenefitsRisks-NOV2022-B.pdf.*

Robinson, M., Sheets Cook, S. and Currie, L.M. (2011). Systemic lupus erythematosus: A genetic review for advanced practice nurses. *Journal of the American Academy of Nurse Practitioners*, 23(12), pp.629–637. doi:https://doi.org/10.1111/j.1745-7599.2011.00675.x.

Rochlani, Y., Pothineni, N.V., Kovelamudi, S. and Mehta, J.L. (2017). Metabolic syndrome: pathophysiology, management, and modulation by natural compounds. *Therapeutic Advances in Cardiovascular Disease*, 11(8), pp.215–225. doi:https://doi.org/10.1177/1753944717711379.

Rodríguez-Olleros Rodríguez, C. and Díaz Curiel, M. (2019). Vitamin K and Bone Health: A Review on the Effects of Vitamin K Deficiency and Supplementation and the Effect of Non-Vitamin K Antagonist Oral Anticoagulants on Different Bone Parameters. *Journal of Osteoporosis*, [online] 2019, pp.1–8. doi:https://doi.org/10.1155/2019/2069176.

Rønn, S.H., Harsløf, T., Pedersen, S.B. and Langdahl, B.L. (2016). Vitamin K2 (menaquinone-7) prevents age-related deterioration of trabecular bone microarchitecture at the tibia in postmenopausal women. *European Journal of Endocrinology*, [online] 175(6), pp.541–549. doi:https://doi.org/10.1530/EJE-16-0498.

Rønn, S.H., Harsløf, T., Pedersen, S.B. and Langdahl, B.L. (2016). Vitamin K2 (menaquinone-7) prevents age-related deterioration of trabecular bone microarchitecture at the tibia in postmenopausal women. *European Journal of*

*Endocrinology*, [online] 175(6), pp.541–549. doi:https://doi.org/10.1530/EJE-16-0498.

Rosamond, W., Flegal, K., Furie, K., Go, A., Greenlund, K., Haase, N., Hailpern, S.M., Ho, M., Howard, V., Kissela, B., Kittner, S., Lloyd-Jones, D., McDermott, M., Meigs, J., Moy, C., Nichol, G., O'Donnell, C., Roger, V., Sorlie, P. and Steinberger, J. (2008). Heart Disease and Stroke Statistics—2008 Update. *Circulation*, 117(4). doi:https://doi.org/10.1161/circulationaha.107.187998.

Rosenthal, M.D., Patel, J., Staton, K., Martindale, R.G., Moore, F.A. and Upchurch, G.R. (2018). Can Specialized Pro-resolving Mediators Deliver Benefit Originally Expected from Fish Oil? *Current Gastroenterology Reports*, 20(9). doi:https://doi.org/10.1007/s11894-018-0647-4.

Ross AC, Taylor CL, Yaktine AL, et al. (2011). *Overview of Calcium*. [online] Nih.gov. Available at: https://www.ncbi.nlm.nih.gov/books/NBK56060/ [Accessed Apr. 2024].

Ruan, X., Seeger, H., Wallwiener, D., Huober, J. and Mueck, A.O. (2014). The ratio of the estradiol metabolites 2-hydroxyestrone (2-OHE1) and 16?-hydroxyestrone (16-OHE1) may predict breast cancer risk in postmenopausal but not in premenopausal women: two case–control studies. *Archives of Gynecology and Obstetrics*, 291(5), pp.1141–1146. doi:https://doi.org/10.1007/s00404-014-3512-1.

Rude, R.K., Singer, F.R. and Gruber, H.E. (2009). Skeletal and hormonal effects of magnesium deficiency. *Journal of the American College of Nutrition*, [online] 28(2), pp.131–41. doi:https://doi.org/10.1080/07315724.2009.10719764.

Rudnicka, E., Kruszewska, J., Klicka, K., Kowalczyk, J., Grymowicz, M., Skórska, J., Pięta, W. and Smolarczyk, R. (2018a). Premature ovarian insufficiency – aetiopathology, epidemiology, and diagnostic evaluation. *Menopausal Review*,

17(3), pp.105–108. doi:https://doi.org/10.5114/pm.2018.78550.

Rupprecht, R. and Holsboer, F. (1999). Neuroactive steroids: mechanisms of action and neuropsychopharmacological perspectives. *Trends in Neurosciences*, 22(9), pp.410–416. doi:https://doi.org/10.1016/s0166-2236(99)01399-5.

Russell, A.S., Dennison, E. and Cooper, C. (2003). Epidemiology and public health impact of osteoporosis. *The Royal Society of Chemistry eBooks*, pp.13–24. doi:https://doi.org/10.1039/9781847551559-00013.

Rybaczyk, L.A., Bashaw, M.J., Pathak, D.R., Moody, S.M., Gilders, R.M. and Holzschu, D.L. (2005). An overlooked connection: serotonergic mediation of estrogen-related physiology and pathology. *BMC Women's Health*, [online] 5(1). doi:https://doi.org/10.1186/1472-6874-5-12.

Rzepecki, A.K., Murase, J.E., Juran, R., Fabi, S.G. and McLellan, B.N. (2019). Estrogen-deficient skin: The role of topical therapy. *International Journal of Women's Dermatology*, 5(2), pp.85–90. doi:https://doi.org/10.1016/j.ijwd.2019.01.001.

Salas-Salvadó, J., Guasch-Ferré, M., Lee, C.-H., Estruch, R., Clish, C.B. and Ros, E. (2015). Protective Effects of the Mediterranean Diet on Type 2 Diabetes and Metabolic Syndrome. *The Journal of Nutrition*, [online] 146(4), pp.920S927S. doi:https://doi.org/10.3945/jn.115.218487.

Saltiel, A.R. and Olefsky, J.M. (2017). Inflammatory mechanisms linking obesity and metabolic disease. *Journal of Clinical Investigation*, [online] 127(1), pp.1–4. doi:https://doi.org/10.1172/jci92035.

Samar, Wang, L., Brooks, M.M., Thurston, R.C., Derby, C.A. and Matthews, K.A. (2016). Increase HDL-C level over the menopausal transition is associated with greater atherosclerotic progression. *Journal of clinical lipidology*, 10(4), pp.962–969. doi:https://doi.org/10.1016/j.jacl.2016.04.008.

Samavat, H. and Kurzer, M.S. (2015). Estrogen metabolism and breast cancer. *Cancer Letters*, [online] 356(2), pp.231–243. doi:https://doi.org/10.1016/j.canlet.2014.04.018.

Sammaritano, L.R. (2012). Menopause in patients with autoimmune diseases. *Autoimmunity Reviews*, 11(6-7), pp.A430–A436. doi:https://doi.org/10.1016/j.autrev.2011.11.006.

Sampson, W.H. (n.d.). *Sampson HW. Alcohol's harmful effects on bone. Alcohol Health Res World. 1998;22(3):190-4. PMID: 15706795; PMCID: PMC6761900..*

Sánchez-Borrego R, von Schacky C, Osorio MJA, Llaneza P, Pinto X, Losa F, Navarro MC, Lubián D, Mendoza N. (2017). Recommendations of the Spanish Menopause Society on the consumption of omega-3 polyunsaturated fatty acids by postmenopausal women. *Maturitas*, [online] 103, pp.71–77. doi:https://doi.org/10.1016/j.maturitas.2017.06.028.

Sandhu, S.K. and Hampson, G. (2011). The pathogenesis, diagnosis, investigation and management of osteoporosis. *Journal of Clinical Pathology*, [online] 64(12), pp.1042–1050. doi:https://doi.org/10.1136/jcp.2010.077842.

Santoro, N. (2016). Perimenopause: From Research to Practice. *Journal of Women's Health*, [online] 25(4), pp.332–339. doi:https://doi.org/10.1089/jwh.2015.5556.

Santoro, N. and Randolph, J.F. (2011). Reproductive Hormones and the Menopause Transition. *Obstetrics and Gynecology Clinics of North America*, [online] 38(3), pp.455–466. doi:https://doi.org/10.1016/j.ogc.2011.05.004.

Santoro, N., Braunstein, G.D., Butts, C.L., Martin, K.A., McDermott, M. and Pinkerton, J.V. (2016). Compounded Bioidentical Hormones in Endocrinology Practice: An Endocrine Society Scientific Statement. *The Journal of Clinical Endocrinology & Metabolism*, 101(4), pp.1318–1343. doi:https://doi.org/10.1210/jc.2016-1271.

Sargis, R.M., Heindel, J.J. and Padmanabhan, V. (2019). Interventions to Address Environmental Metabolism-Disrupting Chemicals: Changing the Narrative to Empower Action to Restore Metabolic Health. *Frontiers in Endocrinology*, 10. doi:https://doi.org/10.3389/fendo.2019.00033.

Sarmento, A.C.A., Costa, A.P.F., Vieira-Baptista, P., Giraldo, P.C., Eleutério, J. and Gonçalves, A.K. (2021). Genitourinary Syndrome of Menopause: Epidemiology, Physiopathology, Clinical Manifestation and Diagnostic. *Frontiers in Reproductive Health*, 3. doi:https://doi.org/10.3389/frph.2021.779398.

Sarraf, P., Parohan, M., Javanbakht, M.H., Ranji-Burachaloo, S. and Djalali, M. (2019). Short-term curcumin supplementation enhances serum brain-derived neurotrophic factor in adult men and women: a systematic review and dose-response meta-analysis of randomized controlled trials. *Nutrition Research (New York, N.Y.)*, [online] 69, pp.1–8. doi:https://doi.org/10.1016/j.nutres.2019.05.001.

Sartori, S.B., Whittle, N., Hetzenauer, A. and Singewald, N. (2012). Magnesium deficiency induces anxiety and HPA axis dysregulation: Modulation by therapeutic drug treatment. *Neuropharmacology*, [online] 62(1), pp.304–312. doi:https://doi.org/10.1016/j.neuropharm.2011.07.027.

Sayón-Orea, C., Santiago, S., Cuervo, M., Martínez-González, M.A., Garcia, A. and Martínez, J.A. (2015). Adherence to Mediterranean dietary pattern and menopausal symptoms in relation to overweight/obesity in Spanish perimenopausal and postmenopausal women. *Menopause*, 22(7), pp.750–757.

doi:https://doi.org/10.1097/gme.0000000000000378.

Schalka, S., Magalhães, W.V., Cazerta, C., Shitara, D., Sufi, B. da S. and Quadros, A. (2017). Nutraceutical compound increases collagen, elastin and hyaluronic acid synthesis. *Surgical & Cosmetic Dermatology*, 9(1). doi:https://doi.org/10.5935/scd1984-8773.201791875.

Schmalenberger, K.M., Tauseef, H.A., Barone, J.C., Owens, S.A., Lieberman, L., Jarczok, M.N., Girdler, S.S., Kiesner, J., Ditzen, B. and Eisenlohr-Moul, T.A. (2021). How to study the menstrual cycle: Practical tools and recommendations. *Psychoneuroendocrinology*, 123(104895), p.104895. doi:https://doi.org/10.1016/j.psyneuen.2020.104895.

Schmelzer, C., Lindner, I., Rimbach, G., Niklowitz, P., Menke, T. and Döring, F. (2008). Functions of coenzyme Q10in inflammation and gene expression. *BioFactors*, 32(1-4), pp.179–183. doi:https://doi.org/10.1002/biof.5520320121.

Schmidt, P.J., Nieman, L.K., Danaceau, M.A., Adams, L.F. and Rubinow, D.R. (1998). Differential Behavioral Effects of Gonadal Steroids in Women with and in Those without Premenstrual Syndrome. *New England Journal of Medicine*, 338(4), pp.209–216. doi:https://doi.org/10.1056/nejm199801223380401.

Schüle, C., Nothdurfter, C. and Rupprecht, R. (2014). The role of allopregnanolone in depression and anxiety. *Progress in Neurobiology*, 113, pp.79–87. doi:https://doi.org/10.1016/j.pneurobio.2013.09.003.

Schwalfenberg, G.K. and Genuis, S.J. (2017). The importance of magnesium in clinical healthcare. *Scientifica*, 2017(1), pp.1–14. doi:https://doi.org/10.1155/2017/4179326.

Schwingshackl, L. and Hoffmann, G. (2014). Monounsaturated fatty acids, olive oil and health status: a systematic review and meta-analysis of cohort studies.

*Lipids in Health and Disease*, [online] 13(1). doi:https://doi.org/10.1186/1476-511x-13-154.

Sealfon, S.C. and Olanow, C.W. (2000). Dopamine receptors: from structure to behavior. *Trends in Neurosciences*, 23, pp.S34–S40. doi:https://doi.org/10.1016/s1471-1931(00)00025-2.

Segerstrom, S.C. and Miller, G.E. (2004). Psychological Stress and the Human Immune System: A Meta-Analytic Study of 30 Years of Inquiry. *Psychological Bulletin*, [online] 130(4), pp.601–630. doi:https://doi.org/10.1037/0033-2909.130.4.601.

Sepkovic, D.W. and Bradlow, H.L. (2009). Estrogen Hydroxylation-The Good and the Bad. *Annals of the New York Academy of Sciences*, 1155(1), pp.57–67. doi:https://doi.org/10.1111/j.1749-6632.2008.03675.x.

Shah, L., Elshaikh, A.O., Lee, R., Joy Mathew, C., Jose, M.T. and Cancarevic, I. (2020). Do Menopause and Aging Affect the Onset and Progression of Rheumatoid Arthritis and Systemic Lupus Erythematosus? *Cureus*. doi:https://doi.org/10.7759/cureus.10944.

Shaver, J.L. and Woods, N.F. (2015). Sleep and menopause. *Menopause*, 22(8), pp.899–915. doi:https://doi.org/10.1097/gme.0000000000000499.

Shaw, L.J., Bairey Merz, C.N., Pepine, C.J., Reis, S.E., Bittner, V., Kelsey, S.F., Olson, M., Johnson, B.D., Mankad, S., Sharaf, B.L., Rogers, W.J., Wessel, T.R., Arant, C.B., Pohost, G.M., Lerman, A., Quyyumi, A.A. and Sopko, G. (2006). Insights From the NHLBI-Sponsored Women's Ischemia Syndrome Evaluation (WISE) Study. *Journal of the American College of Cardiology*, 47(3), pp.S4–S20. doi:https://doi.org/10.1016/j.jacc.2005.01.072.

Shea, B., Adachi, J., Cranney, A., Griffith, L., Guyatt, G., Hamel, C., Ortiz, Z.,

Peterson, J., Robinson, V., Tugwell, P., Wells, G. and Zytaruk, N. (2004). Calcium supplementation on bone loss in postmenopausal women. *Cochrane Database of Systematic Reviews*. doi:https://doi.org/10.1002/14651858.cd004526.pub2.

Shearer, G.C., Savinova, O.V. and Harris, W.S. (2012). Fish oil — How does it reduce plasma triglycerides? *Biochimica et Biophysica Acta (BBA) - Molecular and Cell Biology of Lipids*, [online] 1821(5), pp.843–851. doi:https://doi.org/10.1016/j.bbalip.2011.10.011.

Shekhar, S., Hall, J.E. and Klubo-Gwiezdzinska, J. (2021). The hypothalamic–pituitary–thyroid axis and sleep. *Current Opinion in Endocrine and Metabolic Research*, 17, pp.8–14. doi:https://doi.org/10.1016/j.coemr.2020.10.002.

Shieh, A., Epeldegui, M., Karlamangla, A.S. and Greendale, G.A. (2020). Gut permeability, inflammation, and bone density across the menopause transition. *JCI Insight*, 5(2). doi:https://doi.org/10.1172/jci.insight.134092.

Shulhai, Anna-Mariia Rotondo, R., Maddalena Petraroli, Patianna, V., Predieri, B., Iughetti, L., Esposito, S. and Maria Elisabeth Street (2024). The Role of Nutrition on Thyroid Function. *Nutrients*, [online] 16(15), pp.2496–2496. doi:https://doi.org/10.3390/nu16152496.

Si, H. and Liu, D. (2014). Dietary antiaging phytochemicals and mechanisms associated with prolonged survival. *The Journal of Nutritional Biochemistry*, [online] 25(6), pp.581–591. doi:https://doi.org/10.1016/j.jnutbio.2014.02.001.

Sieghart, W. and Sperk, G. (2002). Subunit Composition, Distribution and Function of GABA-A Receptor Subtypes. *Current Topics in Medicinal Chemistry*, 2(8), pp.795–816. doi:https://doi.org/10.2174/1568026023393507.

Silberstein, S.D. and Merriam, G.R. (2000). Physiology of the Menstrual Cycle. *Cephalalgia*, 20(3), pp.148–154. doi:https://doi.org/10.1046/j.1468-

2982.2000.00034.x.

Simbar, M., Nazarpour, S., KhodaKarami, N., Nasiri, Z., Rashidi Fakari, F., Kiani, Z., Keyvanfar, S. and Alavi Majd, H. (2023). A situation analysis on postmenopausal women's self-care needs and priorities in Tehran: a population-based study. *BMC Public Health*, [online] 23(1). doi:https://doi.org/10.1186/s12889-023-15040-z.

Simon, J.A. and Reape, K.Z. (2009). Understanding the menopausal experiences of professional women. *Menopause*, 16(1), pp.73–76. doi:https://doi.org/10.1097/gme.0b013e31817b614a.

Simopoulos, A.P. (2002). The importance of the ratio of omega-6/omega-3 essential fatty acids. *Biomedicine & Pharmacotherapy*, [online] 56(8), pp.365–379. doi:https://doi.org/10.1016/s0753-3322(02)00253-6.

Simopoulos, A.P. (2003). Importance of the Ratio of Omega-6/Omega-3 Essential Fatty Acids: Evolutionary Aspects. *World Review of Nutrition and Dietetics*, 92, pp.1–22. doi:https://doi.org/10.1159/000073788.

Simopoulos, A.P. (2008). The importance of the omega-6/omega-3 fatty acid ratio in cardiovascular disease and other chronic diseases. *Experimental biology and medicine (Maywood, N.J.)*, [online] 233(6), pp.674–88. doi:https://doi.org/10.3181/0711-MR-311.

Sinclair, R., Patel, M., Dawson, T.L., Yazdabadi, A., Yip, L., Perez, A. and Rufaut, N.W. (2011). Hair loss in women: medical and cosmetic approaches to increase scalp hair fullness. *British Journal of Dermatology*, 165, pp.12–18. doi:https://doi.org/10.1111/j.1365-2133.2011.10630.x.

Singh, M. and Su, C. (2013). Progesterone and neuroprotection. *Hormones and Behavior*, 63(2), pp.284–290. doi:https://doi.org/10.1016/j.yhbeh.2012.06.003.

Slavin, J. and Green, H. (2007). Dietary fibre and satiety. *Nutrition Bulletin*, [online] 32(s1), pp.32–42. doi:https://doi.org/10.1111/j.1467-3010.2007.00603.x.

Slominski, A. (2007). A nervous breakdown in the skin: stress and the epidermal barrier. *Journal of Clinical Investigation*, 117(11), pp.3166–3169. doi:https://doi.org/10.1172/jci33508.

Sluijmer AV, Heineman MJ, Koudstaal J, Theunissen PH, de Jong FH, Evers JL. (1998). Relationship between ovarian production of estrone, estradiol, testosterone, and androstenedione and the ovarian degree of stromal hyperplasia in postmenopausal women. *Menopause*, 5(4). PMID: 9872485. .

Smith, M., Makino, S., Kvetnansky, R. and Post, R. (1995). Stress and glucocorticoids affect the expression of brain-derived neurotrophic factor and neurotrophin-3 mRNAs in the hippocampus. *The Journal of Neuroscience*, 15(3), pp.1768–1777. doi:https://doi.org/10.1523/jneurosci.15-03-01768.1995.

Smith, T. and Contestabile, E. (2002). Executive Summary. *Journal of Obstetrics and Gynaecology Canada*, 24(10), pp.5–11. doi:https://doi.org/10.1016/s1701-2163(17)31074-5.

Society for Endocrinology (2018). *Human Chorionic Gonadotrophin | You and Your Hormones from the Society for Endocrinology*. [online] www.yourhormones.info. Available at: https://www.yourhormones.info/hormones/human-chorionic-gonadotrophin/ [Accessed 4 Jun. 2024].

Soules, M.R., Sherman, S., Parrott, E., Rebar, R., Santoro, N., Utian, W. and Woods, N. (2001). Executive summary: Stages of Reproductive Aging Workshop (STRAW) Park City, Utah, July, 2001. *Menopause*, 8(6), pp.402–407. doi:https://doi.org/10.1097/00042192-200111000-00004.

Sowers, M., Zheng, H., Tomey, K., Karvonen-Gutierrez, C., Jannausch, M., Li,

X., Yosef, M. and Symons, J. (2007). Changes in Body Composition in Women over Six Years at Midlife: Ovarian and Chronological Aging. *The Journal of Clinical Endocrinology & Metabolism*, 92(3), pp.895–901. doi:https://doi.org/10.1210/jc.2006-1393.

Sowers, M.R., Crawford, S., McConnell, D.S., Randolph, J.F., Gold, E.B., Wilkin, M.K. and Lasley, B. (2006). Selected Diet and Lifestyle Factors Are Associated with Estrogen Metabolites in a Multiracial/Ethnic Population of Women. *The Journal of Nutrition*, 136(6), pp.1588–1595. doi:https://doi.org/10.1093/jn/136.6.1588.

Spencer, R.L. and Deak, T. (2017). A users guide to HPA axis research. *Physiology & Behavior*, 178, pp.43–65. doi:https://doi.org/10.1016/j.physbeh.2016.11.014.

Srour, B., Fezeu, L.K., Kesse-Guyot, E., Allès, B., Méjean, C., Andrianasolo, R.M., Chazelas, E., Deschasaux, M., Hercberg, S., Galan, P., Monteiro, C.A., Julia, C. and Touvier, M. (2019). Ultra-processed food intake and risk of cardiovascular disease: prospective cohort study (NutriNet-Santé). *BMJ*, [online] 365(8201), p.l1451. doi:https://doi.org/10.1136/bmj.l1451.

Stachenfeld, N.S. (2008a). Sex Hormone Effects on Body Fluid Regulation. *Exercise and Sport Sciences Reviews*, 36(3), pp.152–159. doi:https://doi.org/10.1097/jes.0b013e31817be928.

Stachowiak, G., Pertyński, T. and Pertyńska-Marczewska, M. (2015). Metabolic disorders in menopause. *Przeglad Menopauzalny = Menopause Review*, [online] 14(1), pp.59–64. doi:https://doi.org/10.5114/pm.2015.50000.

Steiger, A. (2003). Sleep and endocrine regulation. *Frontiers in Bioscience*, 8(6), pp.s358-376. doi:https://doi.org/10.2741/1055.

Steiner, M., Dunn, E. and Born, L. (2003). Hormones and mood: from menarche to menopause and beyond. *Journal of Affective Disorders*, [online] 74(1), pp.67–83. doi:https://doi.org/10.1016/S0165-0327(02)00432-9.

Steptoe, A., O'Donnell, K., Marmot, M. and Wardle, J. (2008). Positive affect, psychological well-being, and good sleep. *Journal of Psychosomatic Research*, 64(4), pp.409–415. doi:https://doi.org/10.1016/j.jpsychores.2007.11.008.

Stránský, M. and Ryšavá, L. (2009). Nutrition as prevention and treatment of osteoporosis. *Physiological Research*, pp.S7–S11. doi:https://doi.org/10.33549/physiolres.931858.

Su, K.-P., Tseng, P.-T., Lin, P.-Y., Okubo, R., Chen, T.-Y., Chen, Y.-W. and Matsuoka, Y.J. (2018). Association of Use of Omega-3 Polyunsaturated Fatty Acids With Changes in Severity of Anxiety Symptoms. *JAMA Network Open*, [online] 1(5), p.e182327. doi:https://doi.org/10.1001/jamanetworkopen.2018.2327.

Suda, K. and Matsuda, K. (2022). How Microbes Affect Depression: Underlying Mechanisms via the Gut–Brain Axis and the Modulating Role of Probiotics. *International Journal of Molecular Sciences*, 23(3), p.1172. doi:https://doi.org/10.3390/ijms23031172.

Sullivan Mitchell, E. and Fugate Woods, N. (2001). Midlife Women's Attributions about Perceived Memory Changes: Observations from the Seattle Midlife Women's Health Study. *Journal of Women's Health & Gender-Based Medicine*, 10(4), pp.351–362. doi:https://doi.org/10.1089/152460901750269670.

Sullivan, S.D., Lehman, A., Nathan, N.K., Thomson, C.A. and Howard, B.V. (2017). Age of Menopause and Fracture Risk in Post-Menopausal Women Randomized to Calcium + Vitamin D, Hormone Therapy, or the combination: Results from the Women's Health Initiative Clinical Trials. *Menopause (New York, N.Y.)*, [online] 24(4), pp.371–378. doi:https://doi.org/10.1097/GME.0000000000000775.

Suri, V. and Suri, V. (2014). Menopause and oral health. *Journal of Mid-life Health*, 5(3), p.115. doi:https://doi.org/10.4103/0976-7800.141187.

Syafitri, D.M., Levita, J., Mutakin, M. and Diantini, A. (2018). A Review: Is Ginger (Zingiber officinale var. Roscoe) Potential for Future Phytomedicine? *Indonesian Journal of Applied Sciences*, 8(1). doi:https://doi.org/10.24198/ijas.v8i1.16466.

Szablewski, L. (2011). Glucose Homeostasis – Mechanism and Defects. *Diabetes - Damages and Treatments*. doi:https://doi.org/10.5772/22905.

Szántó, M., Dózsa, A., Antal, D., Szabó, K., Kemény, L. and Bai, P. (2019). Targeting the gut-skin axis—Probiotics as new tools for skin disorder management? *Experimental Dermatology*, 28(11), pp.1210–1218. doi:https://doi.org/10.1111/exd.14016.

Tachedjian, G., Aldunate, M., Bradshaw, C.S. and Cone, R.A. (2017). The role of lactic acid production by probiotic Lactobacillus species in vaginal health. *Research in Microbiology*, [online] 168(9-10), pp.782–792. doi:https://doi.org/10.1016/j.resmic.2017.04.001.

Tafet, G.E. and Nemeroff, C.B. (2020). Pharmacological Treatment of Anxiety Disorders: The Role of the HPA Axis. *Frontiers in Psychiatry*, 11(443). doi:https://doi.org/10.3389/fpsyt.2020.00443.

Tang, A. C.-W., Huang, S.-T., Wu, S.-Y., & Tang, S. F.-T. (2024). The Clinical and Sonographic Features of Cervical Muscle Involvement in Patients with Frozen Shoulder: A Retrospective Study. *Biomedicines*, *12*(10), 2395. https://doi.org/10.3390/biomedicines12102395

Taraborrelli, S. (2015). Physiology, production and action of progesterone. *Acta Obstetricia et Gynecologica Scandinavica*, 94(S161), pp.8–16. doi:https://doi.

org/10.1111/aogs.12771.

Tardy, A.-L., Pouteau, E., Marquez, D., Yilmaz, C. and Scholey, A. (2020). Vitamins and minerals for energy, fatigue and cognition: A narrative review of the biochemical and clinical evidence. *Nutrients*, [online] 12(1), p.228. doi:https://doi.org/10.3390/nu12010228.

Taylor-Swanson, L., Wong, A.E., Pincus, D., Butner, J.E., Hahn-Holbrook, J., Koithan, M., Wann, K. and Woods, N.F. (2018). The dynamics of stress and fatigue across menopause: attractors, coupling, and resilience. *Menopause (New York, N.Y.)*, [online] 25(4), pp.380–390. doi:https://doi.org/10.1097/GME.0000000000001025.

Tchernof, A. and Després, J.-P. (2013). Pathophysiology of human visceral obesity: an update. *Physiological reviews*, [online] 93(1), pp.359–404. doi:https://doi.org/10.1152/physrev.00033.2011.

Tepper, P.G., Brooks, M.M., Randolph, J.F., Crawford, S.L., El Khoudary, S.R., Gold, E.B., Lasley, B.L., Jones, B., Joffe, H., Hess, R., Avis, N.E., Harlow, S., McConnell, D.S., Bromberger, J.T., Zheng, H., Ruppert, K. and Thurston, R.C. (2016). Characterizing the trajectories of vasomotor symptoms across the menopausal transition. *Menopause*, 23(10), pp.1067–1074. doi:https://doi.org/10.1097/gme.0000000000000676.

Testai, L., Martelli, A., Flori, L., Cicero, A.F.G. and Colletti, A. (2021). Coenzyme Q10: Clinical Applications beyond Cardiovascular Diseases. *Nutrients*, 13(5), p.1697. doi:https://doi.org/10.3390/nu13051697.

Thakur, V.S., Deb, G., Babcook, M.A. and Gupta, S. (2013). Plant Phytochemicals as Epigenetic Modulators: Role in Cancer Chemoprevention. *The AAPS Journal*, 16(1), pp.151–163. doi:https://doi.org/10.1208/s12248-013-9548-5.

Thasneem, K., Kalarani, I.B., Jayaprasad, P., Mohammed, V. and Veerabathiran, R. (2022). Genes linked with early menopause and the pathogenesis of its associated diseases: a systematic review. *Middle East Fertility Society Journal*, 27(1). doi:https://doi.org/10.1186/s43043-021-00093-0.

The Daisy Network (n.d.). *Charity for Women with POI | The Daisy Network*. [online] www.daisynetwork.org. Available at: https://www.daisynetwork.org [Accessed 13 Nov. 2024].

The Emerging Risk Factors Collaboration* (2009). Major Lipids, Apolipoproteins, and Risk of Vascular Disease. *JAMA*, 302(18), p.1993. doi:https://doi.org/10.1001/jama.2009.1619.

The North American Menopause Society (2021). Management of osteoporosis in postmenopausal women: the 2021 position statement of The North American Menopause Society. *Menopause*, 28(9), pp.973–997. doi:https://doi.org/10.1097/gme.0000000000001831.

Theobald, H.E. (2005). Dietary calcium and health. *Nutrition Bulletin*, [online] 30(3), pp.237–277. doi:https://doi.org/10.1111/j.1467-3010.2005.00514.x.

Thomas, M.P. and Potter, B.V.L. (2013). The structural biology of oestrogen metabolism. *The Journal of Steroid Biochemistry and Molecular Biology*, [online] 137, pp.27–49. doi:https://doi.org/10.1016/j.jsbmb.2012.12.014.

Thornton, J. (2007). Effect of estrogens on skin aging and the potential role of SERMs. *Clinical Interventions in Aging*, [online] Volume 2, pp.283–297. doi:https://doi.org/10.2147/cia.s798.

Thurston, R.C., Chang, Y., Buysse, D.J., Hall, M.H. and Matthews, K.A. (2019). Hot flashes and awakenings among midlife women. *Sleep*, 42(9). doi:https://doi.org/10.1093/sleep/zsz131.

Thurston, R.C., Karvonen-Gutierrez, C.A., Derby, C.A., El Khoudary, S.R., Kravitz, H.M. and Manson, J.E. (2018). Menopause versus chronologic aging. *Menopause*, 25(8), pp.849–854. doi:https://doi.org/10.1097/gme.0000000000001143.

Tobin, D.J. (2015). Age-Related Hair Pigment Loss. *Current problems in dermatology*, 47, pp.128–138. doi:https://doi.org/10.1159/000369413.

Toro-Urrego, N., Garcia-Segura, L.M., Echeverria, V. and Barreto, G.E. (2016). Testosterone Protects Mitochondrial Function and Regulates Neuroglobin Expression in Astrocytic Cells Exposed to Glucose Deprivation. *Frontiers in Aging Neuroscience*, 8. doi:https://doi.org/10.3389/fnagi.2016.00152.

Toth, M., Tchernof, A., Sites, C. and Poehlman, E. (2000). Effect of menopausal status on body composition and abdominal fat distribution. *International Journal of Obesity*, 24(2), pp.226–231. doi:https://doi.org/10.1038/sj.ijo.0801118.

Trembling, P.M., Apostolidou, S., Gentry-Maharaj, A., Parkes, J., Ryan, A., Tanwar, S., Burnell, M., Jacobs, I., Menon, U. and Rosenberg, W.M. (2017). Risk of chronic liver disease in post-menopausal women due to body mass index, alcohol and their interaction: a prospective nested cohort study within the United Kingdom Collaborative Trial of Ovarian Cancer Screening (UKCTOCS). *BMC Public Health*, 17(1). doi:https://doi.org/10.1186/s12889-017-4518-y.

Trüeb, R. (2016). Serum biotin levels in women complaining of hair loss. *International Journal of Trichology*, 8(2), p.73. doi:https://doi.org/10.4103/0974-7753.188040.

Trueb, R.M. (2005). Aging of hair. *Journal of Cosmetic Dermatology*, 4(2), pp.60–72. doi:https://doi.org/10.1111/j.1473-2165.2005.40203.x.

Tsuchiya, Y., Nakajima, M. and Yokoi, T. (2005). Cytochrome P450-mediated metabolism of estrogens and its regulation in human. *Cancer Letters*, [online] 227(2), pp.115–124. doi:https://doi.org/10.1016/j.canlet.2004.10.007.

Tucker, K.L. (2009). Osteoporosis prevention and nutrition. *Current Osteoporosis Reports*, 7(4), pp.111–117. doi:https://doi.org/10.1007/s11914-009-0020-5.

Turakitwanakan, W. and Mekseepralard, C. (n.d.). *Effects of mindfulness meditation on serum cortisol of medical students. J Med Assoc Thai. 2013 Jan;96 Suppl 1:S90-5. PMID: 23724462.*

Valimaa, H., Savolainen, S., Soukka, T., Silvoniemi, P., Makela, S., Kujari, H., Gustafsson, J. and Laine, M. (2004). Estrogen receptor-beta is the predominant estrogen receptor subtype in human oral epithelium and salivary glands. *Journal of Endocrinology*, 180(1), pp.55–62. doi:https://doi.org/10.1677/joe.0.1800055.

Velarde, M.C. (2013). Pleiotropic actions of estrogen: a mitochondrial matter. *Physiological Genomics*, 45(3), pp.106–109. doi:https://doi.org/10.1152/physiolgenomics.00155.2012.

Veldhorst, M., Smeets, A., Soenen, S., Hochstenbach-Waelen, A., Hursel, R., Diepvens, K., Lejeune, M., Luscombe-Marsh, N. and Westerterp-Plantenga, M. (2008). Protein-induced satiety: Effects and mechanisms of different proteins. *Physiology & Behavior*, 94(2), pp.300–307. doi:https://doi.org/10.1016/j.physbeh.2008.01.003.

Ventura, M., Melo, M. and Carrilho, F. (2017). Selenium and thyroid disease: From pathophysiology to treatment. *International Journal of Endocrinology*, [online] 2017(1), pp.1–9. doi:https://doi.org/10.1155/2017/1297658.

Verdier-Sevrain, S., Bonte, F. and Gilchrest, B. (2006). Biology of estrogens in skin: implications for skin aging. *Experimental Dermatology*, 15(2), pp.83–94. doi:https://doi.org/10.1111/j.1600-0625.2005.00377.x.

Vetrani, C., Barrea, L., Rispoli, R., Verde, L., De Alteriis, G., Docimo, A., Auriemma, R.S., Colao, A., Savastano, S. and Muscogiuri, G. (2022). Mediterranean Diet: What Are the Consequences for Menopause? *Frontiers in Endocrinology*, [online] 13(13). doi:https://doi.org/10.3389/fendo.2022.886824.

Vigil, P., Lyon, C., Flores, B., Rioseco, H. and Serrano, F. (2017). Ovulation, a sign of health. *The Linacre Quarterly*, [online] 84(4), pp.343–355. doi:https://doi.org/10.1080/00243639.2017.1394053.

Wada, T., Hori, S., Sugiyama, M., Fujisawa, E., Nakano, T., Tsuneki, H., Nagira, K., Saito, S. and Sasaoka, T. (2010). Progesterone inhibits glucose uptake by affecting diverse steps of insulin signaling in 3T3-L1 adipocytes. *American Journal of Physiology-Endocrinology and Metabolism*, 298(4), pp.E881–E888. doi:https://doi.org/10.1152/ajpendo.00649.2009.

Wakabayashi I. Associations of Smoking and Drinking with New Lipid-Related Indices in Women with Hyperglycemia. Womens Health Rep (New Rochelle). 2021 Jan 29;2(1):23-31. doi: 10.1089/whr.2020.0100. PMID: 33786527; PMCID: PMC7957949Wallace, T.C., Blusztajn, J.K., Caudill, M.A., Klatt, K.C. and Zeisel, S.H. (2019). Choline: The Neurocognitive Essential Nutrient of Interest to Obstetricians and Gynecologists. *Journal of Dietary Supplements*, 17(6), pp.733–752. doi:https://doi.org/10.1080/19390211.2019.1639875.

Walters, D.G. (2004). Cruciferous vegetable consumption alters the metabolism of the dietary carcinogen 2-amino-1-methyl-6-phenylimidazo[4,5-b]pyridine (PhIP) in humans. *Carcinogenesis*, 25(9), pp.1659–1669. doi:https://doi.org/10.1093/carcin/bgh164.

Walton, C., Godsland, I.F., Proudler, A.J., Wynn, V. and Stevenson, J.C. (1993). The effects of the menopause on insulin sensitivity, secretion and elimination in non-obese, healthy women. *European Journal of Clinical Investigation*, 23(8), pp.466–473. doi:https://doi.org/10.1111/j.1365-2362.1993.tb00792.x.

Wang, R., Li, Y.-H., Xu, Y., Li, Y.-B., Wu, H.-L., Guo, H., Zhang, J.-Z., Zhang, J.-J., Pan, X.-Y. and Li, X.-J. (2010). Curcumin produces neuroprotective effects via activating brain-derived neurotrophic factor/TrkB-dependent MAPK and PI-3K cascades in rodent cortical neurons. *Progress in Neuro-Psychopharmacology and Biological Psychiatry*, 34(1), pp.147–153. doi:https://doi.org/10.1016/j.pnpbp.2009.10.016.

Wang, X., Ha, D., Yoshitake, R., Chan, Y.S., Sadava, D. and Chen, S. (2021). Exploring the Biological Activity and Mechanism of Xenoestrogens and Phytoestrogens in Cancers: Emerging Methods and Concepts. *International Journal of Molecular Sciences*, [online] 22(16), p.8798. doi:https://doi.org/10.3390/ijms22168798.

Wang, Y., Xu, D. Effects of aerobic exercise on lipids and lipoproteins. *Lipids Health Dis* **16**, 132 (2017). https://doi.org/10.1186/s12944-017-0515-5

Ward, R.J., Zucca, F.A., Duyn, J.H., Crichton, R.R. and Zecca, L. (2014). The role of iron in brain ageing and neurodegenerative disorders. *The Lancet Neurology*, [online] 13(10), pp.1045–1060. doi:https://doi.org/10.1016/s1474-4422(14)70117-6.

Warren, J.M., Smith, N. and Ashwell, M. (2017). A Structured Literature Review on the Role of mindfulness, Mindful Eating and Intuitive Eating in Changing Eating behaviours: Effectiveness and Associated Potential Mechanisms. *Nutrition Research Reviews*, [online] 30(2), pp.272–283. doi:https://doi.org/10.1017/s0954422417000154.

Watkins, B. (2001). Bioactive fatty acids: role in bone biology and bone cell function. *Progress in Lipid Research*, 40(1-2), pp.125–148. doi:https://doi.org/10.1016/s0163-7827(00)00016-3.

Wautier, M.-P., Guillausseau, P.-J. and Wautier, J.-L. (2017). Activation of the receptor for advanced glycation end products and consequences on health. *Diabetes & Metabolic Syndrome: Clinical Research & Reviews*, 11(4), pp.305–309. doi:https://doi.org/10.1016/j.dsx.2016.09.009.

Weaver, C.M., Gordon, C.M., Janz, K.F., Kalkwarf, H.J., Lappe, J.M., Lewis, R., O'Karma, M., Wallace, T.C. and Zemel, B.S. (2016). The National Osteoporosis Foundation's position statement on peak bone mass development and lifestyle factors: a systematic review and implementation recommendations. *Osteoporosis International*, [online] 27(4), pp.1281–1386. doi:https://doi.org/10.1007/s00198-015-3440-3.

Weber, M.T., Rubin, L.H. and Maki, P.M. (2013). Cognition in perimenopause: the effect of transition stage. *Menopause (New York, N.Y.)*, [online] 20(5), pp.511–517. doi:https://doi.org/10.1097/gme.0b013e31827655e5.

Wei, J.-J., William, J. and Bulun, S. (2011). Endometriosis and Ovarian Cancer. *International Journal of Gynecological Pathology*, 30(6), pp.553–568. doi:https://doi.org/10.1097/pgp.0b013e31821f4b85.

Weiland, N.G. and Orchinik, M. (1995). Specific subunit mRNAs of the GABAA receptor are regulated by progesterone in subfields of the hippocampus. *Molecular Brain Research*, 32(2), pp.271–278. doi:https://doi.org/10.1016/0169-328x(95)00087-9.

West, S.L. (2008). Prevalence of Low Sexual Desire and Hypoactive Sexual Desire Disorder in a Nationally Representative Sample of US Women. *Archives of Internal Medicine*, 168(13), p.1441. doi:https://doi.org/10.1001/archinte.168.13.1441.

Wever, M.C.M., van Meer, F., Charbonnier, L., Crabtree, D.R., Buosi, W., Giannopoulou, A., Androutsos, O., Johnstone, A.M., Manios, Y., Meek, C.L., Holst, J.J. and Smeets, P.A.M. (2021). Associations between ghrelin and leptin and neural food cue reactivity in a fasted and sated state. *NeuroImage*, [online] 240, p.118374. doi:https://doi.org/10.1016/j.neuroimage.2021.118374.

White, D.J., Cox, K.H.M., Hughes, M.E., Pipingas, A., Peters, R. and Scholey, A.B. (2016). Functional Brain Activity Changes after 4 Weeks Supplementation with a Multi-Vitamin/Mineral Combination: A Randomized, Double-Blind, Placebo-Controlled Trial Exploring Functional Magnetic Resonance Imaging and Steady-State Visual Evoked Potentials during Working Memory. *Frontiers in Aging Neuroscience*, 8. doi:https://doi.org/10.3389/fnagi.2016.00288.

Williams, P.T. and Thompson, P.D. (2013). Walking versus running for hypertension, cholesterol, and diabetes mellitus risk reduction. *Arteriosclerosis, thrombosis, and vascular biology*, [online] 33(5), pp.1085–91. doi:https://doi.org/10.1161/ATVBAHA.112.300878.

Wilson, P.W.F., D'Agostino, R.B., Parise, H., Sullivan, L. and Meigs, J.B. (2005). Metabolic Syndrome as a Precursor of Cardiovascular Disease and Type 2 Diabetes Mellitus. *Circulation*, 112(20), pp.3066–3072. doi:https://doi.org/10.1161/circulationaha.105.539528.

Womens Health Concern (n.d.). *womens-health-concern.org/wp-content/uploads/2023/11/25-WHC-FACTSHEET-VaginalDryness-OCT2023-B.pdf.*

Woods, N.F., Mitchell, E.S. and Landis, C. (2005). Anxiety, hormonal changes, and vasomotor symptoms during the menopause transition. *Menopause*, 12(3), pp.242–245. doi:https://doi.org/10.1097/01.gme.0000161054.45892.01.

World Health Organisation (1994). *Assessment of fracture risk and its application to screening for postmenopausal osteoporosis : report of a WHO study group [meeting held in Rome from 22 to 25 June 1992].* [online] *iris.who.int.* World Health Organization. Available at: https://iris.who.int/handle/10665/39142 [Accessed 13 Oct. 2024].

World Health Organisation (2020). *Economic and financing considerations of self-care interventions for sexual and reproductive health and rights.* [online] Who.int. Available at: https://www.who.int/publications/i/item/WHO-SRH-20.2 [Accessed 7 Dec. 2024].

World Health Organization (2021). Research on the menopause in the 1990s : report of a WHO scientific group. *Who.int.* [online] doi:https://doi.org/924120866X.

Wright, V. J., Schwartzman, J. D., Itinoche, R., & Wittstein, J. (2024). The musculoskeletal syndrome of menopause. *Climacteric, 27*(5), 466–472. https://doi.org/10.1080/13697137.2024.2380363

Wu, G. (2016). Dietary Protein Intake and Human Health. *Food & Function*, [online] 7(3), pp.1251–1265. doi:https://doi.org/10.1039/c5fo01530h.

Xu, Y. and López, M. (2018). Central regulation of energy metabolism by estrogens. *Molecular Metabolism*, [online] 15, pp.104–115. doi:https://doi.org/10.1016/j.molmet.2018.05.012.

Xu, Z.-X., Liu, J., Gu, L.-P., Huang, B. and Pan, X.-J. (2017). Biological effects of xenoestrogens and the functional mechanisms via genomic and nongenomic pathways. *Environmental Reviews*, 25(3), pp.306–322. doi:https://doi.org/10.1139/er-2016-0075.

Yamaguchi, A., Stanger, L., Freedman, C., Prieur, A., Thav, R., Tena, J., Holman, T.R. and Holinstat, M. (2022). Supplementation with omega-3 or omega-6 fatty acids attenuates platelet reactivity in postmenopausal women. *Clinical and Translational Science.* doi:https://doi.org/10.1111/cts.13366.

Yan, H., Yang, W., Zhou, F., Li, X., Pan, Q., Shen, Z., Han, G., Newell-Fugate, A., Tian, Y., Majeti, R., Liu, W., Xu, Y., Wu, C., Allred, K., Allred, C., Sun,

Y. and Guo, S. (2018). Estrogen Improves Insulin Sensitivity and Suppresses Gluconeogenesis via the Transcription Factor Foxo1. *Diabetes*, 68(2), pp.291–304. doi:https://doi.org/10.2337/db18-0638.

Yang, J. (2012). Effect of dietary fiber on constipation: A meta analysis. *World Journal of Gastroenterology*, [online] 18(48), p.7378. doi:https://doi.org/10.3748/wjg.v18.i48.7378.

Yokoi, K. and Konomi, A. (2017). Iron deficiency without anaemia is a potential cause of fatigue: meta-analyses of randomised controlled trials and cross-sectional studies. *British Journal of Nutrition*, 117(10), pp.1422–1431. doi:https://doi.org/10.1017/s0007114517001349.

Zaghlool, S., Shehata, B., Abo-Seif, A. and Abd El-Latif, H. (2015). Protective effects of ginger and marshmallow extracts on indomethacin-induced peptic ulcer in rats. *Journal of Natural Science, Biology and Medicine*, [online] 6(2), p.421. doi:https://doi.org/10.4103/0976-9668.160026.

Zailani, H., Satyanarayanan, S.K., Liao, W.-C., Liao, H.-F., Huang, S.-Y., Gałecki, P., Su, K.-P. and Chang, J.P.-C. (2023). Omega-3 Polyunsaturated Fatty Acids in Managing Comorbid Mood Disorders in Chronic Obstructive Pulmonary Disease (COPD): A Review. *Journal of Clinical Medicine*, 12(7), p.2653. doi:https://doi.org/10.3390/jcm12072653.

Zampelas, A. and Magriplis, E. (2019). New Insights into Cholesterol Functions: A Friend or an Enemy? *Nutrients*, [online] 11(7), p.1645. doi:https://doi.org/10.3390/nu11071645.

Zárate, S., Stevnsner, T. and Gredilla, R. (2017). Role of Estrogen and Other Sex Hormones in Brain Aging. Neuroprotection and DNA Repair. *Frontiers in Aging Neuroscience*, 9. doi:https://doi.org/10.3389/fnagi.2017.00430.

Zhang, X., Shu, X.-O., Xiang, Y.-B., Yang, G., Li, H., Gao, J., Cai, H., Gao, Y.-T. and Zheng, W. (2011). Cruciferous vegetable consumption is associated with a reduced risk of total and cardiovascular disease mortality. *The American Journal of Clinical Nutrition*, 94(1), pp.240–246. doi:https://doi.org/10.3945/ajcn.110.009340.

Zhou, M., Han, S., Zhang, W. and Wu, D. (2022). Efficacy and safety of vitamin K2 for postmenopausal women with osteoporosis at a long-term follow-up: meta-analysis and systematic review. *Journal of Bone and Mineral Metabolism*. doi:https://doi.org/10.1007/s00774-022-01342-6.

Zhou, Q., Xue, S., Zhang, L. and Chen, G. (2022). Trace elements and the thyroid. *Frontiers in Endocrinology*, [online] 13, p.904889. doi:https://doi.org/10.3389/fendo.2022.904889.

Zhu, B.T. and Conney, A.H. (1998). Functional role of estrogen metabolism in target cells: review and perspectives. *Carcinogenesis*, [online] 19(1), pp.1–27. doi:https://doi.org/10.1093/carcin/19.1.1.

Zhu, F., Du, B. and Xu, B. (2017). Anti-inflammatory effects of phytochemicals from fruits, vegetables, and food legumes: A review. *Critical Reviews in Food Science and Nutrition*, 58(8), pp.1260–1270. doi:https://doi.org/10.1080/10408398.2016.1251390.

Zierau, O., Zenclussen, A.C. and Jensen, F. (2012). Role of female sex hormones, estradiol and progesterone, in mast cell behavior. *Frontiers in Immunology*, [online] 3. doi:https://doi.org/10.3389/fimmu.2012.00169.

Zou, L., Sasaki, J., Wei, G.-X., Huang, T., Yeung, A., Neto, O., Chen, K. and Hui, S. (2018). Effects of Mind–Body Exercises (Tai Chi/Yoga) on Heart Rate Variability Parameters and Perceived Stress: A Systematic Review with Meta-Analysis of Randomized Controlled Trials. *Journal of Clinical Medicine*, [online] 7(11), p.404. doi:https://doi.org/10.3390/jcm7110404.

## Reference list - Jane Kerridge (The Balanced Health clinic)

Asltoghiri, M. and Ghodsi, Z. (2012). The effects of Reflexology on sleep disorder in menopausal women. *Procedia - Social and Behavioral Sciences*, 31, pp.242–246. doi:https://doi.org/10.1016/j.sbspro.2011.12.049.

Cagnacci, A., Cannoletta, M., Caretto, S., Zanin, R., Xholli, A. and Volpe, A. (2011). Increased cortisol level. *Menopause*, 18(3), pp.273–278. doi:https://doi.org/10.1097/gme.0b013e3181f31947.

Gozuyesil, E. and Baser, M. (2016). The effect of foot reflexology applied to women aged between 40 and 60 on vasomotor complaints and quality of life. *Complementary Therapies in Clinical Practice*, [online] 24, pp.78–85. doi:https://doi.org/10.1016/j.ctcp.2016.05.011.

Mahdavipour, F., Rahemi, Z., Sadat, Z. and Ajorpaz, N.M. (2019). The effects of foot reflexology on depression during menopause: A randomized controlled clinical trial. *Complementary Therapies in Medicine*, [online] 47, p.102195. doi:https://doi.org/10.1016/j.ctim.2019.102195.

Printed in Dunstable, United Kingdom

79383087R00251